Analog Circuits and Signal Processing

The *Analog Circuits and Signal Processing* book series, formerly known as the *Kluwer International Series in Engineering and Computer Science* , is a high level academic and professional series publishing research on the design and applications of analog integrated circuits and signal processing circuits and systems. Typically per year we publish between 5-15 research monographs, professional books, handbooks, and edited volumes with worldwide distribution to engineers, researchers, educators, and libraries.The book series promotes and expedites the dissemination of new research results and tutorial views in the analog field. There is an exciting and large volume of research activity in the field worldwide. Researchers are striving to bridge the gap between classical analog work and recent advances in very large scale integration (VLSI) technologies with improved analog capabilities. Analog VLSI has been recognized as a major technology for future information processing. Analog work is showing signs of dramatic changes with emphasis on interdisciplinary research efforts combining device/circuit/technology issues. Consequently, new design concepts, strategies and design tools are being unveiled. Topics of interest include: Analog Interface Circuits and Systems; Data converters; Active-RC, switched-capacitor and continuous-time integrated filters; Mixed analog/digital VLSI; Simulation and modeling, mixed-mode simulation; Analog nonlinear and computational circuits and signal processing; Analog Artificial Neural Networks/Artificial Intelligence; Current-mode Signal Processing; Computer-Aided Design (CAD) tools; Analog Design in emerging technologies (Scalable CMOS, BiCMOS, GaAs, heterojunction and floating gate technologies, etc.); Analog Design for Test; Integrated sensors and actuators; Analog Design Automation/Knowledge-based Systems; Analog VLSI cell libraries; Analog product development; RF Front ends, Wireless communications and Microwave Circuits; Analog behavioral modeling, Analog HDL.

Ebrahim Ghafar-Zadeh • Saghi Forouhi
Tayebeh Azadmousavi

Advanced CMOS Biochips

Design and Fabrication

Springer

Ebrahim Ghafar-Zadeh
Biologically Inspired Sensors and Actuators (BioSA), Department of Electrical Engineering and Computer Science
Lassonde School of Engineering, York University
Toronto, ON, Canada

Saghi Forouhi
Department of Electrical Engineering (ISY) (Division of Electronics and Computer Engineering (ELDA))
Linköping University
Linköping, Östergötlands Län, Sweden

Tayebeh Azadmousavi
Department of Electrical Engineering
University of Bonab
Bonab, Iran

ISSN 1872-082X ISSN 2197-1854 (electronic)
Analog Circuits and Signal Processing
ISBN 978-94-007-0098-7 ISBN 978-94-007-0099-4 (eBook)
https://doi.org/10.1007/978-94-007-0099-4

This Springer imprint is published by the registered company Springer Nature B.V.
The registered company address is: Van Godewijckstraat 30, 3311 GX Dordrecht, The Netherlands

Contents

List of Frequently Used Acronyms and Abbreviations

Explanation	Acronym/ Abbreviation
Above Thermal Drain Voltage	AVT
Action Potential	AP
Active Pixel Sensor	APS
Address Event Representation	AER
Adenosine Triphosphate	ATP
Advanced Photo System Type-C	APS-C
Age-Related Macular Degeneration	AMD
Alternating Current	AC
Aluminum	Al
Aluminum Oxide	Al_2O_3
Always-On	AO
Amplified Metal-Oxide-Semiconductor Imager	AMI
Amplitude-Locked Loop	ALL
Amplitude-Shift Keying	ASK
Analog Front End	AFE
Analog-to-Digital Converter	ADC
Anisotropic Magnetoresistance	AMR
Anti-Aliasing Filter	AAF
Application-Specific Integrated Circuit	ASIC
Artificial Intelligence	AI
Auto-Balanced Bridge	ABB
Automatic Light Control	ALC
Back-End-Of-Line	BEOL
Barium Titanate	BTO
Base Stored Image Sensor	BASIS
Beats Per Minute	BPM
$Bi_{0.5}Na_{0.5}TiO_3$	BNT

(continued)

Biological/Chemical Field-Effect Transistor	Bio/ChemFET
Biotin-Bovine Serum Albumin	BSA
Bipolar Junction Transistor	BJT
Bisphenol A	BPA
Bulk Charge Modulated Device	BCMD
Capacitance-to-Digital Converter	CDC
Capacitance-to-Frequency Converter	CFC
Capacitance-to-Voltage Converter	CVC
Capacitive Coupled Device	CCD
Capacitive Digital to Analog Converter	CDAC
Capacitive-Feedback Transimpedance Amplifier	CF-TIA
Capacitive Transimpedance Amplifier	CTIA
Carbon Nanotube	CNT
Cardiovascular Disease	CVD
Carr Purcell Meiboom Gill	CPMG
Cerebral Blood Flow	CBF
Charge and Discharge Circuit	C&DC
Charge Modulation Device	CMD
Charge-Based Capacitance Measurement	CBCM
Chemically Controlled Ring Oscillator	CCRO
Chromium	Cr
Chronoamperometry	CA
Clock Data Recovery	CDR
CMOS Image Sensor	CIS
Common Mode Rejection Ratio	CMRR
Complementary Metal-Oxide-Semiconductor	CMOS
Complementary to Absolute Temperature	CTAT
Concurrent Dual-Frequency	CDF
Constant Frequency	CTF
Constant Phase Shift	CTP
Constant-Voltage Constant-Current	CVCC
Continuous-Time Phase-Domain Delta-Sigma Modulator	CT-PDΣΔM
Continuous-Time Sigma-Delta Modulator	CTΣΔM
Copper	Cu
Correlated Double Counting	CdC
Correlated Double Sampling	CDS
Counter Electrode	CE
Cross-Sectional Area	CSA
Crystal Violet Lactone	CVL
Current Conveyor	CC
Current-Controlled Oscillator	CCO
Current-Controlled Stimulation	CCS
Current-to-Frequency	I-to-F
Current-to-Voltage	I-to-V
Current-Voltage Mirror	CVM

(continued)

Cyclic Voltammetry	CV
Data Acquisition	DAQ
Delta-Sigma	ΔΣ
Delta-Sigma Modulator	ΔΣM
Deoxyribonucleic Acid	DNA
Differential Capacitive Transimpedance Amplifier	DCTIA
Differential Difference Amplifier	DDA
Differential Stacked Coil	DSC
Diffuse Speckle Contrast Flowmetry	DSCF
Digital Signal Processing	DSP
Digital Silicon Photomultiplier	dSiPM
Digital-to-Analog Converter	DAC
Digital-to-Capacitance Converter	DDC
Direct Current	DC
Direct Current Integration	DCI
Direct Digital Synthesizer	DDS
Discrete Fourier Transform	DFT
Dopamine	DA
Drive Right Leg	DRL
Duty-Cycle Resistors	DCR
Duty-Cycle-Modulated	DCM
Dynamic Element Matching	DEM
Dynamic Nuclear Polarization	DNP
Dynamic Threshold Metal-Oxide-Semiconductor Field-Effect Transistor	DTMOS
Electrocardiogram	ECG
Electrochemical Impedance Spectroscopy	EIS
Electroencephalography	EEG
Electroless Nickel Immersion Gold	ENIG
Electrolyte-Gated OFET	EGOFET
Electromyography	EMG
Electron Spin Resonance	ESR
Electrooculography	EOG
Electrothermal Filter	ETF
Extracellular-Action-Potential	EAP
Fast-Scan Cyclic Voltammetry	FSCV
Fast-Settling Miller Compensation	FSMC
Fiber-Optic faceplate	FOF
Field-Programmable Gate Array	FPGA
Finite Impulse Response	FIR
Finite State Machine	FSM
Finite-Difference Time-Domain	FDTD
Floating Diffusion	FD
Foreign Body Reaction	FBR
Frequency Division Multiplexing	FDM

(continued)

Frequency Locked Loop	FLL
Frequency Response Analysis	FRA
Frequency Shift Keying	FSK
Giant Magnetoresistance	GMR
Gold	Au
Graphene Field-Effect Transistor	GFET
Heart Rate	HR
High Density-Microelectrode Array	HD-MEA
High Frequency Structural Simulator	HFSS
High-Frequency Interference Rejection	HFIR
High-Pass Filter	HPF
human Chorionic Gonadotropin	hCG
Human Serum Albumin	HSA
Imageur Moléculaire Intra Cérébral	IMIC
Inductor-Capacitor	LC
Injection-Locked Oscillator	ILO
Inner Helmholtz Plane	IHP
Input Dynamic Range	IDR
Input-Referred Noise	IRN
Instrumentation Amplifier	IA
Integrated Circuit	IC
Inter Layer Dielectric	ILD
Interdigitated Electrode	IDE
Intermediate Frequency	IF
Ion-Sensitive Field-Effect Transistor	ISFET
Lab-on-Chip	LoC
Layer-By-Layer	LBL
Light-Emitting Diode	LED
Light-to-Digital Converter	LDC
Limit of Detection	LoD
Local Field Potential	LFP
Low-Dropout	LOD
Low-Noise Amplifier	LNA
Low-Path Filter	LPF
Machine Learning	ML
Magnetic Correlated Double Sampling	MCDS
Magnetic Flow Cytometer	MFC
Magnetic Immunoassay	MIA
Magnetic Nanoparticles	MNP
Magnetic Resonance Imaging	MRI
Magnetomyography	MMG
Magneto-Relaxometry	MRX
Magnetoresistive	MR
Magnetoresistive Correlated Double Sampling	MRCDS
Mean Absolute Error	MAE

(continued)

Metal-Insulator-Metal	MIM
Metal-Oxide-Semiconductor	MOS
Metal-Oxide-Semiconductor Field-Effect Transistor	MOSFET
Micro-Capillary Electrophoresis	μCE
Micro-Controller Unit	MCU
Microelectrode Array	MEA
Micro-Electromechanical Systems	MEMS
Monolithic Active Pixel Sensor	MAPS
Multiply-Accumulate	MAc
N-Channel Metal-Oxide Semiconductor	NMOS
Near-Infrared Spectroscopy	NIRS
Negative-Feedback Transimpedance Amplifier	NF-TIA
Neuromorphic Sensing System	NSS
Nickel	Ni
Noise Efficiency Factor	NEF
Noise Figure	NF
Non-Return-to-Zero	NRZ
Nuclear Magnetic Resonance	NMR
Numerically Controlled Oscillator	NCO
On–Off Keying	OOK
Opamp	OP
Operational Amplifier	OpAmp
Operational Transconductance Amplifier	OTA
Organic Field-Effect Transistor	OFET
Outer Helmholtz Plane	OHP
Output Differential Amplifier	ODA
Palladium	Pd
Paraffin Wax	PW
Parts Per Million	ppm
Passive Pixel Sensor	PPS
P-Channel Metal-Oxide Semiconductor	PMOS
Personal Computer	PC
Phase Shifter	PS
Phase-Domain Delta-Sigma Modulator	PDΔΣM
Phase-Locked Loop	PLL
Photomultiplier Tube	PMT
Photoplethysmogram	PPG
Photo-Shooting	PS
Plasma-Enhanced Atomic Layer Deposition	PEALD
Plasma-Enhanced Chemical Vapor Deposition	PECVD
Platinum	Pt
Point-of-Care	PoC
Polydimethylsiloxane	PDMS
Polyelectrolyte Multilayer	PEM
Polymerase Chain Reaction	PCR

(continued)

Poly-Phase Filter	PPF
Polysomnography	PSG
Power Amplifier	PA
Power Management Unit	PMU
Power Supply Rejection Ratio	PSRR
Power-on-Reset	POR
Printed Circuit Board	PCB
Programmable Gain Amplifier	PGA
Programmable Gate	PG
Proportional Integral	PI
Proportional to Absolute Temperature	PTAT
Pseudo-Reference Electrode	PRE
Pulmonary Arterial Pressure	PAP
Pulse Pause Encoding	PPE
Pulse Rate	PR
Pulse Width Modulation	PWM
Pulse-Frequency Modulation	PFM
Quadrature Voltage-Controlled Oscillator	QVCO
Quantum Efficiency	QE
Quasi-Interdigitated Electrode	quasi-IDE
Radio Frequency	RF
Radio Frequency Identification	RFID
Random-Access Memory	RAM
Reactive Ion Etching	RIE
Readout Integrated Circuit	ROIC
Receiver	RX
Reference Electrode	RE
Reference Field-Effect Transistor	REFET
Region of Interest	ROI
relative CBF	rCBF
Resistance-to-Digital Converter	RDC
Resistive-Feedback Transimpedance Amplifier	RF-TIA
Retinitis Pigmentosa	RP
Reverse Transcription Polymerase Chain Reaction	RT-PCR
Ring Oscillator	RO
Self-Assembled Monolayer	SAM
Serial Stacked Coil	SSC
Shallow Trench Isolation	STI
Signal-to-Noise Ratio	SNR
Signal-to-Noise-and-Distortion Ratio	SNDR
Silicon	Si
Silicon Large-Scale Integration	Si-LSI
Silicon Nanowire	SiNW
Silicon-On-Insulator	SOI
Simultaneous Neural Active Pixel Sensor	SiNAPS

(continued)

Single-Instruction Multiple-Data	SIMD
Single-Photon Avalanche Photodiode	SPAD
Sodium Chloride	NaCl
Spin-Valve	SV
Standard Deviation	SD
Static Induction Transistor	SIT
Static Random-Access Memory	SRAM
Sub-Thermal drain Voltage	STV
Successive Approximation Register	SAR
Switch Matrix	SM
Switch-Capacitor Stimulation	SCS
Switched-Capacitor Loop Filter	SCLF
System-On-a-Chip	SoC
Tantalum	Ta
Temperature Coefficient	TC
Temperature-to-Frequency Converter	TFC
Time Division Multiplexing	TDM
Time-Domain Near-Infrared Spectroscopy	TD-NIRS
Time-to-Digital Converter	TDC
Timing Control Module	TCM
Titanium Nitride	TiN
Titanium-Tungsten	TiW
Transceiver	TRX
Transimpedance Amplifier	TIA
Transmitter	TX
Tunnel Magnetoresistance	TMR
Ultrasound	US
Ultraviolet	UV
Vapor-Liquid-Solid	VLS
Voltage/Current-Controlled Stimulation	V/CCS
Voltage-Controlled Oscillator	VCO
Voltage-Frequency Converter	VFC
Voltage-to-Current	V-to-I
Working Electrode	WE
Zinc	Zn

Chapter 1
Introduction to CMOS Sensors

CMOS (Complementary Metal-Oxide-Semiconductor) technology is at the forefront of sensor integration, enabling the development of a diverse array of sensors on a single chip. These sensors include capacitive [1–5], impedimetric [6] optical [7], nuclear magnetic resonance (NMR) [8], magnetic hall effect [9], thermal [10], and mechanical [11] types, each designed to detect specific physical changes. CMOS technology facilitates the miniaturization and integration of these sensors, along with their interface circuits, onto a compact and cost-effective platform. This integration allows for the detection of minute electrical changes, which are then processed through on-chip analog circuits, converting analog signals into digital data that is transferred to an external data acquisition (DAQ) system, as illustrated in Fig. 1.1.

Figure 1.1 depicts a CMOS chip consisting of an array of sensors (interdigitated electrodes) with on-chip circuitry, assembled on a printed circuit board (PCB). The PCB includes a DAQ system that communicates with external devices such as a computer or cloud-based systems. The graphical user interface displays the droplet evaporation profile, which serves as a fingerprint of the droplet's alcohol content, as reported in [12].

Advanced CMOS sensors can be equipped with on-chip processors, enabling efficient data preprocessing, control, and analog-to-digital signal conversion. This integration is crucial for real-time applications where sensors generate, process, and convert signals instantaneously. Emerging CMOS sensors are also incorporating artificial intelligence (AI) directly on the chip, allowing for intelligent data analysis and decision-making at the sensor level. These advancements pave the way for autonomous systems in fields such as medical diagnostics, environmental monitoring, and industrial automation.

Figure 1.2 illustrates an advanced CMOS sensor system on a single chip. This chip features a recognition element (e.g., catalyst material or antibody) that converts chemical or biological properties into physical changes (e.g., optical or dielectric). Physical sensors (e.g., FET, capacitive, impedimetric, optical, magnetic, thermal,

E. Ghafar-Zadeh et al., *Advanced CMOS Biochips*, Analog Circuits and Signal Processing, https://doi.org/10.1007/978-94-007-0099-4_1

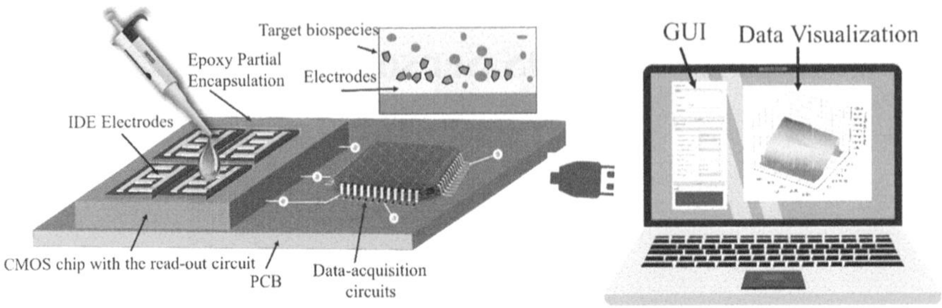

Fig. 1.1 Illustration of a CMOS sensing platform consisting of a CMOS chip integrated on a PCB, connected to a computer through a DAQ system, and operated using a GUI running on the computer

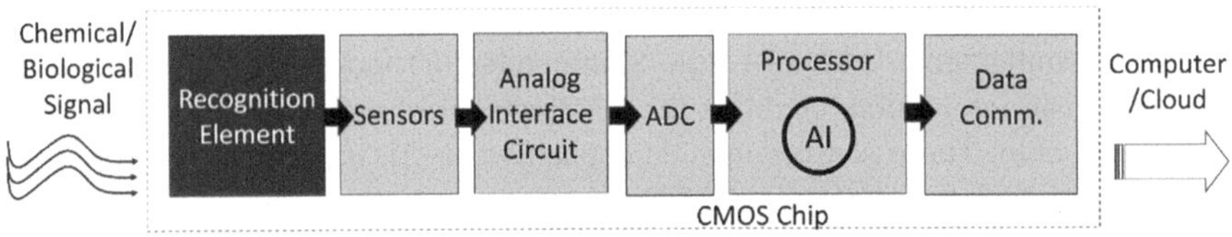

Fig. 1.2 Illustration of an advanced CMOS sensor system on a single chip

and mechanical sensors) measure these physical changes and convert them into electrical signals. The analog interface circuit detects minute changes in the electrical signal and converts them into current or voltage. An analog-to-digital converter efficiently processes these signals with high resolution and maximum dynamic range. A processor, microcontroller, or signal logic circuit then manages the data process and transfer to a computer after preprocessing. The data can be sent to the cloud or other workstations to train AI or ML models for pattern extraction or sensitivity enhancement. These models can be deployed to interpret unknown signals or run directly within a processor embedded inside the CMOS sensor chip.

1.1 CMOS Sensing Devices for Life Science Applications

CMOS sensors are increasingly used for point-of-care diagnostics in various forms, including handheld systems, implantable sensors for measuring specific biomarkers, and wearable sensors for monitoring electrophysiological signals. For example, CMOS sensors can detect biomarkers such as physiological signals (e.g., Electrocardiogram (ECG)), specific molecules (e.g., glucose or cortisol in sweat), or other substances. For the separation of large molecules or cells in body fluids, microfluidic devices are employed. Microfluidics enhances the efficiency of the diagnostic process by separating large molecules or cells from whole body fluid samples [2, 13].

The goal of developing point-of-care diagnostic technologies is to measure biomarkers non-invasively. For instance, CMOS sensors can directly detect biomarkers in materials such as sweat, saliva, urine, and blood. CMOS sensors, coupled with microfluidics and recognition elements, are designed to measure these biomarkers effectively.

1.2 CMOS Technology

CMOS technology involves multiple thin film layers, including polysilicon, used to develop the transistor channels. The silicon oxide layer above polysilicon, located between metal layers, plays a crucial role and acts as an isolation layer. While the metal material inside the chip is generally not crucial for sensing, the materials on top of the CMOS are essential. Typically, the top layer, often aluminum (e.g. M6 in below Fig. 1.3), is covered with anodized aluminum oxide. The thickness of the material layer on top is vital for developing the sensing electrode and affects the measurement of biological or chemical materials.

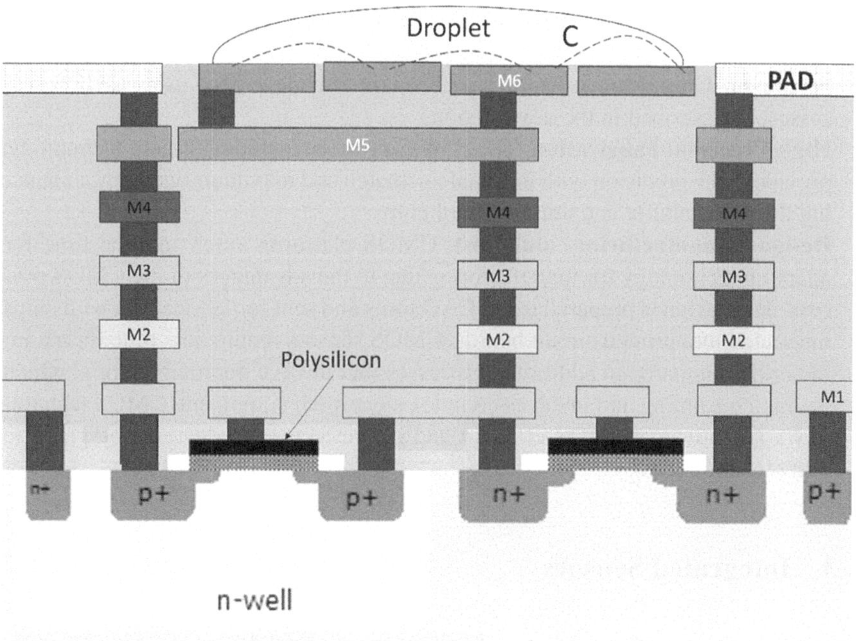

Fig. 1.3 Illustration of the CMOS layers used in creating CBCM-based sensors on top of the CMOS chip

As seen in Fig. 1.3 the CMOS chip can be developed to create two transistors for charge-based capacitance measurement (CBCM) to measure the capacitance (C) between the interdigitated electrodes on the top of the CMOS chip exposed to a droplet [16]. This figure illustrates the metal layers, vias, and pads used for connecting the transistors to the top-layer sensor and for providing electrical supplies.

1.2.1 Why CMOS?

CMOS processes, traditionally used for developing electronic devices and CPUs with millions of transistors operating at high speeds (e.g., 100 GHz), are now being applied to sensor technology. CMOS technology represents a new frontier in integrated circuit design, with substantial investment and reliability making it the most advanced platform for developing electronic sensors for life science applications such as DNA sequencing [14].

- **Documented Analog and Digital Integrated Circuits**: CMOS technology supports both analog and digital integrated circuits, such as multiplexers and operational amplifiers. Analog front-end circuits for capacitive sensors, current and charge amplifiers for measuring small currents or charges (e.g., in DNA nanopore sensors), and sensors sensitive to capacitance are developed using CMOS technology
- **Sensor-on-Chip**: Many sensors have been directly developed using CMOS processes, as described in the next section
- **High-Precision Fabrication**: The CMOS process, including 22 nm technology, provides high precision with minimal mismatch and maximum accuracy, enhancing the repeatability and uniformity of chips.
- **Design, Manufacturing, and Cost**: CMOS platforms offer minimal time for adapting technology for manufacturing due to the advantages of the CMOS process. The design is prepared using CAD tools and sent for fabrication, with chips integrated into printed circuit boards. CMOS sensors require less time for manufacturing compared to additional processes that involve microfabrication, which is time-consuming and involves complex cleanroom equipment. CMOS technology's key advantage is its efficient and cost-effective production compared to other technologies.

1.3 Integrated Sensors

Integrated sensors within CMOS technology are physical devices designed to measure various physical changes such as charge, dielectric properties, impedance, optical, magnetic, or thermal variations. Coated with specific sensitive materials, these sensors can transduce chemical or biological phenomena into detectable physical changes, making them versatile tools in biosensing and chemical detection.

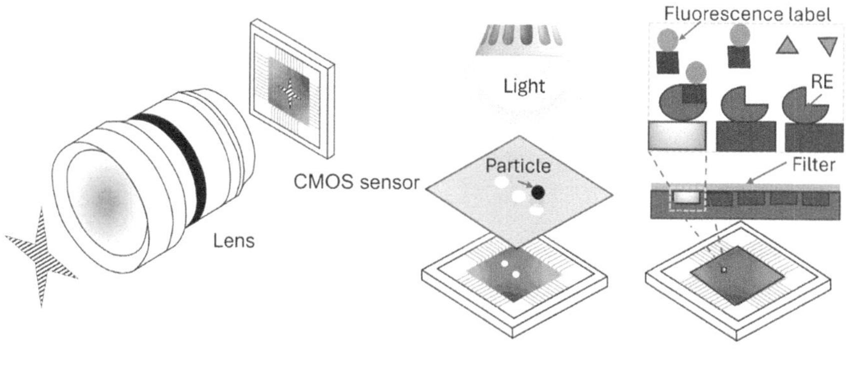

(a) (b) (c)

Fig. 1.4 Illustration of optical sensors: (**a**) CMOS imager, (**b**) near-field bright field optical sensor, (**c**) near-field fluorescence sensor

1.3.1 Optical Sensors

Optical sensors in CMOS technology are among the most advanced and widely used, particularly as CMOS image sensors as shown in Fig. 1.4a. These image sensors consist of millions of photodiodes, each responsible for capturing light across different colors, enabling high-resolution imaging. These sensors can also be adapted for near-field detection as seen in Fig. 1.4b, with each pixel capable of detecting and differentiating between nanoscale particles [15]. Optical sensors can be configured for fluorescence detection with appropriate filters and dyes, playing a crucial role in bioassays where target molecules are labeled with fluorescent dyes (see Fig. 1.4c) [16].

1.3.2 Field-Effect Transistor (FET) Sensors

Field-effect transistor (FET) sensors, developed using CMOS technology, are pivotal in applications such as DNA sequencing (See Figs. 1.5a and b). For example, the CMOS-based DNA sequencing system by Ion Torrent incorporates millions of FET sensors to detect DNA sequences [17]. These sensors measure charge changes resulting from biochemical reactions, such as nucleotide binding, which leads to detectable pH changes. FET sensors are valuable in medical diagnostics, including infectious disease detection. Designed with a gate above the channel, these sensors create a double-layer capacitance due to a metal thin layer exposed to biochemical electrolytes. The resulting current fluctuations are measured with high sensitivity and selectivity.

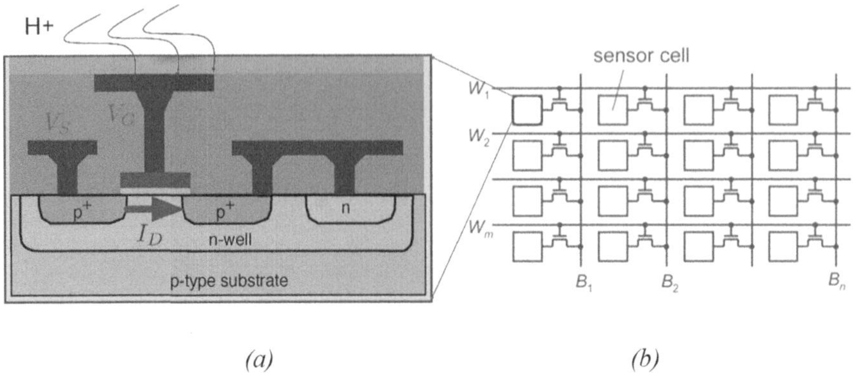

Fig. 1.5 ISFET sensor array (**a**) a single cell, (**b**) array of sensing cells

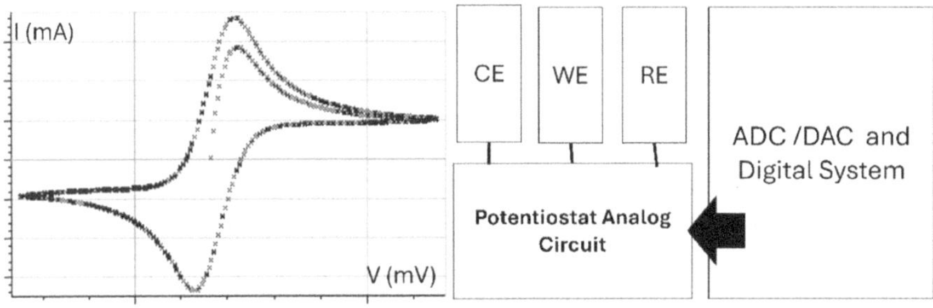

Fig. 1.6 Principle of CMOS Electrochemical system

1.3.3 Electrochemical Sensors

Electrochemical sensors on CMOS chips are used for applications such as cellular monitoring and drug studies. These sensors measure capacitive, resistive, or impedance properties, often using two or three-electrode configurations. The three-electrode setup, including working (WE), counter (CE), and reference (RE) electrodes, allows for measuring electrical variations by applying DC or AC signals through the sample. These sensors are employed in biosensing for DNA hybridization monitoring, drug studies, and cellular analysis, making them essential in both research and clinical settings. Figure 1.6 The main electronic blocks of an electrochemical interface circuit and a typical cyclic voltammetry (CV) method, which are widely used in biological and chemical sensors [18].

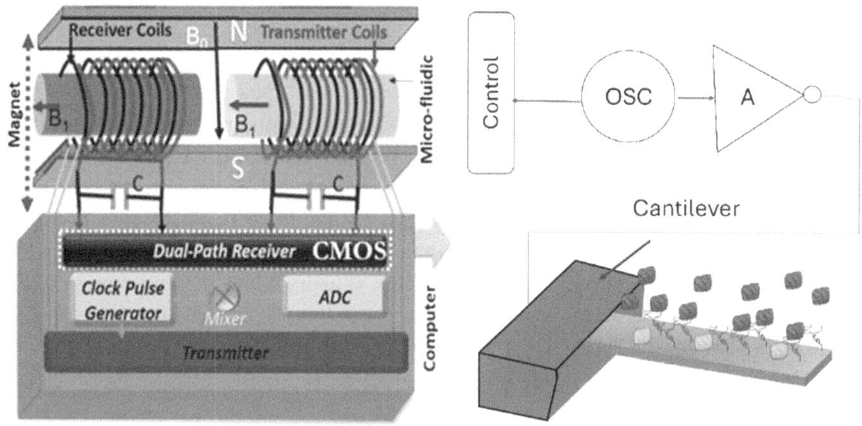

(a) (b)

Fig. 1.7 Illustration of magnetic and cantilever based sensor (**a**) CMOS dual path CMOS NMR including two external micro coils controlled CMOS consisting of ADC, Mixer and pulse generator and (**b**) Cantilever sensor integrable on CMOS using an oscillator (OSC) for actuation

1.3.4 Magnetic Sensors

Magnetic sensors in CMOS technology detect magnetic beads used as substrates for molecular attachment. This capability enables the identification of unknown molecules by detecting these beads. Magnetic sensors can detect micro and nano-sized beads, sensitive to magnetic fields, indicating the presence of target molecules or cells. Miniaturized nuclear magnetic resonance (NMR) sensors integrated onto CMOS platforms have gained attention for their potential in various applications. These palm-sized dual path NMR sensors (Fig. 1.7a) operate at lower frequencies than standard systems, suitable for portable and accessible diagnostics [19].

1.3.5 Thermal and Mechanical Sensors

Thermal sensors, or temperature sensors, are critical for ensuring that bioassays or sensors operate within specific temperature ranges. CMOS technology allows the fabrication of electronic temperature sensors, such as bipolar transistors, used for monitoring chip temperature, especially under high power consumption. CMOS technology also supports the development of specialized sensors using post-CMOS processes, such as micro-machining. Cantilevers (see Fig. 1.7b) are fabricated on CMOS chips and integrated with circuitry to generate signals through oscillators, converting them to pulses via Schmitt trigger circuitry, as shown in Fig. 1.7b. These are used in biosensing applications or to create accelerometers for various uses, such as triggering airbags or fall detection systems [20].

1.4 Summary and Organization

CMOS technology's ability to integrate diverse sensor types onto a single chip has revolutionized the sensor industry. The ongoing development of CMOS sensors, including those with on-chip AI capabilities and specialized post-CMOS processes, promises to enhance the precision, functionality, and application range of these sensors. As CMOS technology advances, it will continue to drive innovation in fields such as medical diagnostics and environmental monitoring. This book's chapters include: Chap. 2 on design strategies for CMOS sensors; Chaps. 3 and 4 on sensors and circuits used in CMOS sensing platforms; Chap. 5 on advanced electronic technologies beyond CMOS; and Chap. 6 on future work and state-of-the-art technologies.

References

1. Sun F, Tang S (2024) A CMOS front-end circuit for capacitive sensors with zero adjustment. Eng Res Express 3(3):035353
2. Ghafar-Zadeh E, Sawan M, Ghafar-Zadeh E, Sawan M (2010) CMOS capacitive sensors for lab-on-chip applications. Springer
3. Laborde C, Pittino F, Verhoeven H, Lemay S, Selmi L, Jongsma M et al (2015) Real-time imaging of microparticles and living cells with CMOS nanocapacitor arrays. Nat Nanotechnol 10:791–795
4. Forouhi S, Dehghani R, Ghafar-Zadeh E (2019) CMOS based capacitive sensors for life science applications: A review. Sensors Actuators A Phys 297:111531
5. Osouli Tabrizi H, Forouhi S, Azadmousavi T, Ghafar-Zadeh E (2024) A multidisciplinary approach toward CMOS capacitive sensor array for droplet analysis. Micromachines 15:232
6. Hedayatipour A, Aslanzadeh S, McFarlane N (2019) CMOS based whole cell impedance sensing: Challenges and future outlook. Biosens Bioelectron 143:111600
7. Hosseini Y, Kaler KV (2010) Integrated CMOS optical sensor for cell detection and analysis. Sensors Actuators A Phys 157:1–8
8. Krüger D, Zhang A, Aghelnejad B, Hinton H, Arnal VM, Song Y-Q et al (2023) A portable CMOS-based spin resonance system for high-resolution spectroscopy and imaging. IEEE J Solid State Circuits 58:1838–1849
9. Zou H, Lei K-M, Martins RP, Mak P-I (2023) A CMOS hall sensors Array with integrated readout circuit resilient to local magnetic interference from current-carrying traces. IEEE Sensors J 23:16145–16153
10. Xu W, Li Z, Fang Z, Wang B, Hong L, Yang G et al (2023) A sub-5mW Monolithic CMOS-MEMS thermal flow sensing SoC with $\pm $6 m/s linear range. IEEE J Solid State Circuits 99:1–11
11. Bausells J, Carrabina J, Merlos A, Bota S, Samitier J (1997) Mechanical sensors integrated in a commercial CMOS technology. Sensors Actuators A Phys 62:698–704
12. Forouhi S, Tabrizi HO, Panahi A, Magierowski S, Ghafar-Zadeh E (2023) Novel CMOS thermo-capacitive sensing method for lab-on-chip applications. IEEE Biomed Circuits Syst Conf (BioCAS) 2023:1–5
13. Carrara S (2023) Bio/CMOS interfaces for capacitance sensing. In: Bio/CMOS interfaces and co-design. Springer, pp 405–429
14. Garrido-Cardenas JA, Garcia-Maroto F, Alvarez-Bermejo JA, Manzano-Agugliaro F (2017) DNA sequencing sensors: an overview. Sensors 17:588

15. Seiler ST, Rich IS, Lindquist NC (2016) Direct spectral imaging of plasmonic nanohole arrays for real-time sensing. Nanotechnology 27:184001
16. Patounakis G, Shepard KL, Levicky R (2006) Active CMOS array sensor for time-resolved fluorescence detection. IEEE J Solid State Circuits 41:2521–2530
17. Magierowski S, Huang Y, Wang C, Ghafar-Zadeh E (2016) Nanopore-CMOS interfaces for DNA sequencing. Biosensors 6:42
18. Hosseini S-N, Das PS, Lazarjan VK, Gagnon-Turcotte G, Bouzid K, Gosselin B (2023) Recent advances in CMOS electrochemical biosensor design for microbial monitoring: review and design methodology. IEEE Trans Biomed Circuits Syst 17:202–228
19. Pourmodheji H, Ghafar-Zadeh E, Magierowski S (2017) A CMOS differential receiver dedicated to nuclear magnetic resonance applications. Analog Integr Circ Sig Process 91:97–109
20. Kirstein K-U, Li Y, Zimmermann M, Vancura C, Volden T, Song WH et al (2005) Cantilever-based biosensors in CMOS technology. In: Design, automation and test in Europe. IEEE, pp 1340–1341

Chapter 2
CMOS Sensors' Design Strategies

In designing a CMOS sensor, several critical factors must be carefully considered, including the application, sensing mechanism, CMOS chip design, electrical and chemical characterization procedures, and final test procedures. Each of these elements must be meticulously planned and integrated with practical considerations.

2.1 CMOS Chip Design

The design of the CMOS chip encompasses standard CMOS chip design and fabrication, post-CMOS fabrication procedures, interface system design, and graphical User Interface (GUI) system design.

As illustrated in Fig. 2.1, as an example, the counting of oral neutrophil cells for periodontal applications through a CMPOS chip has been chosen. This application is described in Sect. 2.4.1.1. After the completion of the chip design, post-CMOS fabrication, and implementation of the interface system and GUI, as detailed in Appendix A, characterization and application (e.g. Oral Periodontal) should follow a plan that requires attention from the initial stages of chip development.

2.1.1 Critical Questions to Be Addressed

Before starting the design of a CMOS chip, the following critical questions should be addressed:

E. Ghafar-Zadeh et al., *Advanced CMOS Biochips*, Analog Circuits and Signal Processing, https://doi.org/10.1007/978-94-007-0099-4_2

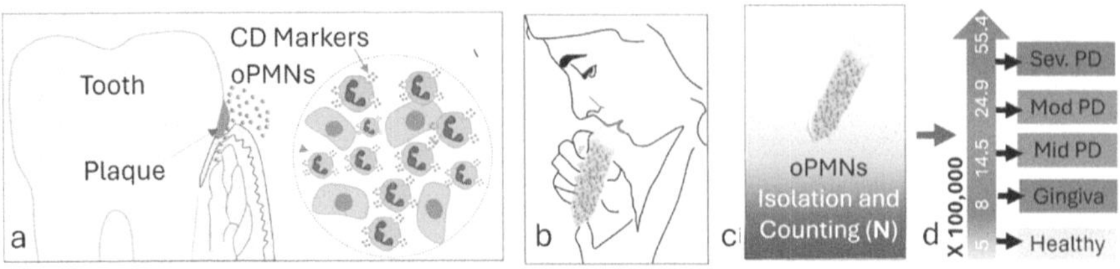

Fig. 2.1 Illustration of oral neutrophil (**a**) generation, (**b**) collection, (**c**) counting, and (**d**) diagnostics

2.1.1.1 Main Application and Purpose

What should be sensed by the integrated CMOS sensor and circuit? It is essential to consider the application's requirements and the external motivations driving the use of CMOS technology. For instance, urgent needs like those arising from the COVID-19 pandemic have highlighted CMOS's advantages due to its low design-to-market time, mass production capabilities, and cost reduction. The applicant should have a promising market to justify these benefits.

- *Uniqueness of CMOS for Specific Applications*: Developing a CMOS sensor is most advantageous when the integration of the sensor and circuitry provides unique benefits, such as the following:
- *Large Array of Sensors*: CMOS is ideal for applications requiring a large number of sensors, such as hundreds of millions of FETs for DNA sequencing. Other technologies might struggle with the extensive wiring needed to connect these sensors to interface circuits. CMOS facilitates the integration of a large array of sensors with their corresponding circuits.
- *Extremely Small Sensor and Circuit*: For applications requiring tiny sensors, such as those in wearable devices or smart endoscopy capsules, CMOS technology's low power consumption, low cost, and miniaturization capabilities are crucial. Integration of the sensor and circuitry on the same chip is important for achieving high precision and efficient data transfer.
- *Measurement of Extremely Small Changes*: If the application involves measuring very small changes, such as femtofarad variations due to cell attachment on the chip's surface, CMOS enables the integration of very small sensors with the circuit on the same chip.

2.1.2 Main Application and Post-CMOS Processes

To choose the appropriate application to be addressed using CMOS technology, the following questions must be raised and addressed by the designer:

- What should the post-CMOS processes be to prepare the CMOS chip for chemical or biological sensing, particularly for label-free or highly selective sensing applications?

- Are the suggested post-CMOS processes compatible with CMOS technology, or are they too harsh and likely to damage the device?
- What is the required size of the sensing area that can be adapted to the post-CMOS processes, considering mask alignment (if needed) and other requirements?
- Should we develop microfluidic devices on top of the CMOS chip? Should the integration or post-CMOS processes be performed on the wafer before dicing?

To answer these questions, we need to clarify which applications are best suited to CMOS-compatible processes. For example, if the CMOS chip will experience very high temperatures that might affect its performance, the post-CMOS processes must be compatible with CMOS technology to avoid damage and maintain functionality.

2.2 Sensing Mechanisms

While CMOS technology can support various multimodal sensing modules, including capacitive, impedimetric, magnetic, thermal, electrochemical, and mechanical techniques, the key question is determining the most suitable sensing mechanism for specific applications. For example, in detecting a virus, one might consider detecting a specific gene, such as the N-Gene. This could be achieved through DNA hybridization detection, which is challenging for longer genes, or by using an ion-sensitive field-effect transistor (ISFET) to detect pH changes resulting from DNA hybridization and amplification. In the first case, a capacitive sensor could be employed, while the second approach might utilize an ISFET. As illustrated, selecting the appropriate sensing mechanism is crucial in deploying a CMOS sensing platform. In this chapter, we present a CMOS capacitive sensor for cellular monitoring as a case study.

2.3 Plan for Testing and Characterization

To verify the design of the CMOS sensor and circuitry, computer-aided design (CAD) tools, such as Cadence, are employed. After fabrication, the electrical functionality of the chip can be validated by assessing the electrical input/output signals to ensure the chip is operational. The next step involves introducing chemicals after encapsulating the chip to prevent direct contact between the wires and the liquid. The chemical solution should be selected based on the specific application. For instance, dielectric chemical solutions such as deionized water (DI) and ethanol can be used for characterizing a capacitive sensor. For biological characterization, the device should be tested after following proper sample preparation and coating the surface with materials that enhance biocompatibility, such as those used for cellular analysis.

2.4 Design and Implementation of a CMOS Sensor

In this section, a CMOS sensor is designed and implemented for a life science application. The materials presented serve as an example to illustrate the design strategy and practical considerations.

2.4.1 Periodontal Application

To investigate the advantages of CMOS technology for developing sensors and circuits for periodontal applications, let's begin with an introduction to the importance of periodontal health. We will then explore how CMOS technology can address specific challenges related to periodontal applications.

2.4.1.1 Why Is Early Detection of Periodontal Disease Important?

Recent periodontal research studies have found a correlation between gum diseases and other conditions such as diabetes, osteoporosis, and human immunodeficiency virus (HIV) [1–3]. For instance, it is well documented that patients with severe osteoporosis will likely experience periodontal breakdown [4]. There are also reports regarding the increased populations of periodontal-related bacteria in patients with HIV [5, 6]. Moreover, there is a high risk of heart diseases in people with unhealthy gums which is a result of bacterial infection in the bloodstream [7, 8]. Also, the recent studies show a link between the salivatory oral cells such as Oral Polymorphonuclear Neutrophils (oPMNs) and gum diseases (Fig. 2.1) [9–11]. Indeed, the quantification and analysis of oral cells can improve our understanding of the cellular activities in saliva and might deliver a clear picture of oral health. For example, it has been verified that the number of oPMNs in patients with periodontitis is 4 times higher in comparison to healthy individuals [12]. The presence of an excessive number of oPMNs might have a negative impact on the oral tissue's integrity [13]. As a result of periodontitis and chronic activation of oral neutrophils, there might be damage to the periodontal connective tissue which leads to the loss of attachment, alveolar bone, and tooth loss [14]. Another example is a link between the epithelial cells derived from oral cavities and oral health. As per recent studies, epithelial cells contain biomarkers for oral diseases such as oral cancer [15, 16]. These research findings further show the importance of oral cell analysis using advanced sensing technologies to improve our understanding of the role of salivary cells in the gum and other inflammatory diseases [17, 18]. Until now, there has been no already-established sensing platform for analyzing oral cellular activities. Researchers employ standard methods such as fluorescence microscopic and flow cytometry [19]. These methods need specialized equipment with tens of thousands of dollars, a costly service contract, and trained staff to operate them. Therefore, their use is restricted to well-funded laboratories [20]. The question that arises is how CMOS sensors can be utilized to monitor oral cell activities.

2.4.2 *Sensing Mechanism*

Capacitive sensors are one of the popular CMOS biosensors reported to be advantages for studying growth and other cellular activities [21]. In these applications, the cells are firmly attached to the surface through integrin-containing multi-protein structures [22]. But, there are some challenges related to studying oral cells and doing research on them [23]. Unlike other cells, oral cells have very low culture ability, thus, they have less affinity to the surface even if they are in a culture medium [24–26]. Although researchers have made some efforts to culture oral cells in the saliva medium or other similar mediums, it has not been quite successful [23]. In many experiments for culturing neutrophils, the cells have undergone apoptosis and died after less than an hour and their morphology has changed [23]. In most tests on periodontal diseases, normal saline was used to take samples and study saliva cells without culturing them. Oral cells should be studied in the most similar material to saliva in order to be alive during the experiments [27]. These cells cannot be cultured in an in-vitro environment because they have a concise life span [28]. It is worth mentioning that since oral neutrophils have been activated during their migration from blood circulation to the oral cavity, they cannot be divided anymore. So, they are in the last stage of their life cycle, and their nucleus cannot do cytokines as well [28]. There are different types of CD markers on the surface of neutrophil cells that might be responsible for cell attachment. According to the literature, the essential CD markers accountable for cell attachment are Mac-1 (CD 11b and CD18) [25, 28]. These CD markers may increase the affinity of cells to the hydrophilic surface of the silicon oxide or aluminum oxide above the CMOS chip. This section addresses the challenge of monitoring the hydrophilic adhesion using the CMOS capacitive sensing platform.

2.4.2.1 Novelty of Using Capacitive Sensors for Oral Cell Monitoring

To date, many papers have reported the advantages of CMOS capacitive sensors for monitoring the growth and proliferation of various cell types, with some state-of-the-art examples presented in Table 2.1. These capacitive sensors have achieved high resolution and sensitivity. However, they are limited by a low dynamic range and suffer from parasitic capacitances caused by debris and other remnants accumulating above the sensor. In this chapter, we employ the CMOS capacitive sensor proposed in Chap. 2 for oral cell monitoring for the first time, examining different

Table 2.1 Capacitive sensing electrodes for cellular monitoring

CMOS Technology	Type of cell	Electrode material	Resolution	IDR (fF)	Reference
0.5 μm	hBC	Al/1pass	0.1 fF	25	[31]
0.35 μm	hOC	Al/SiO_2/Si_3N_4	14.4 aF	12	[32, 33]
0.25 μm	*S.epidermidis*	Al/Al_2O_3	10 fF	NA	[34]
0.25 μm	*S.epidermidis*	Al/Al_2O_3	450 aF	57	[35]
0.18 μm	*E.Coli*	Al/wPass	10 aF	7	[36]
0.35 μm	hLC	Al/PEM	10 aF	6	[21]
90 nm	hBC	AuCu	10 aF	1	[37]
0.35 μm	Oral cells	Al/A_2O_3	416 aF	400	This work

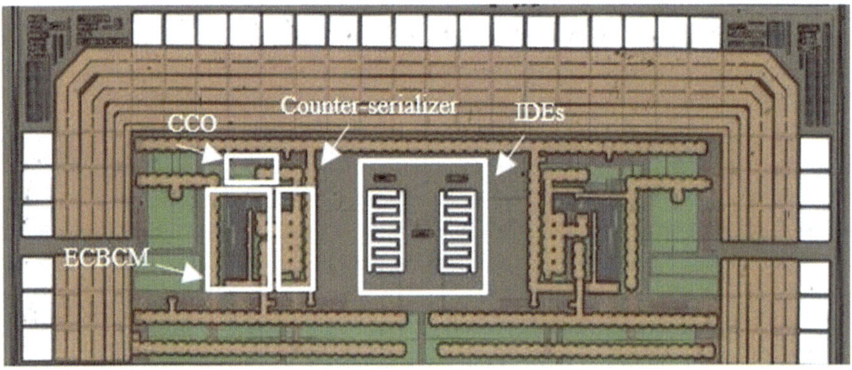

Fig. 2.2 Microscopic image of a CMOS capacitive interface and two IDEs

oral cell types within the sample. Additionally, the sensing electrodes used in this chapter, as well as in other reported studies, consist of metal or metal oxides, which demonstrate hydrophilic properties. These properties are suitable for measuring hydrophilic materials such as oral neutrophils that attach to the electrodes [29, 30].

2.4.3 *Integrated Capacitive Circuits and Sensors*

To date, many papers have reported the design of CMOS capacitive sensors for cellular monitoring. A CMOS capacitive interface circuit typically consists of a capacitive sensor, a current or voltage converter (also known as Enhanced Capacitance-Based Measurement, ECBCM), and an Analog-to-Digital Converter (ADC) for converting analog signals to digital. This setup uses a Controlled Current Oscillator (CCO) and Integrated Electrodes (IDE), as illustrated in Fig. 2.2 [38].

2.4.4 Computer -CMOS Sensor Interface System and Encapsulation

The connection between the capacitive interface circuit and the computer requires an electronic board that transfers digital numbers to the computer. This hardware is matched with graphical user interface (GUI) software, as described in Appendix A. Figure 2.3 shows an interface system and the encapsulated CMOS chip.

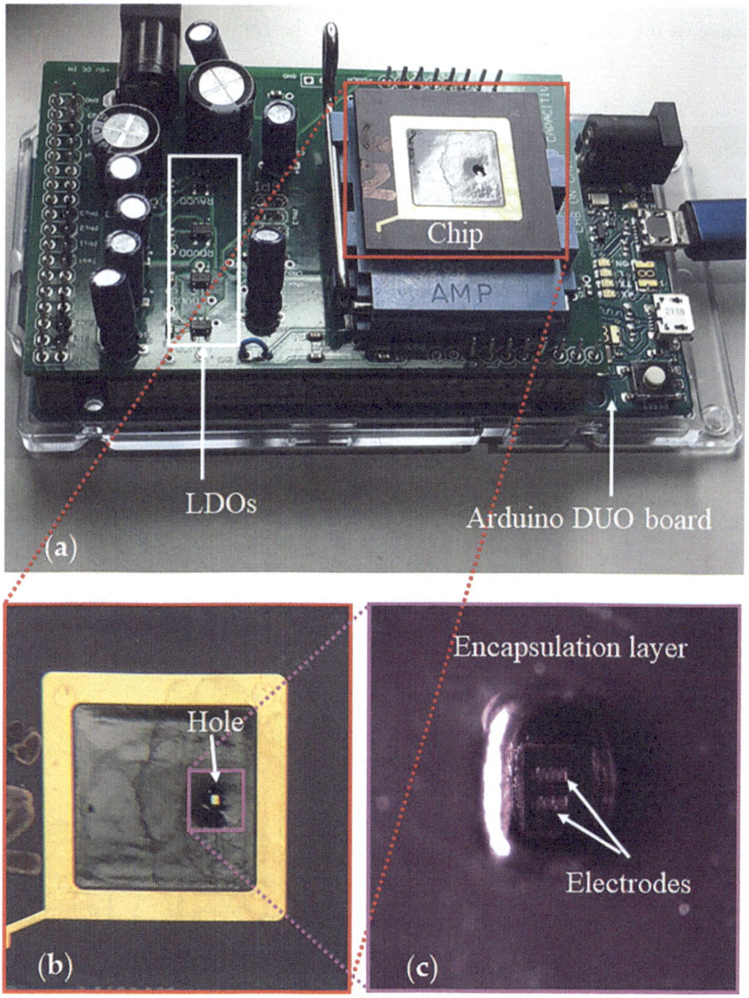

Fig. 2.3 (**a**) An Arduino DUE microcontroller board together with a custom-made electronic board holding the chip, (**b**) The chip, (**c**) The microscopic image of the two electrodes and the surrounding encapsulation layer with a hole for the non-passivated sensing electrodes

2.4.5 Characterization: Electrical/Chemical/Biological

The characterization of the CMOS sensor includes both electrical and chemical tests following Cadence simulation, as reported in [39]. Additionally, to demonstrate the functionality of the proposed CMOS sensor for oral cell monitoring, the sensor was tested with oral cells prepared according to the protocol in [14]. The process involved exposing the cells to the CMOS sensor, as shown in the microscopic image in Fig. 2.4, oral ells with various concentrations were introduced into the CMOS chip, corresponding to the results shown in samples 2–4. These results are corroborated by the microscopic images in Fig. 2.4b–e. Figure 2.4a and f depict the surface of the chip before washing and after the removal of oral neutrophils.

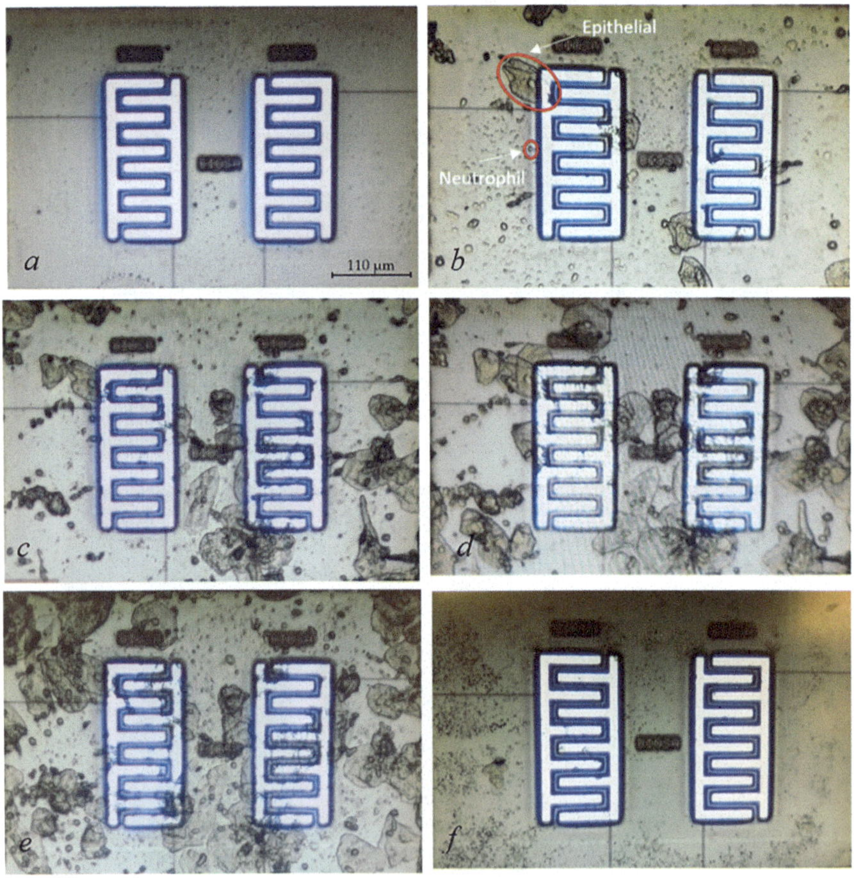

Fig. 2.4 Illustrates the microscopic images of oral cells on the chip at various stages: (**a**) before cell introduction, (**b**) after the first trial, (**c**) with doubled cell concentration, (**d**) tripled cell concentration, (**e**) quadrupled cell concentration, and (**f**) post-cleaning

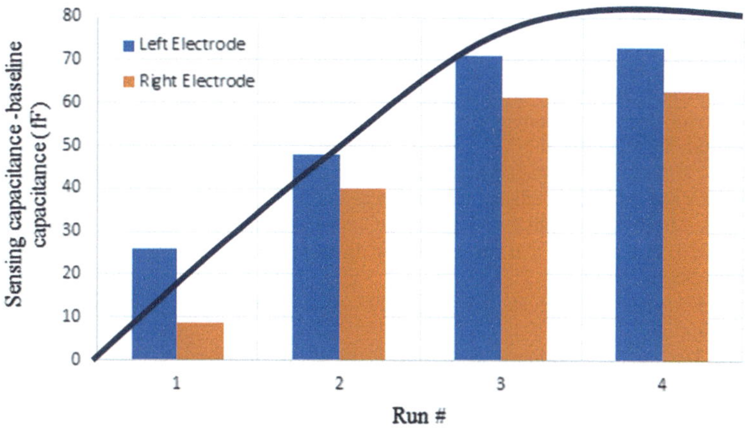

Fig. 2.5 Oral neutrophil measurement results using the CMOS capacitive sensor

Figure 2.5 shows that the capacitive sensor output increases with higher cell concentrations, although the relationship is nonlinear due to non-uniform cell distribution and other non-idealities associated with the bipolar electrodes on the chip.

2.5 Summary

In this chapter, design strategies for CMOS sensors are presented, emphasizing the selection criteria for applications and leveraging CMOS advantages, such as the ability to develop large sensor arrays, low power consumption, and integration of sensors with circuitry. The chapter includes a detailed example demonstrating the design, implementation, and characterization of a CMOS capacitive sensor. The results showcase the sensor's performance and effectiveness, illustrating its potential for various applications.

References

1. Llambés F, Arias-Herrera S, Caffesse R (2015) Relationship between diabetes and periodontal infection. World J Diabetes 6:927–935
2. Wang C-W, McCauley LK (2016) Osteoporosis and periodontitis. Curr Osteoporos Rep 14:284–291
3. Pólvora TLS, Nobre ÁVV, Tirapelli C, Taba M Jr, Macedo LDD, Santana RC et al (2018) Relationship between human immunodeficiency virus (HIV-1) infection and chronic periodontitis. Expert Rev Clin Immunol 14:315–327
4. Hajishengallis G, Moutsopoulos NM, Hajishengallis E, Chavakis T (2016) Immune and regulatory functions of neutrophils in inflammatory bone loss. Semin Immunol 28(2):146–158

5. Levine AM, Karim R, Mack W, Gravink DJ, Anastos K, Young M et al (2006) Neutropenia in human immunodeficiency virus infection: Data from the women's interagency HIV study. Arch Intern Med 166:405–410
6. Perez Rosero E, Heron S, Jovel J, O'Neil CR, Turvey SL, Parashar P et al (2021) Differential signature of the microbiome and neutrophils in the oral cavity of HIV-infected individuals. Front Immunol 12:780910
7. Liccardo D, Cannavo A, Spagnuolo G, Ferrara N, Cittadini A, Rengo C et al (2019) Periodontal disease: A risk factor for diabetes and cardiovascular disease. Int J Mol Sci 20:1414
8. Sanz M, Marco del Castillo A, Jepsen S, Gonzalez-Juanatey JR, D'Aiuto F, Bouchard P et al (2020) Periodontitis and cardiovascular diseases: Consensus report. J Clin Periodontol 47:268–288
9. Fine N, Glogauer M, Perio D. The neutrophil in oral health and disease: The new diagnostic biomarker.
10. Fine N, Hassanpour S, Borenstein A, Sima C, Oveisi M, Scholey J et al (2016) Distinct oral neutrophil subsets define health and periodontal disease states. J Dent Res 95:931–938
11. Çetin Özdemir E, Bilen E, Yazar FM (2022) Can the delta neutrophil ındex be used as a preliminary biomarker ın the evaluation of periodontal disease: A pilot study. J Appl Oral Sci 30:e20210555
12. Nicu EA, Rijkschroeff P, Wartewig E, Nazmi K, Loos BG (2018) Characterization of oral polymorphonuclear neutrophils in periodontitis patients: A case-control study. BMC Oral Health 18:1–9
13. Hirschfeld J (2020) Neutrophil subsets in periodontal health and disease: A mini review. Front Immunol 10:3001
14. Khoury W, Glogauer J, Tenenbaum HC, Glogauer M (2020) Oral inflammatory load: Neutrophils as oral health biomarkers. J Periodontal Res 55:594–601
15. Akbari E, Epstein JB, Samim F (2024) Unveiling the hidden links: periodontal disease, Fusobacterium Nucleatum, and cancers. Curr Oncol Rep:1–10
16. Farhad SZ, Karbalaeihasanesfahani A, Dadgar E, Nasiri K, Esfahaniani M, Nabi Afjadi M (2024) The role of periodontitis in cancer development, with a focus on oral cancers. Mol Biol Rep 51:814
17. Rijkschroeff P, Jansen ID, Van Der Weijden FA, Keijser BJ, Loos BG, Nicu EA (2016) Oral polymorphonuclear neutrophil characteristics in relation to oral health: A cross-sectional, observational clinical study. Int J Oral Sci 8:191–198
18. Rijkschroeff P, Loos BG, Nicu EA (2018) Oral polymorphonuclear neutrophil contributes to oral health. Curr Oral Health Rep 5:211–220
19. McKinnon KM (2018) Flow cytometry: An overview. *Curr Protoc Immunol* 120:5.1. 1–5.1. 11
20. Vembadi A, Menachery A, Qasaimeh MA (2019) Cell cytometry: Review and perspective on biotechnological advances. Front Bioeng Biotechnol 7:147
21. Nabovati G, Ghafar-Zadeh E, Letourneau A, Sawan M (2018) Smart cell culture monitoring and drug test platform using CMOS capacitive sensor array. IEEE Trans Biomed Eng 66:1094–1104
22. Burridge K (2017) Focal adhesions: A personal perspective on a half century of progress. FEBS J 284:3355–3361
23. Li R, Wang Z, Huang J, He S, Peng Y, Wan Y et al (2022) Neutrophils culture in collagen gel system. Front Immunol 13:816037
24. Southgate J, Williams H, Trejdosiewicz L, Hodges G (1987) Primary culture of human oral epithelial cells. Lab Investig 56:211–223
25. Oda D, Watson E (1990) Human oral epithelial cell culture I. Improved conditions for reproducible culture in serum-free medium. In Vitro Cell Dev Biol 26:589–595
26. Sheth R, Neale MH, Shortt AJ, Massie I, Vernon AJ, Daniels JT (2015) Culture and characterization of oral mucosal epithelial cells on a fibrin gel for ocular surface reconstruction. Curr Eye Res 40:1077–1087

27. Yang Y, Knight R, Stephens P, Zhang Y (2020) Three-dimensional culture of oral progenitor cells: Effects on small extracellular vesicles production and proliferative function. J Oral Pathol Med 49:342–349
28. Amulic B, Cazalet C, Hayes GL, Metzler KD, Zychlinsky A (2012) Neutrophil function: From mechanisms to disease. Annu Rev Immunol 30:459–489
29. Nussbaum G, Shapira L (2011) How has neutrophil research improved our understanding of periodontal pathogenesis? J Clin Periodontol 38:49–59
30. Bae J, Samek IA, Stair PC, Snurr RQ (2019) Investigation of the hydrophobic nature of metal oxide surfaces created by atomic layer deposition. Langmuir 35:5762–5769
31. Prakash SB, Abshire P (2008) Tracking cancer cell proliferation on a CMOS capacitance sensor chip. Biosens Bioelectron 23:1449–1457
32. Senevirathna B, Lu S, Dandin M, Basile J, Smela E, Abshire P (2019) High resolution monitoring of chemotherapeutic agent potency in cancer cells using a CMOS capacitance biosensor. Biosens Bioelectron 142:111501
33. Bunnfors K, Abrikossova N, Kilpijärvi J, Eriksson P, Juuti J, Halonen N et al (2020) Nanoparticle activated neutrophils-on-a-chip: A label-free capacitive sensor to monitor cells at work. Sensors Actuators B Chem 313:128020
34. Couniot N, Bol D, Poncelet O, Francis LA, Flandre D (2014) A capacitance-to-frequency converter with on-chip passivated microelectrodes for bacteria detection in saline buffers up to 575 MHz. IEEE Trans Circuits Syst II: Express Briefs 62:159–163
35. Couniot N, Francis LA, Flandre D (2015) A 16 × 16 CMOS capacitive biosensor array towards detection of single bacterial cell. IEEE Trans Biomed Circuits Syst 10:364–374
36. Ghafar-Zadeh E, Sawan M, Chodavarapu VP, Hosseini-Nia T (2010) Bacteria growth monitoring through a differential CMOS capacitive sensor. IEEE Trans Biomed Circuits Syst 4:232–238
37. Widdershoven F, Cossettini A, Laborde C, Bandiziol A, van Swinderen PP, Lemay SG et al (2018) A CMOS pixelated nanocapacitor biosensor platform for high-frequency impedance spectroscopy and imaging. IEEE Trans Biomed Circuits Syst 12:1369–1382
38. Tabrizi HO, Forouhi S, Farhanieh O, Bozkurt A, Magierowski S, Ghafar-Zadeh E (2021) Calibration-free CMOS capacitive sensor for life science applications. IEEE Trans Instrum Meas 70:1–12
39. Tabrizi HO, Forouhi S, Ghafar-Zadeh M, Farhanieh O, Shaffaf T, Magierowski S et al (2022) CMOS capacitive dry DNA storage monitoring: Design, implementation and experimental results. IEEE Sensors J 22:5521–5530

Chapter 3
Sensing Elements

This chapter provides an overview of the sensing mechanisms and transducers utilized in various types of CMOS biosensors, which are critical for detecting and measuring biological signals and chemical reactions. It offers a comprehensive exploration of various sensing mechanisms central to CMOS microelectrode systems and related technologies, including voltammetric, impedimetric, capacitive, optical, magnetic, and temperature sensors. The chapter details the electrode-electrolyte system, CMOS microelectrode structures, and fabrication, and explores microelectrode arrays (MEAs) for neural applications. It also examines Biological/Chemical Field-Effect Transistors (Bio/ChemFETs), their physics, operational regions, and fabrication, followed by a discussion on optical and magnetic sensing mechanisms. Additionally, it covers Nuclear Magnetic Resonance (NMR) principles and various temperature sensing methods, providing a deep understanding of their roles in different sensing environments.

3.1 Voltammetric, Impedimetric, and Capacitive Sensing Mechanism

Electrochemical sensing detects and measures chemical compounds and biological species in solutions by assessing their interaction with electrodes and the sensing layer or recognition elements on top of the electrodes. Various types of sensors exist, like voltammetric, impedimetric, and capacitive sensors, each with distinct mechanisms and uses. Such sensors rely on electrodes to convert bio-chemical signals into measurable signals. Figure 3.1a, b show the cross-sectional view of a CMOS electrode used for these biosensing techniques.

Voltammetric and impedimetric sensors operate based on electron transfer, generating current or voltage output through electrochemical cell reactions. Voltammetric sensors work based on applying varying potentials and measuring

E. Ghafar-Zadeh et al., *Advanced CMOS Biochips*, Analog Circuits and Signal Processing, https://doi.org/10.1007/978-94-007-0099-4_3

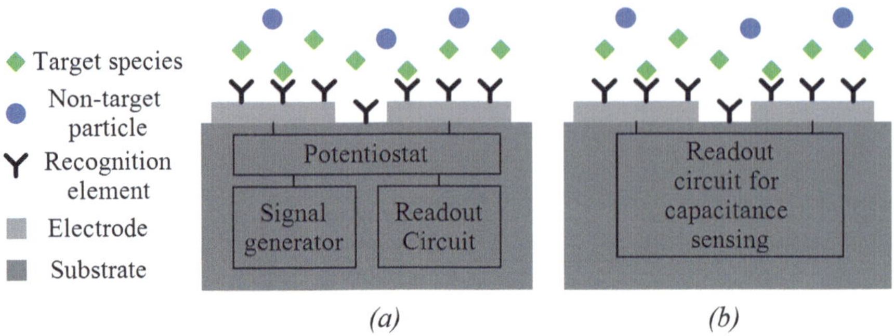

Fig. 3.1 Cross-sectional view of (**a**) An electron transfer-based system for voltammetric and impedimetric sensing, (**b**) a capacitive sensor

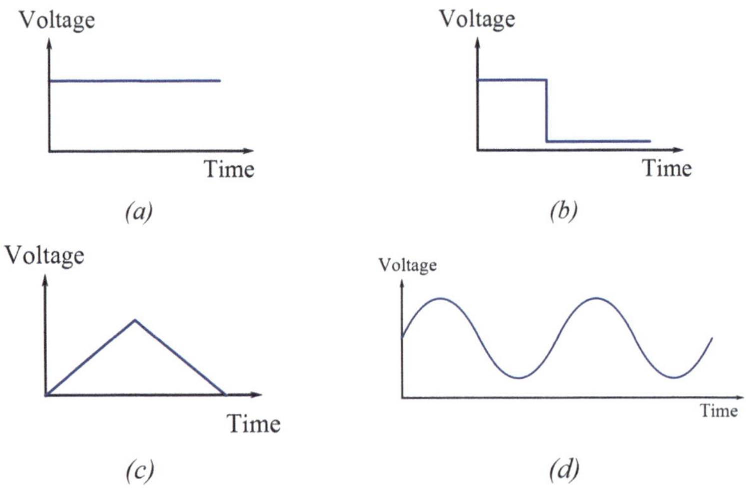

Fig. 3.2 Electrode voltage waveform for (**a**) Amperometry, (**b**) CA, (**c**) CV, (**d**) impedance spectroscopy

resulting currents, encompassing techniques like cyclic voltammetry (CV) and amperometry, which are among the techniques that can be easily integrated using CMOS processes [1]. Figure 3.2a–c show voltage waveforms for various voltammetric methods: Amperometry with constant potential, Chronoamperometry (CA) with step potential application, and CV wherein the potential is linearly increased over time until reaching a set point, followed by reversal to return to the initial potential. The biological sensing mechanism of voltammetric sensors involves the detection of analytes through electrochemical reactions at the electrode surface, where the current generated is proportional to the concentration of the analyte. On the other hand, impedimetric sensors evaluate electrode impedance using a sinusoidal stimulus voltage, preserving the bio-recognition layer integrity and finding utility in diverse applications [2]. Figure 3.2d depicts the voltage waveform for impedance spectroscopy in impedimetric sensors, representing sinusoidal stimulus voltage by frequency. The biological sensing mechanism of impedimetric sensors involves detecting changes in impedance caused by biomolecular interactions at the sensor's surface.

Capacitive biosensors detect biological molecules by measuring changes in capacitance. They include an electrode and a biorecognition element, like enzymes or antibodies, immobilized on the electrode surface. When the target biomolecule interacts with this element, it alters the electrode's dielectric properties or surface charge density, changing capacitance. This change is then measured to determine the presence or concentration of the target analyte.

In this section, we commence by elucidating the equivalent circuit representation of an electrode-electrolyte system. This connection binds various occurrences at the electrode-electrolyte interface to the components of an equivalent circuit. Then, this section introduces two prevalent on-chip electrode types applicable in life science and bio-chemical applications. Subsequently, various CMOS microelectrode structures are reviewed.

3.1.1 Electrode-Electrolyte System

In general, electrochemical interactions can be categorized as either Faradaic or non-Faradaic, depending on the magnitude of the direct current flowing within the system. When it comes to non-Faradaic interactions the interface capacitance assumes a crucial role. Conversely, for Faradaic interactions the pivotal role is taken on by the charge-transfer resistance [3]. In this subsection, after introducing the circuit model for an electrode-electrolyte system, a short overview of these two interaction types will be provided.

3.1.1.1 Equivalent Circuit Model of an Electrode-Electrolyte System

In Fig. 3.3a, a widely utilized schematic model representing the electrode-electrolyte system is depicted [4–6]. This model incorporates the resistance of the solution bulk (R_B) aligned in series with the impedance of the electrode-electrolyte junction. This impedance encompasses the charge transfer resistance (R_{CT}) parallel with the double-layer capacitance (C_{DL}). The charge transfer resistance emerges from interactions between solution ions and electrode electrons, facilitating current flow. This process entails bidirectional charge movement between the electrode and the electrolyte [4]. Meanwhile, the C_{DL} is associated with the distribution of ions in the vicinity of the electrode-electrolyte interface.

As previously noted, electrochemical reactions fall into Faradaic or non-Faradaic categories, contingent on the magnitude of the DC current flowing across the interface. Non-Faradaic reactions involve negligible DC current, emphasizing the

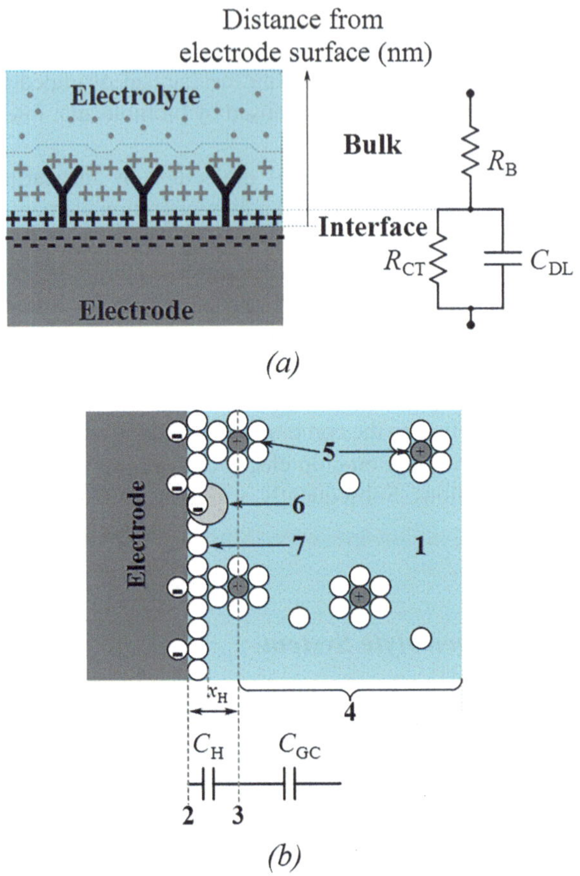

Fig. 3.3 (**a**) Equivalent Circuit Model of an Electrode-Electrolyte System, (**b**) Charge profile near electrode-electrolyte interface: 1. Electrolyte, 2. IHP, 3. OHP, 4. Diffuse layer, 5. Solvated ions (cations), 6. Specifically adsorbed ions, 7. Molecules of the electrolyte solvent

pivotal role of C_{DL} in shaping the impedance response. Conversely, Faradaic reactions involve substantial DC currents, where R_{CT} becomes a key determinant in the system's behavior [3].

3.1.1.2 Non-Faradaic Interactions

Close to the point where the voltage difference at the interface of the electrode and electrolyte is zero, it exhibits capacitor-like behavior [4]. The electrical charge residing on the metal electrode is counterbalanced by ions in the adjacent electrolyte, near the interface. When charge transfer reactions are not occurring, the Gouy-Chapman-Stern model offers a foundational structure for comprehending the electric double layer present at the interface between the metal and electrolyte. Per this model, the dual-layer capacitance is illustrated through the connection of two capacitors in series. The first capacitor known as Helmholtz capacitance (C_H), is conventionally linked with ions having limited entry (while in a hydrated state) to reach the surface of the electrode. C_H accounts for electronic surface effects, polarization, and solvent characteristics, contingent on the types of anions, cations, and the electrode's charge [7]. The Helmholtz (or Stern) layer comprises two distinct planes: the inner Helmholtz plane (IHP) and the outer Helmholtz plane (OHP). OHP encompasses solvated ions near the metal electrode, establishing pairs with charged surface sites. Conversely, the IHP is delineated by the centers of specifically adsorbed ions in direct contact with the electrode (see Fig. 3.3b) [4]. The second capacitor is the diffuse layer capacitance (C_{GC}), also termed Gouy–Chapman capacitance. C_{GC} is anticipated to remain unaffected by the specific ion species, instead depending solely on the charges of the ions, the strength of the ionic solution, and the applied voltage. The equations representing these capacitances are as follows [7]:

$$C_H = \frac{\varepsilon_0 \varepsilon_r}{x_H} \tag{3.1}$$

$$C_{GC} = \frac{\varepsilon_0 \varepsilon_r}{L_D} \cosh\left(\frac{z\psi_0}{2V_T}\right) \tag{3.2}$$

where ε_0 denotes the vacuum permittivity, ε_r stands for the solvent's relative permittivity. x_H identifies the distance between the OHP and the metal electrode. L_D stands for the Debye length. ψ_0 is the potential applied to the electrode. The charge of the involved ionic species is denoted by z. V_T denotes the thermal voltage that is $V_T = k_B T/q$, where T represents the temperature, k_B stands for the Boltzmann constant, and q denotes the electronic charge. The overall interfacial C_{DL} is represented by the reciprocal of the sum of the reciprocals of C_H and C_{GC}:

$$\frac{1}{C_{DL}} = \frac{1}{C_H} + \frac{1}{C_{GC}} \tag{3.3}$$

C_H is relatively constant with concentration and predominantly determined by the metal electrode type and electrolyte ions. Typically, this capacitance value surpasses the diffuse layer capacitance by 4–5 times [3].

Electrodes lacking passivation generally exhibit lower impedance in comparison to electrodes with passivation. However, in capacitive sensors aiming to minimize faradaic current, non-passivated electrodes often undergo a modification with a semi-passivated layer, such as a thin layer of chemicals or biomolecules. This additional layer acts as an insulator, introducing a capacitance denoted as C_{ins}. The thickness of the electric double layer varies depending on the thicknesses of the OHP, IHP, and diffuse layer. Introducing an insulating layer alters the electrode configuration, effectively increasing the distance between the plates. Upon specific binding events between probes and targets, this distance further extends, consequently affecting the overall capacitance observed at the interface.

3.1.1.3 Faradaic Interactions

Let us explore a simplified electrochemical reaction where species Re and Ox are involved in transferring n electrons at the interface:

$$Ox + ne^{-} \leftrightharpoons \mathrm{Re} \tag{3.4}$$

Under equilibrium, the concentrations of Ox and Re, denoted as C^{*}_{Ox} and C^{*}_{Re} respectively, are equal ($C^{*}_{Ox} = C^{*}_{\mathrm{Re}}$), with C^{*} representing the concentration in the bulk. When the forward and reverse reaction rate constants are k_1 and k_2, respectively, reaching equilibrium implies $k_1 = k_2$, and this leads to a potential difference denoted as E^0 between the electrode and the bulk solution, known as the standard equilibrium potential. The equilibrium rate constant, k^0, is defined at E^0, while the rate constants at other potentials (E) are expressed exponentially with respect to the overpotential ($\eta = E - E^0$):

$$k_1 = k^0 \exp\left(-\alpha\left(\frac{n}{V_T}\right)\eta\right) \tag{3.5}$$

$$k_2 = k^0 \exp\left(\left(1-\alpha\right)\left(\frac{n}{V_T}\right)\eta\right) \tag{3.6}$$

where α represents the transfer coefficient and is determined based on energy considerations. The Butler-Volmer formulation describes the current as a function of overpotential, considering oxidized ($C_{Ox}(0,t)$) and reduced ($C_{Re}(0,t)$) species concentrations over time:

$$i(t) = FAk^0\left[C_{Ox}(0,t)\exp\left(-\alpha\left(\frac{n}{V_T}\right)\eta\right) - C_{\mathrm{Re}}(0,t)\exp\left(\left(1-\alpha\right)\left(\frac{n}{V_T}\right)\eta\right)\right] \tag{3.7}$$

where A represents the electrode's surface area and F denotes Faraday's constant. At equilibrium, the overall current is zero, and the electrode attains a stable potential set by the bulk concentrations, C^{*}_{Re} and C^{*}_{Ox}. This exchange current is directly linked to k^0, and when $C^{*}_{Ox} = C^{*}_{\mathrm{Re}} = C$, it equates to:

$$i_0 = FAk^0 C \tag{3.8}$$

When the potential deviates from the equilibrium point, the Faradaic current transitions into a non-linear relationship with the applied potential. When there is a slight overpotential, $e^x \approx 1 + x$, enabling the current to be characterized as:

$$i = -i_0 \left(\frac{n}{V_T} \right) \eta \tag{3.9}$$

The ratio of $-n/i$ can be represented as an equivalent resistor and is denoted as R_{CT}:

$$R_{CT} = \frac{V_T}{i_0} \tag{3.10}$$

This approach, incorporating the Butler-Volmer formulation and R_{CT}, provides a circuit-based interpretation of Faradaic processes, useful for analyzing Electrochemical Impedance Spectroscopy (EIS) data [3].

3.1.2 Common Structures of CMOS Microelectrodes

In traditional electrode setups, the working electrode (WE) is submerged within a solution, forming a connection with the electrolyte, while the reference electrode (RE) is grounded at a hypothesized infinite distance. In CMOS technology, the WE is constructed from the uppermost metal layer, and the RE is a grounded wire linked via a bonding pad. For example, Prakash et al. [8] applied this arrangement to monitor the behavior of living cells and cell growth.

An alternative electrode design is an interdigitated electrode (IDE) (as shown in Fig. 3.4a), which features comb-like fingers that interlock, providing a substantial surface area for interactions with the environment. Integrated into CMOS technology, IDEs offer improved sensing performance, reduced polarization effects, and efficient charge transfer. Their versatility makes them suitable for various applications, such as dopamine detection [9], drug testing [10], and bacterial growth monitoring [11]. The interdigitated structure enhances sensitivity, signal-to-noise ratios (SNRs), and overall performance, establishing IDEs as a preferred choice for diverse sensing needs.

Another design, which is commonly reported for CMOS capacitive gas sensors [12–14], is quasi-interdigitated electrode (quasi-IDE), illustrated in Fig. 3.4b. Quasi-IDEs offer the advantage of being able to utilize the top two metallic layers without requiring passivation layers. In this configuration, the electrode located below serves as the reference point, while the upper electrodes function as the active WEs. Through the implementation of a pad-etching technique, the passivation layers on IDEs are eliminated, leading to an enhancement in the electric field surrounding the electrode and consequently boosting sensitivity [13, 15–17].

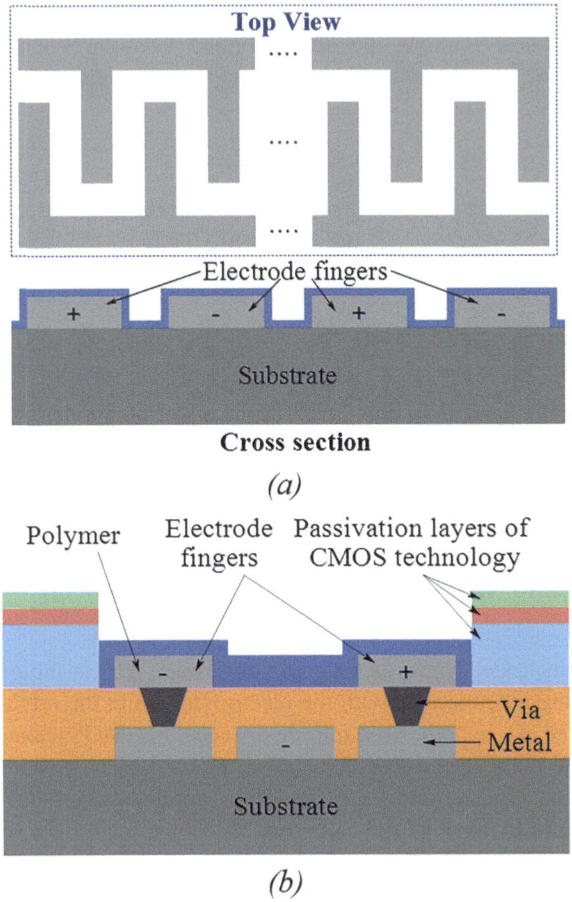

Fig. 3.4 (**a**) Top view and cross-sectional view of an IDE, (**b**) Cross sectional view of a Quasi-IDE

3.1.3 *Fabrication of CMOS Microelectrodes*

This section explores integrating sensing electrodes across diverse applications, utilizing standard CMOS structures and post-CMOS processing techniques. In conventional CMOS technology, the uppermost metal layer typically contains aluminum (Al) with silicon (Si) impurities, particularly in the 0.18 μm process, where Al incorporates a 1% Si composition [18]. Following this, protective coatings consisting of SiO_2, Si_3N_4, and polyimide are layered on top of the uppermost metallic layer. The electrode designs are divided into seven classes, which consist of passivated electrodes, Al/Al_2O_3-electrodes, high-sensitivity passivated electrodes, polymer-coated electrodes, platinum (Pt)-coated electrodes, gold (Au)-coated electrodes, and titanium nitride (TiN) electrodes. These configurations serve various CMOS sensors, enabling impedimetric, capacitive, voltammetry, and biopotential recording techniques.

3.1.3.1 Passivated Electrodes

The passivated electrode structure, depicted in Fig. 3.5a, represents a prevalent configuration wherein the passivation layers of CMOS metal layers are preserved. This design has found application in various fields such as cell growth monitoring [8, 19–21] and dopamine (DA) detection [9].

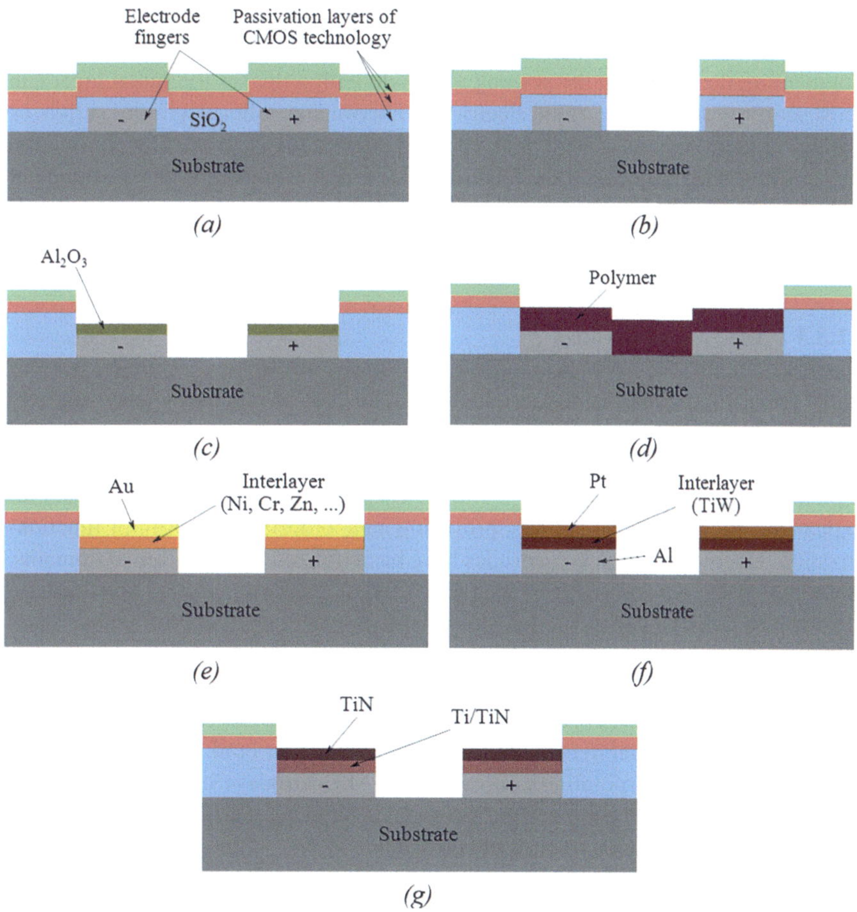

Fig. 3.5 Cross-section of (**a**) a passivated IDE, (**b**) a passivated IDE featuring a window situated between its fingers, (**c**) a bare IDE, (**d**) a polymer-coated IDE, (**e**) an Au-coated IDE, (**f**) a Pt-coated IDE, (**g**) a TiN-coated IDE

Reducing the thickness of the protective passivation layer leads to an increase in the parasitic capacitance, affecting the overall capacitance measurement and improving sensitivity. However, achieving this requires a particular procedure [20]. While passivated electrodes might improve sensitivity by reducing the passivation layer thickness, they might not meet the requirements for applications involving the immobilization of particular biological particles and recognition components over the electrodes.

3.1.3.2 Sensitivity-Enhanced Passivated Electrodes

To enhance sensitivity between electrode connectors, removing the passivation layer using a pad-etching method can increase the electric field, as illustrated in Fig. 3.5b. However, given the electrodes' smaller size compared to the pad, it's essential to run simulations to assess design rule violations with Cadence software. Augmenting the height of the sensing electrode with a thicker top metal layer can boost sensor performance, as the electric field between parallel electrodes surpasses that above them. Ghafar-Zadeh et al. [22, 23] utilized this approach by eliminating the passivation layer between the fingers of IDEs, requiring precise mask alignment with the finger gap. These electrodes were employed for detecting chemical solvents [24] and monitoring bacteria growth by the research team [11].

3.1.3.3 Al/Al_2O_3 Electrodes

Al is prone to oxidation, posing challenges in CMOS processes when directly exposing Al electrodes to samples. However, when in contact with air, a natural aluminum oxide (Al_2O_3) layer develops on the exposed Al electrode surface, as depicted in Fig. 3.5c [25]. The Al_2O_3 layer acts as an insulating barrier against biological and chemical surroundings, providing an appropriate platform for functionalization. Uncovered or bare electrodes have been utilized across different domains, including DNA detection [26], chemical solvent monitoring [25], and bacteria growth monitoring [27]. A method for establishing a sensing region amidst electrodes involves incorporating thick upper metal layers and substantial gaps between electrodes, facilitated by the adoption of a specific mask for pad-etching [28]. As an example, Nikkhoo et al. [27] employed a method involving two electrodes separated by a trench for bacterial detection. Additionally, Couniot et al. [29, 30] utilized a similar approach, incorporating non-passivated Al electrodes (SiO_2 and Si_3N_4) with a thin layer of Al_2O_3 deposited on the top metal layer using plasma-enhanced atomic layer deposition (PEALD) to prevent corrosion.

3.1.3.4 Polymer-Coated Electrodes

Polymeric membranes are frequently applied to boost sensitivity for gaseous samples on sensing electrodes, as depicted in Fig. 3.5d [12–14]. Additionally, polymer coatings display considerable potential in augmenting biocompatibility, as observed by Nabovati and colleagues [31] applied poly(dimethylsiloxane) (PDMS) layers via spin-coating onto bare Al electrodes, facilitating cell growth screening. In another study [10], they proposed using polyelectrolyte multilayer (PEM) coatings through the layer-by-layer (LBL) technique, enhancing cell adhesion on Al electrodes. Remarkably, specific bioactive coating strategies relying on PEMs have demonstrated success in drug delivery [32] and glucose detection [33, 34]. Furthermore, researchers utilized an 8 × 8 grid of electrodes in both studies [10, 31]. In a separate study, Kummer and colleagues [15] utilized a Quasi-IDE equipped with a polymer coating to identify volatile organic compounds in the surrounding environment.

3.1.3.5 Gold-Coated Electrodes

Au, a noble metal known for its biocompatibility and stability [28, 35], is widely employed across various biosensing applications, including DNA detection [36–38] and anti-Rubella [39], due to its excellent electron conductivity. Au demonstrates the ability to create self-assembled monolayers (SAMs) between electrodes [28], facilitating the immobilization of biorecognition components such as DNA oligonucleotides [40] and glucose oxidase [41]. Nonetheless, constructing Au electrodes above the CMOS chip necessitates post-processing steps, and Au can be deposited on various substrates such as Al, Pt, copper (Cu), palladium (Pd), and nickel (Ni) [42, 43]. To enhance adhesion on Al, an interlayer of Ni, chromium (Cr), or zinc (Zn) is often applied [35], as depicted in Fig. 3.5e. Various methods, such as photolithography and electroless deposition processes, are utilized to apply Au onto Al electrodes within CMOS technology [39, 42, 44]. Guiducci et al. [38] employed photolithography for DNA sensing, incorporating tantalum (Ta) as an intermediate layer between Al and Au [71]. In other studies, electroless nickel immersion gold (ENIG) plating was used to fabricate Au IDEs for an electrochemical biosensor array [39] and to engineer biocompatible Au microelectrodes for DNA and protein detection [45]. Widdershoven et al. [46–48] investigated nanoelectrodes for high-frequency impedance spectroscopy and imaging, connecting them to a vertical structure composed of four stacked Cu vias from CMOS technology, resulting in the creation of Au/Cu nanoelectrodes characterized by a reduced electrode size.

3.1.3.6 Platinum-Coated Electrodes

Pt, similar to Au in its inertness but less resistant to oxidation, needs post-CMOS processing for electrode fabrication. Deposition and pattern formation of Pt commonly entail photolithographic methods, often necessitating the inclusion of a titanium-tungsten (TiW) adhesion layer between Al and Pt [35] (Fig. 3.5f). Pt electrodes are frequently employed for stimulating, measuring impedance, and capturing electrical activity in electroactive cells like neurons or cardiomyocytes [49–52]. In [49, 50, 52], the deposition of Pt onto Al electrodes is accomplished using a straightforward post-processing technique with only two masks, succeeded by sputter-deposition and lift-off procedures. A Si_3N_4/SiO_2 passivation alternation, formed via plasma-enhanced chemical vapor deposition (PECVD), and reactive ion etching (RIE) are utilized to determine the shape and dimensions of the electrodes. For instance, research conducted by Dragas et al. [49] and Frey et al. [50, 53] involved the utilization of Pt electrode arrays for diverse purposes like extracellular communication and neuronal stimulation, while a separate investigation [54] focused on densely populated Pt-microelectrodes within a sensing area measuring 4.5×2.5 mm^2.

3.1.3.7 TiN Electrodes

TiN electrodes, as shown in Fig. 3.5g, have also been utilized in biosensing [55, 56]. For example, in a study led by Lopez et al. [56], a chip was described incorporating 16,384 TiN-electrodes, crafted utilizing 0.13 μm Al CMOS technology and employing a six-metal-layer Al back-end-of-line (BEOL) configuration. The fabrication process involved passivating the top layer of the last BEOL metal layer (M_6) with SiO_2 through PECVD, adding an additional layer of SiO_2 for adequate passivation thickness, and then creating via holes in the passivation layer using RIE to access the M_6 contacts. A seed layer of Ti/TiN was deposited, succeeded by the application of a TiN layer via reactive physical vapor deposition, and patterned with RIE. The chip's capabilities for neuro-electrophysiological investigations were showcased in [55], displaying electrodes of varying dimensions from 2.5×3.5 μm^2 to 11×11 μm^2.

3.2 Microelectrode Array (MEA) for Neural Stimulation/Recording

To study and manipulate neural processes for functional brain analysis, advanced tools are needed [57]. Bioelectric activity in neurons can be measured intracellularly or extracellularly using microelectrodes. External action potentials (APs), reflecting membrane depolarizations, have waveforms between 100 Hz and 10 kHz, with 50 μVpp to 500 μVpp amplitudes for extracellular measurements [58]. Intracellular APs, around 70 mVpp, involve penetrating the neuron's membrane but face limitations due to cell death [57]. Local field potentials (LFPs), with mHz to 200 Hz frequencies and 500 μVpp to 5 mVpp amplitudes, offer insights and are detected extracellularly [59, 60]. While intracellular APs provide robust signals, extracellular APs, and LFPs offer the potential for chronic utilization [57–60].

The findings suggest that while intracellular AP measurements offer strong signals, their long-term viability is limited. On the other hand, extracellular LFP and AP measurements capture weaker signals but show promise for chronic applications. Electroencephalography (EEG) share similarities with LFPs, although the former is less invasive. Carbon fiber [61, 62] or iridium oxide microelectrodes [63] can be utilized for neurotransmitter measurement employing approaches such as voltammetry or amperometry, with fast-scan cyclic voltammetry (FSCV) being a preferred method due to its real-time monitoring capability on a shorter time scale. Analysis of chemicals involves minimal redox currents but holds considerable promise for long-term use. Conversely, patch-clamping techniques manage larger currents but are less suitable for chronic applications [64].

Recent research focusing on neural signals and network behavior has seen a rise in the popularity of CMOS-based high density-microelectrode arrays (HD-MEAs) [50]. These devices are increasingly utilized to observe extracellular electrical activity in laboratory settings, capturing localized alterations in charge distribution due to neural activity. Such activity induces a voltage discrepancy between the microelectrode and the reference bath potential, which is supplied by a reference electrode [65]. Within existing literature, three main types of readout strategies have been utilized: passive pixel sensors (PPS), active pixel sensors (APS), and switch matrix (SM) sensors.

Passive pixel CMOS arrays were designed with a passive layout and fixed wiring, lacking active circuitry like amplifiers [66]. (Fig. 3.6a). Each electrode in these arrays directly connects to an external signal pad via wiring, necessitating external equipment for signal conditioning. While passive MEAs offer a relatively simple manufacturing process and enable access to all electrodes simultaneously, they are hindered by wiring limitations and the geometric configuration of electrodes. Typically, they can support fewer than 300 electrodes with approximately 30 μm spatial accuracy [67, 68]. Despite historical advancements, including the development of multielectrode arrays by pioneers like Robinson [69], Thomas et al. [70], Gross et al. [71], Pine [72], Regehr et al. [73], and Taketani and Kawana et al. [74, 75], passive MEAs face challenges such as high noise and low sensitivity due to significant capacitance. These challenges impede their ability to detect axonal signals or accurately distinguish overlapping neuron signals [76, 77].

Conversely, active pixel arrays integrate an amplifier within each pixel alongside on-chip multiplexers (Fig. 3.6b). APS technology offers significant advantages over traditional capacitive coupled devices (CCDs), including lower cost, reduced power consumption, and enhanced dynamic range pixels [78]. Integrating active transistors within every pixel unit enhances APS technology, offering advantages like greater scalability for expansive array configurations and reduced noise during readout in contrast to PPS [79]. Various APS technologies, including the charge modulation device (CMD) [80], amplified metal-oxide-semiconductor imager (AMI) [80], base stored image sensor (BASIS) [53], bulk charge modulated device (BCMD) [81], and static induction transistor (SIT) [82] have been adapted for MEAs, resulting in the formation of active electrodes or pixels. Despite advancements,

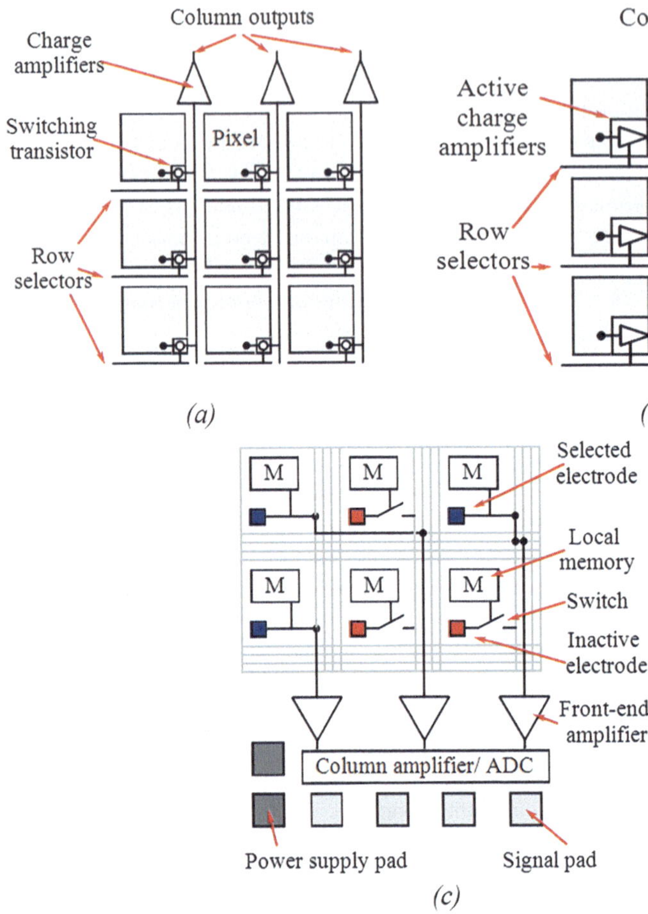

Fig. 3.6 (**a**) PPS- MEA, (**b**) APS- MEA, (**c**) SM-MEA

challenges remain in designing low-noise circuitry due to the limited area near each electrode, leading to higher levels of noise and reduced spatial resolution [83–85]. Introduced in 2001, the APS-MEA platform transformed in vitro neural recording by facilitating simultaneous recordings with minimal inter-electrode distances across a broad surface. Widely employed for both in vivo and in vitro neural recording, APS MEAs, including HD-MEAs, strive to augment overall electrode quantity and spatial precision to fulfill the requirements of progressively demanding applications, albeit encountering drawbacks like increased noise levels and compromises in spatial resolution due to limitations in power consumption and restricted pixel area [65, 83–85].

To attain excellent spatial precision and accommodate intricate shapes, specific sensors employ an analog SM method. In this configuration, every pixel in the array comprises only static random-access memory (SRAM) cells and toggles (see Fig. 3.6c) [50]. In the SM approach, transistors within the array serve as switches, enabling the transmission of signals from electrodes to external readout circuits located beyond the electrode array. The SM's routing process is static, with electrode selection dictated by the opening or closing of switches, ensuring that recordings begin without changing electrode selection. This setup enhances the SNR by optimizing amplifiers situated external to the array [86]. Ballini et al. [50] presented a CMOS-based SM MEA setup that maintains precise spatial resolution across a wide sensing area, featuring 1024 channels for high-speed recording at 20 kS/s. They attained improved noise performance by optimizing circuit design and resolving challenges related to crossover distortions and variations in channel length [87]. Different SM MEA systems have demonstrated varying degrees of versatility in their routing functionalities. Some have employed uncomplicated methods based on selecting rows and columns [66]. For in vivo applications, enhanced electrode selection freedom has been achieved [88, 89]. Frey et al. [53] showcased intricate routing, averaging 1.2 memory cells for each electrode. Building upon this, Ballini et al. [50] significantly extended the possibilities by utilizing 2.2 memory cells for each electrode, enabling broader subset choices. Enhancing versatility further, Viswam et al. [90] raised the bits per electrode to beyond 3, essentially allowing for unrestricted subset selections.

3.3 Biological/Chemical Field-Effect Transistors (Bio/ChemFETs) Sensing Mechanism

Bio/ChemFETs, like ion-sensitive field-effect transistors (ISFETs), share a structure akin to metal-oxide-semiconductor FETs (MOSFETs), consisting of a gate electrode, insulating layer, and semiconductor substrate. However, in Bio/ChemFETs, the gate electrode is coated with a material sensitive to specific ions or molecules (see Fig. 3.7a), enabling the device to respond to changes in their concentration. This modification induces electrical property changes in the transistor, detectable as shifts in voltage or current. Bio/ChemFETs are valuable for diverse analytical applications, including biotechnology and environmental monitoring, as they can detect various biological or chemical targets. These sensors operate based on ISFET principles, introduced in the 1970s, by removing the metal layer atop the oxide layer of MOSFETs [91]. In this device, the fluidic gate manipulation of the oxide layer's surface potential allows for target species detection. The charge induced by the presence and concentration of the target species alters the sensor's surface potential, resulting in detectable electron currents in the conductive channel. Subsequently, various ISFET structures emerged for different biological and chemical samples, leading to the evolution of Bio/ChemFET structures [92].

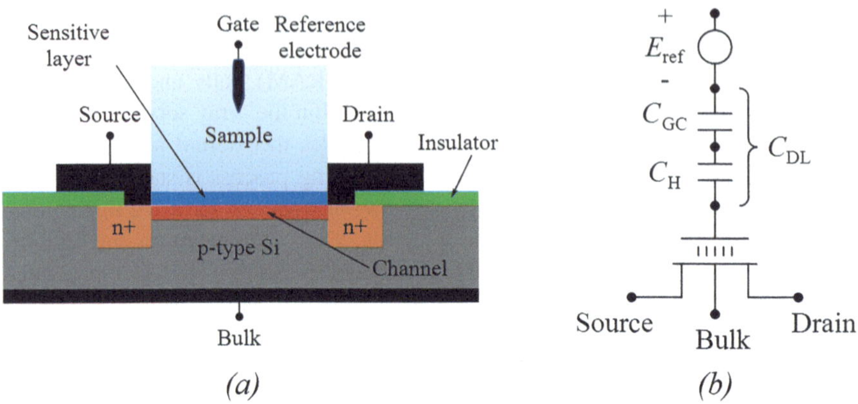

Fig. 3.7 (**a**) Standard structure of an n-channel ISFET, (**b**) Equivalent electric circuit of ISFET structure

3.3.1 *Physics of Bio/ChemFETs*

The integration of Bio/ChemFETs into CMOS technology enables the miniaturization of these devices alongside essential readout circuits, providing significant advantages for biosensors. In 1999, Bausells et al. [93] showcased the possibility of producing ISFETs using a conventional CMOS procedure, similar to the steps for fabricating MOSFETs. They employed physico-chemical models integrated into SPICE to analyze ISFETs, with specific emphasis on the interplay between the ion-sensitive membrane and the analyte, as detailed in subsequent studies [94–99].

As illustrated in Fig. 3.7a, b, the interaction between ions and the oxide layer induces the creation of double-layer capacitance (C_{DL}) near the oxide layer, which appears atop the channel. The decrease in charge resulting from absorbed surface charges leads to another capacitance, affected by electron/hole movement within the channels and surface charge density. The influence of charge on the surface of the oxide layer triggers the drain-source current, which can be mathematically represented as Eq. (3.11) for the unsaturated (linear) region ($V_{DS} < V_{GS}$—$V_{th(ISFET)}$):

$$I_D = \mu C_{ox} \frac{W}{L} \left\{ \left[V_{GS} - V_{th(ISFET)} \right] V_{DS} - \frac{1}{2} V_{DS}^{\ 2} \right\} \tag{3.11}$$

where μ represents the average mobility within the channel; L and W correspondingly indicate the length and width of the gate; V_{DS} and V_{GS} represent the voltage across the drain and source, and the voltage across the gate and source, respectively; C_{ox} stands for the gate oxide capacitance. $V_{th(ISFET)}$ denotes the ISFET's threshold voltage, which can be articulated as:

$$V_{th(ISFET)} = E_{ref} - \Psi_o + \chi^{sol} - \frac{\Phi_{Si}}{q} - \frac{Q_{ox} + Q_{ss}}{C_{ox}} - \frac{Q_B}{C_{ox}} + 2\Phi_f \tag{3.12}$$

where E_{ref} signifies the reference electrode's potential; χ^{sol} represents the surface dipole potential of the solution, while Φ_{Si} signifies the work function of silicon electrons. The variable q denotes the elementary charge; Q_{ox}, Q_{ss}, and Q_B represent charges within the oxide, surface, and interface states, and the depletion charge, respectively. Additionally, Φ_f identifies the difference in potential between the Fermi levels of intrinsic and doped silicon. Ψ_o characterizes the potential difference between the electrolyte and the insulator, indicating the disparity between the oxide surface potential Ψ_S and the bulk potential of the solution Ψ_B ($\Psi_o = \Psi_S - \Psi_B$). With the exception of Ψ_o, all parameters in eqs. (3.11) and (3.12) remain constant, highlighting Ψ_o 's influence on the oxide layer and its impact on the $V_{th(ISFET)}$. Changes in the ionic solution and its biomolecular composition alter the threshold voltage, thereby influencing the current flow in the channel.

A slight change in the electrolyte ion concentration, either due to biochemical processes within a biological sample or the presence of charged substances in the solution, can impact the surface potential. Generally, the introduction of an analyte at a particular level induces a pH change in the solution, which correlates with the surface potential. As a result, this modification affects the current flowing between the drain and source in the conductive pathway. Consequently, the threshold voltage of an ISFET can be described as [100–102]:

$$V_{th(ISFET)} = V_{th(MOS)} + \left(\gamma + 2.3\alpha V_T pH\right) \tag{3.13}$$

The constant parameter α, ranging between 0 and 1, is heavily influenced by intrinsic buffer capacity and the differential capacitance [100]. Here, γ stands for a pH-independent aggregation of chemical potentials, V_T is the thermal voltage calculated as K_BT/q, while K_B represents the Boltzmann constant, and T signifies the absolute temperature; $V_{th(MOS)}$ denotes the threshold voltage of a conventional MOSFET. These principles are universally applicable to semiconductor-oxide-electrolyte Bio/ChemFETs, yet they may not hold for certain nanomaterial-based counterparts, like carbon nanotubes (CNTs) and graphene, due to limitations of the site-bonding theory in describing ion-complexation behavior on such surfaces. The complexities in mathematically modeling molecular interactions at oxide or nitride surfaces preclude accurate prediction of surface potential as outlined by the site-bonding theory. Atomistic molecular dynamics simulations have recently been employed to investigate ion complexation and evaluate surface potential, providing fresh perspectives on molecular interactions at channel surfaces and double-layer capacitance that are beyond the capabilities of existing models [103–105].

3.3.2 Operational Regions of ISFETs

The operational states of ISFETs are divided into four categories: (1) the triode or linear region represented by Eq. (3.11), (2) strong inversion or saturation, (3) weak inversion or subthreshold, and (4) velocity saturation. Equation (3.11) characterizes the drain current within the triode or linear region, whereas for the saturation region ($V_{DS} > V_{GS}—V_{th(ISFET)}$), the drain current of an ISFET follows a different expression:

$$I_D = \mu C_{ox} \frac{W}{L} \left(V_{GS} - V_{th(ISFET)} \right)^2 \left(1 + \lambda V_{DS} \right) \tag{3.14}$$

where λ represents the channel length modulation factor. When maintaining constant I_D and V_{DS}, adjustments in V_{GS} occur to offset variations in $V_{th(ISFET)}$.

In the weak inversion region, by considering $V_{DS} > 4V_T$ and zero bulk-source voltage, ISFET operation can be described [106]:

$$I_D = I_0 \frac{W}{L} \exp\left(\frac{V_{GS} - V_{th(ISFET)}}{nV_T} \right) \tag{3.15}$$

where n stands for the subthreshold slope parameter and I_0 denotes a positive constant current.

The behavior of the device in the velocity saturation region, as described in [107], can be represented by:

$$I_D = v_{sat} C_{ox} W \left(V_{GS} - V_{th(ISFET)} - V_{D,sat} \right) \tag{3.16}$$

where v_{sat} represents the saturated carrier velocity and $V_{D,sat}$ indicates the stage when the drain current reaches saturation.

3.3.3 Structures and Fabrication of Bio/ChemFET-Based Sensors

Pioneered by Piet Bergveld in the early 1970s, the ISFET technology was first evaluated for pH assessment in solutions containing sodium chloride (NaCl). Since then, various configurations have emerged, categorized based on their design and functionality including (1) single-gate, (2) extended gate, (3) dual-gate, and (4) nanostructure-based Bio/ChemFETs.

3.3.3.1 Single-Gate Bio/ChemFETs

The conventional ISFET integrates a MOSFET with the substitution of the metal gate by a dielectric membrane, which acts as the sensing layer, typically crafted from silicon oxide. The capacitance of this layer (C_{ox}) plays a direct role in sensitivity, affecting the induced charge for each modification in potential [108]. These ISFETs embody a sole gate and represent the most fundamental structure [109–111]. Figure 3.8a illustrates the straightforward layout of a single-gate ISFET.

Like conventional ISFETs, researchers are investigating high-*k* materials like Ta_2O_5 and HfO_2 as substitutes for the gate oxide layer to serve as alternative sensing membranes due to their increased capacitance and compact structure (see Fig. 3.8b). This exploration aims to enhance performance by improving sensitivity and mitigating drifting. High-*k* dielectrics offer superior charge coupling and stability, making them well-suited for challenging sensing applications [109].

3.3.3.2 Extended Gate Bio/ChemFETs

A different arrangement of Bio/ChemFET is the extended-gate design, which separates the gate dielectric from the solution. Instead, it incorporates a gate metal extension to the top passivation layer of the device, simplifying post-processing steps. However, this introduces a serial capacitor made of passivation material such as silicon nitride, that diminishes the overall sensitivity of the sensor [109] (see Fig. 3.8b). This configuration simplifies the fabrication process by allowing the sensing area to align with the fluidic section's design requirements. Traditional FET biosensor designs encounter challenges related to surface chemistry, ion complexations, and subsequent ion trapping, resulting in signal noise. Extended-gate Bio/ChemFETs tackle these challenges and have undergone thorough examination for diverse uses, encompassing pH assessments and biological interfaces. Compared to conventional ISFETs, extended gate FETs offer improved stability against chemical, thermal, and light disturbances, along with heightened sensitivity [92, 112, 113].

3.3.3.3 Dual-Gate Bio/ChemFETs

The dual-gate ISFET incorporates a back gate opposite the active channel, such as a thin-film semiconductor or silicon substrate (see Fig. 3.8c). Previous research indicates that the sensitivity of dual-gate ISFET can surpass the Nernstian limit of 59 mV/pH to around 1 V/pH [114–118]. This enhanced sensitivity is achieved through the optimization of sensitivity regions by bottom-gate and top-gate matrices. The increased pH sensitivity stems from the capacitance asymmetry between the bottom and top gate oxide layers. Experimental investigations entail varying the bias of the lower gate while keeping the fluid-gate bias constant, defining sensitivity

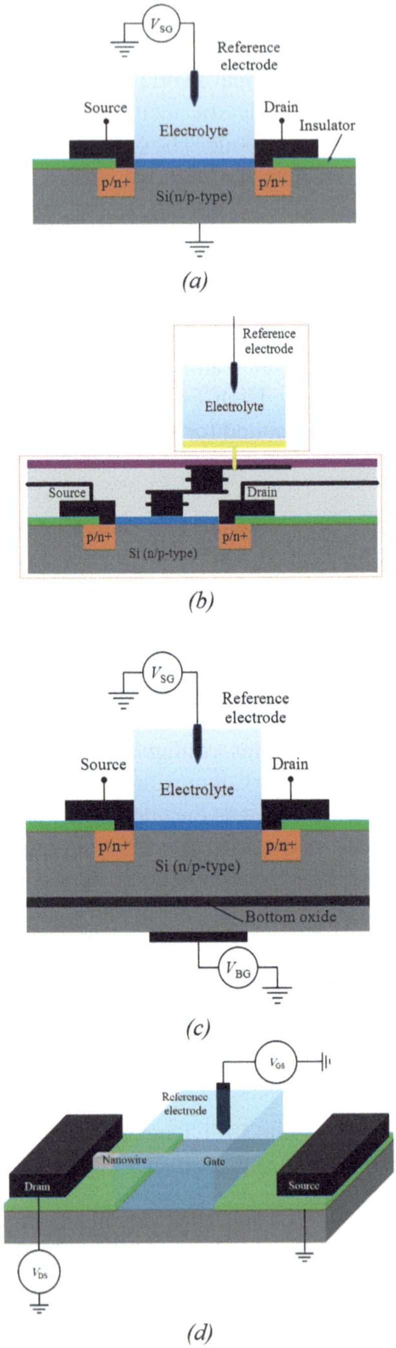

Fig. 3.8 The cross section of (**a**) Conventional ISFET, (**b**) Extended gate ISFET, (**c**) Dual-gate ISFET, (**d**) SiNW ISFET

as the voltage shift at the threshold caused by alterations in pH. The modification in drain current conductance induced by the lower gate bias voltage is employed to counterbalance alterations in pH or the concentration of substances on the sensor's surface.

Huang et al. [119] effectively integrated the dual-gate ISFET into CMOS technology. Their setup, fabricated on a silicon-on-insulator (SOI) base with a high-*k* sensing insulator, demonstrated significant improvements in signal clarity, stability over time, and responsiveness.

3.3.3.4 Nanostructure-Based Bio/ChemFETs

Utilizing nanostructures such as CNTs or graphene, these Bio/ChemFETs offer enhanced sensitivity and selectivity. The unique properties of nanostructures enable improved interaction with analytes, making them suitable for advanced sensing applications (see Fig. 3.8d).

Silicon nanowire (SiNW), an exceedingly sensitive solid-state biosensor, was initially introduced by Cui et al. [120]. SiNWs have demonstrated remarkable capabilities in detecting nucleic acid [121–125], proteins [126–129], and viruses [130] with unparalleled limits of detection (LoD). Typically, a SiNW biosensor features a slender structure resembling a wire, forming an intricate pathway either through crystalline or poly-silicon material, with connections linking drain and source electrodes at its edges. Two main varieties of SiNW sensors exist: one functions as a resistor, while the other, is a transistor type, that integrates an extra gate at its base to facilitate transistor-like behavior. The fabrication of SiNW-based sensing tools employs two distinct methods: one begins from the bottom, while the other starts from the top.

The bottom-up technique, led by Cui et al. [120], involves SiNW growth on a substrate through chemical vapor deposition using the vapor-liquid-solid (VLS) method, succeeded by the deposition of drain and source metals for connecting purposes. Conversely, the top-down approach [131], demonstrated by lithographic methods, generates SiNWs using processes such as E-beam lithography on SOI substrates, followed by RIE to establish a three-dimensional wire structure. The top-down approach has gained popularity due to its compatibility with standard CMOS processes, facilitating integration with interface circuits and offering the potential for mass production and cost-effectiveness [109].

In addition to SiNWs, other nano-structured FETs such as organic field-effect transistors (OFETs) and graphene field-effect transistors (GFETs) also offer remarkable sensing capabilities [132]. OFETs utilize organic semiconductors, providing flexibility and compatibility with flexible substrates. Operating in accumulation mode, OFETs are modifiable by immersing them in an electrolyte surrounding, allowing the device to be regulated through a reference electrode acting as the solution gate electrode. This configuration, known as electrolyte-gated OFET (EGOFET), has shown promising results in detecting various analytes such as glucose, DNA, and proteins, with detection limits reaching down to the picomolar regime [132–136].

GFETs, conversely, utilize graphene's outstanding attributes, including its high electron mobility and mechanical robustness. These FETs display ambipolar features, enabling drain current generation with both negative and positive gate voltages. They can be structured with either a single or double-gate design, offering promising functionality even in liquid environments. GFET biosensors have demonstrated high sensitivity in detecting various analytes, including pH, proteins, IgE, DNA, glucose, and living cells [137–139].

Additionally, novel field-effect transistors, such as SiNW tunneling FETs, offer tunable characteristics for enhanced biosensing capabilities. Strategies such as opposite doping and multi-gate field-effect designs have been explored to improve sensitivity and dynamic range. Compound semiconductors like AlGaN/GaN are also emerging as promising candidates for FET-based biosensors, offering high mobility characteristics for detecting biomarkers [140, 141].

3.4 Optical Sensing Mechanism

3.4.1 Biological Sensing

The optical biosensors identify biological interactions by analyzing changes in the properties of light, which are directly correlated to the concentration of a particular analyte. Generally, optical biosensors are classified into two groups: label-based sensors, which bring in a labeling process during detection, and label-free sensors, which do not require labeling [142]. Labeled biosensing relies on the attachment of a label to the analyte, where the label acts as an indirect indicator of the presence of a specific analyte as illustrated in Fig. 3.9a [143]. Label-free affinity biosensing relies on a receptor attached to a transducer that responds to affinity binding between

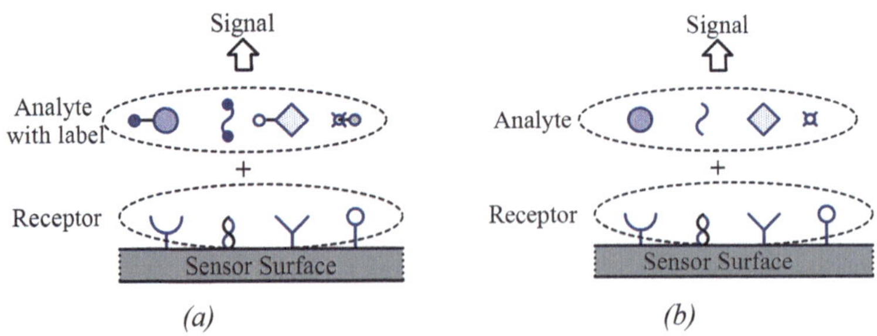

Fig. 3.9 Scheme of typical biosensors (**a**) label-based and (**b**) label-free

receptor and analyte (see Fig. 3.9b) [144]. Changes in the properties of light can happen in the emission, polarization, absorbance, or luminescence decay time of the receptor [142].

Various optical biosensor structures that have the potential for use in clinical diagnosis that are documented in the literature including fluorescence [145–152], bioluminescence [153–155], absorption photometry [156–158], silicon photonics [159–165], surface-enhanced raman scattering [166, 167], and plasmon biosensors [168–172]. Among the mentioned methods, the ones that are particularly well-suited for implementation in CMOS technology include fluorescence, bioluminescence, and evanescent wave approaches, which will be discussed in the following.

3.4.1.1 Principles of Fluorescence Sensing

Figure 3.10 illustrates the sensing principles of fluorescence biosensors. During this lable-based method, the fluorophores (labels of the targets) absorb excitation light photons generated by an excitation source at a particular wavelength and after capturing by probes, which are immobilized on a surface, emit photons in a different wavelength [173]. As a result, the reactions between the target and probe produce an optical signal, which can be detected by photosensitive elements after passing a filter to eliminate the background excitation light.

3.4.1.2 Principles of Bioluminescence Sensing

The sensing principles of bioluminescence biosensors (label-based) are shown in Fig. 3.11. In these biosensors, signal photoemission is triggered by a chemical reaction instead of an excitation source. Also, background emission is ignorable

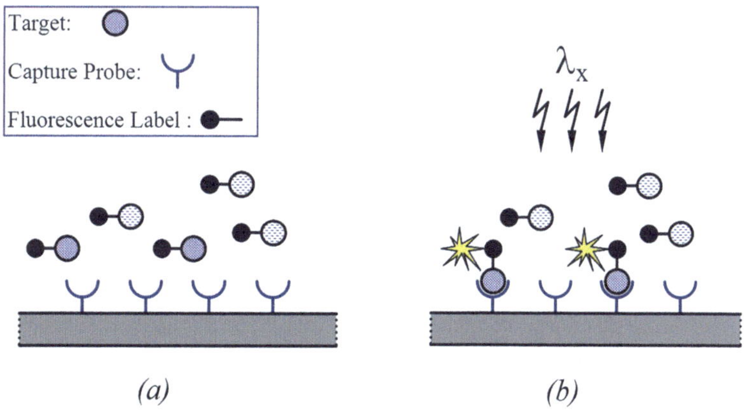

Fig. 3.10 Fluorescence sensing principle (**a**) before sensing (**b**) after sensing

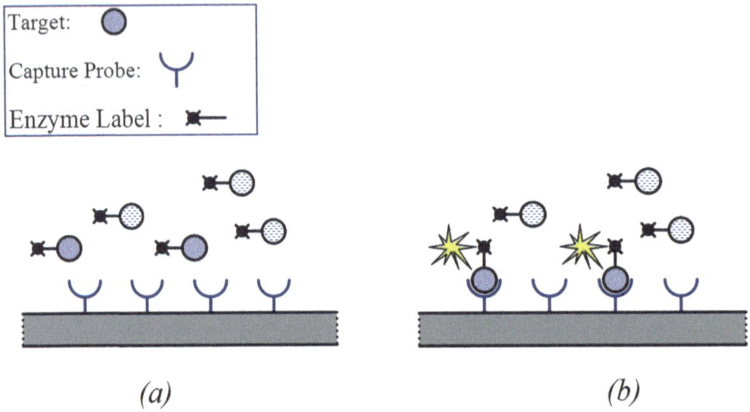

Fig. 3.11 Bioluminescence sensing principle (**a**) before sensing (**b**) after sensing

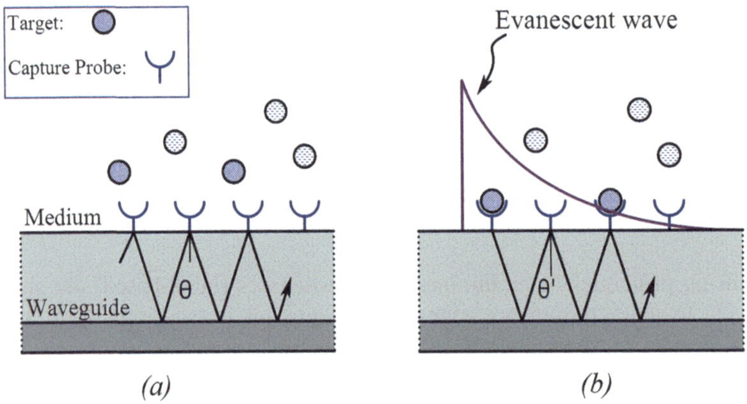

Fig. 3.12 Evanescent field sensing principle (**a**) before sensing (**b**) after sensing

which implies the filter is not necessary. Therefore, bioluminescence can offer a cost-effective and easily integrated solution for lab-on-a-chip (LoC) applications, compared to fluorescence methods.

3.4.1.3 Principles of Evanescent Field Sensing

The evanescent field detection is one of the widely used label-free sensing methods for optical biosensors [174–180], which allows real-time monitoring of molecular interactions [181]. In this sensing method (see Fig. 3.12), a receptor layer is immobilized onto the waveguide surface in which the refractive index of the waveguide is higher than the dielectric medium. If a light with an incidence angle (θ) greater than the critical angle (θ_c, see equation (see Eq. (3.17)) is launched into the waveguide, the electromagnetic field called the "evanescent wave" penetrates at a small distance from the interface into the lower index medium [177, 179]. The interaction between the receptor and analyte is identified through the evanescent field of the guided light. The evanescent field has a very limited reach, enabling the biosensor to interact solely with the material directly adjacent to its surface. This means that unbound materials suspended in solution do not affect the biosensor. The silicon photonic biosensors are one of the most employed evanescent-field sensing methods, which can be implemented with CMOS technology [176, 181].

$$\theta_c = \sin^{-1}\left(n_{medium} / n_{waveguide}\right) \tag{3.17}$$

3.4.2 Physical Sensing

In optical biosensors, the produced light signals arising from the analyte-bioreceptor interaction comprise the analyte information [182]. Also, this signal contains some undesirable background light. So, in the front-end of the optical biosensors, a filter is required to eliminate background light and ensure accurate biological data acquisition and a photosensitive element to detect the optical signals, which are briefly discussed below.

3.4.2.1 Optical Filtering

As mentioned above, a filter is utilized in the biosensing system to eliminate background light in most optical biosensing methods, especially in fluorescence-based sensing [183–185]. There have been attempts to incorporate a monolithic filter as an on-chip component. Nonetheless, the process necessitates complex post-processing steps to fabricate the optical filter structures, thereby increasing both the cost and complexity of the system [186–189].

To our knowledge, Hong et al. [190] introduced the first integrated nanoplasmonic filter, utilizing a 65 nm CMOS process. The filters are implemented using copper-based bottom five metal layers and four via layers. The plasmonic filters effectively direct the fluorescence signals emitted by the Qdot 800 fluorophores on the chip surface toward the on-chip detectors. These filters can achieve an extinction ratio of over 51 dB (or 63 dB, as determined by finite-difference time-domain (FDTD) simulation) [191]. This advancement enables angle and scattering-insensitive filtering, opening the doors for the implementation of fully integrated fluorescence biosensors without the need for post-processing and external optical elements (only for an excitation source).

In another work by Hong et al. [192], to design a filter the metal and via layers between M_4 and M_7 in CMOS processes is utilized to manipulate and redirect light in a controlled manner. This enables the detection and analysis of spectrum information within the range of 500 nm to 830 nm. In another effort, Jiang et al. [193] demonstrated a CMOS image sensor integrated with a nano-filter employed the technique presented by Hong et al. [190] for filter implementation. This filter is constructed with stacked and periodically patterned nano-scale copper lines, including fifth and 2th metal layers. The nano-filter exhibited a measured rejection ratio of 24.2 dB for excitation light and emission light of 467 nm and 820 nm, respectively.

Worth mentioning, that in fluorescence sensors in addition to intensity, other properties of the emission light, such as its lifetime, are also measured, which provides filterless fluorescence biosensing. Lifetime represents the average duration during which a fluorophore remains excited before reverting to the ground state. This parameter can be quantified using techniques like time-resolved fluorescence [194]. This time-resolved fluorescence detection technique offers several profits, including enhanced rejection of background signals, even without the use of optical filtering [195–201].

3.4.2.2 Photodetectors

Previously, employing a photomultiplier tube (PMT) for light detection was widespread. However, this approach had limitations as it made the system complex, bulky, and expensive, thus limiting its application. In the last decades, to address this issue, the PMT has been replaced with optical detectors implemented in CMOS technology. The most employed photosensitive element in CMOS technology are photodiodes, which will be discussed in the following.

The fundamental structure of photodiodes is comprised of a P-type and an N-type semiconductor that is specially designed to function under reverse bias conditions, resulting in a depletion region formed between the N and P layers, where free carriers are absent. When the diode is illuminated with light, photons carrying sufficient energy can enter the depletion region and collide with atoms. This collision generates a pair of mobile electron-hole pairs, which in turn induces a photocurrent in the photodiode.

Several types of photodiodes have been explored in literature such as PN photodiode, PIN photodiode, and avalanche photodiode [202–207]. The most essential performance specifications of photodiodes in CMOS optical biosensors include quantum efficiency (QE), and dark current. QE is a measure of the probability that an incident photon will generate an electron-hole pair, thus contributing to the detection signal. The QE is influenced by the material properties and device geometry of the photodiode. Dark current refers to the smallest level of reverse current that exists in the lack of light illumination. It is an undesired current that arises from thermally excited electrons or current leakage along the current path. Dark current is a significant source of noise in photodiodes.

3.5 Magnetic Sensing Mechanism

Biological entities typically exhibit a non-magnetic characteristic, so magnetic microbeads and magnetic nanoparticles (MNPs) are widely used as labels for detection [208]. The magnetic particles can be classified based on magnetic size or magnetism. The sizes of the magnetic particles range from a few micrometers to tens of nanometers, influencing both sensitivity and magnetic moment. Magnetic particles demonstrate different types of magnetism, including diamagnetism [209], paramagnetism [210], ferromagnetism [211], ferrimagnetism [212], antiferromagnetism [213], and superparamagnetism [214], depending on their properties and how they respond to externally applied magnetic fields.

In magnetic sensors, the diagnosis process is carried out in two stages including biological sensing and physical detection. During biological sensing, the magnetic labels are functionalized with specific probes. Then under an external magnetic field magnetic nanoparticles can selectively bind to target analytes and become magnetized which induces a net magnetic moment. Next, in the physical detection process, the induced net magnetic moment can be detected by a circuit of the sensor. These processes will be briefly examined in the following.

3.5.1 *Biological Sensing*

MNPs labeling is a critical part of magnetic sensing, which converts biological information into detectable signals through different types of assay configurations. These assays comprised clustering assay, direct labeling assay, magnetic amplification assay, and sandwich assay, which are briefly illustrated following [215]. Figure 3.13a illustrates the clustering assay that utilizes magnetic particles with multivalent affinity ligands to bind to a single target molecule. This binding leads to particle aggregation, which can be easily detected. This assay is particularly useful for detecting small molecules, nucleic acids, and proteins in suspension without the need for washing steps [64]. Moreover, the clustering assay offers a faster alternative to surface-based detection methods, as the reaction occurs throughout the entire sample volume.

The direct labeling assay is shown in Fig. 3.13b. In this assay, magnetic particles label the entire target, suitable for large biological entities that cannot be easily surface-immobilized. Moreover, as unbound particles can be eliminated based on their size difference compared to target cells, it can offer high sensitivity [216, 217].

In the assay of magnetic amplification, depicted in Fig. 3.13c, a series of magnetic layers can be generated by successively applying magnetic particles linked to distinct binding partners [218]. This sequential process enhances magnetic signals, enabling the identification of elusive molecular targets and thereby enhancing the overall detection sensitivity [219].

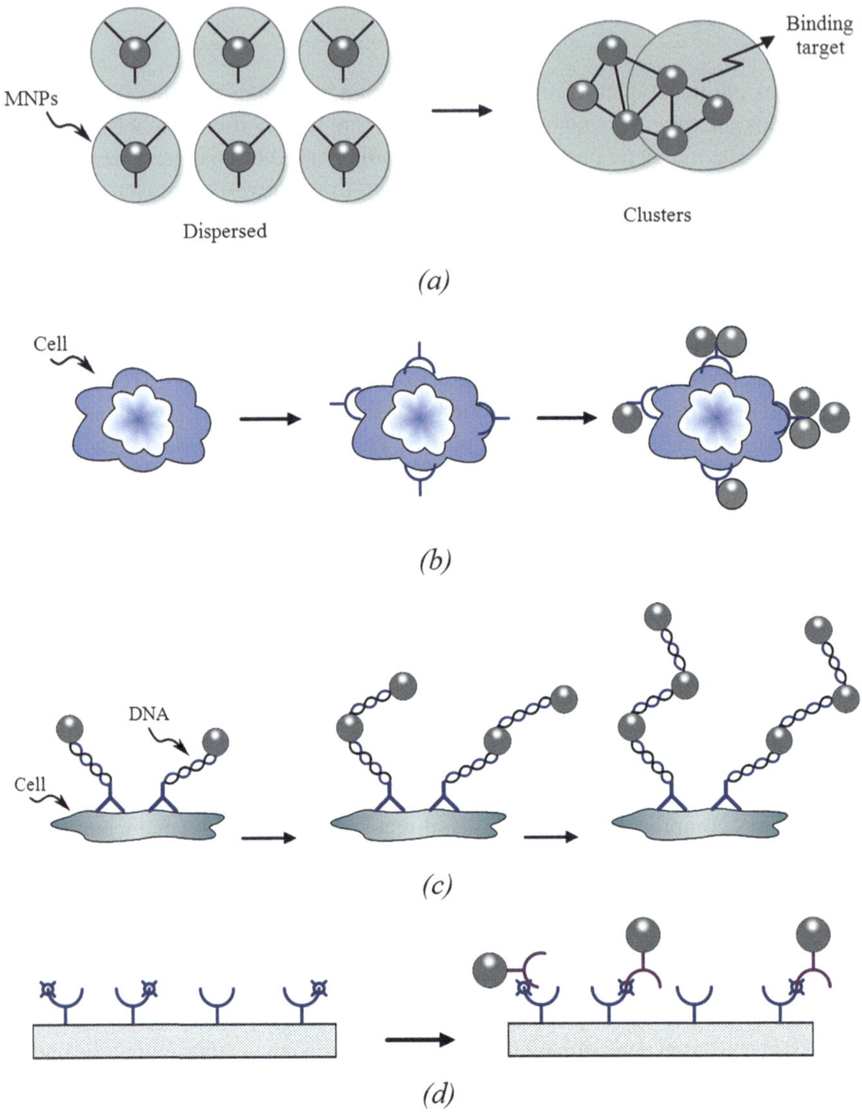

Fig. 3.13 Labeling technique: (**a**) clustering. When binding targets are present, multivalent MNPs tend to aggregate due to cross-linking. This aggregation results in alterations to the organizational state of the MNPs, which can be quantified through methods such as NMR relaxometry or Brownian relaxation measurements. Notably, these techniques allow for measurement without requiring any additional washing steps., (**b**) direct. to label large biological entities, the entire target can first be tagged with affinity ligands and then later marked with MNPs, (**c**) magnetic amplification, Amplification of magnetic signals for detecting rare molecular targets can be achieved by sequentially applying multiple layers of MNPs to a target. This process involves using MNPs that are modified with orthogonal binding partners, allowing for enhanced labeling, (**d**) sandwich, in a sandwich labeling approach, a solid substrate is functionalized with affinity ligands to enrich small molecular targets from a complex biological mixture. Following this initial capture, secondary labeling with MNPs is performed

The most widely used magnetic assay is an affinity-based sandwich (see Fig. 3.13d). In this approach, through the functionalization of a solid substrate with affinity ligands, the effective enrichment of small molecular targets is achieved amidst a complex biological background. Following the initial capture, the introduction of secondary MNPs labeling serves to bring MNPs into proximity with the sensor surface, enhancing the overall detection sensitivity.

3.5.2 *Physical Sensing*

In this section, the fundamental principle operation of magnetic sensors based on Hall-effect, inductive, and giant magnetoresistance (GMR) will be briefly examined.

3.5.2.1 The Operating Principles of Hall-Effect Biosensors

When a thin and elongated conducting plate with voltage (or current) biasing is subjected to a perpendicular magnetic field (B_{Ext}), the Lorentz force causes the deviation of carriers (electrons in this instance) from their trajectories. This deviation results in the generation of a Hall voltage (V_H) between the electrical contacts at the periphery of the plate (see Fig. 3.14). This phenomenon is referred to as the Hall effect and serves as a fundamental principle in the design of Hall-effect sensors [220]. Notably, the Hall plate is biased with voltage or current. The magnitude of V_H of the Hall plate with voltage and current biasing are represented by the following equations:

$$V_H = G_H \frac{W}{L} \mu_H B_{Ext} V_{Bias} \tag{3.18}$$

$$V_H = G_H \frac{r_H}{n.e.t} B_{Ext} I_{Bias} \tag{3.19}$$

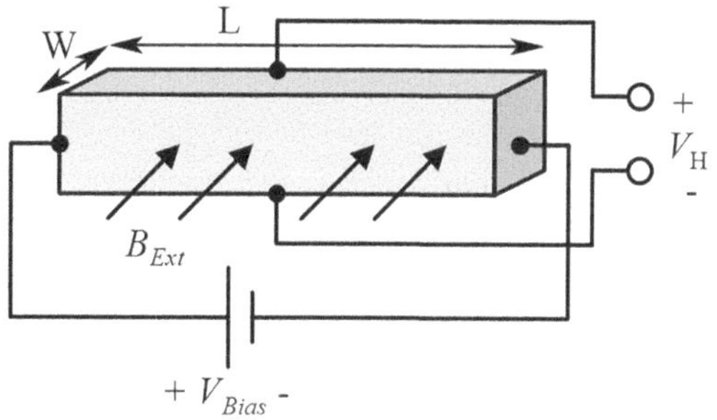

Fig. 3.14 The operational principle of a Hall plate

where G_H is the geometrical correcting factor, W and L are the width and length of the Hall plate, μ_H is the Hall mobility of the majority carriers, V_{Bias} is the biasing voltage, I_{Bias} is the biasing current, r_H is the Hall scattering factor, n is the carrier concentration, e is the electron charge, and t is the thickness of the n-well implantation. By combining the vertical components of B_{Ext} and the induced magnetic field from the MNPs (B_{MNP}), the Hall sensor transforms them into an alternating voltage signal of V_H magnitude [221]. This signal is then distributed across two opposite sense contacts on the Hall sensor.

As indicated in eqs. (3.18) and (3.19), V_H exhibits linearity with both the magnetic field and the biasing voltage (current). Hence, the sensitivity parameter for a Hall-effect sensor, referred to as voltage-related sensitivity and current-related sensitivity can be formally defined by (3.20) and (3.21)

$$S_V = G_H \mu_H \left(W / L \right) \tag{3.20}$$

$$S_I = G_H \frac{r_H}{n.e.t} \tag{3.21}$$

The voltage-related sensitivity (S_V), relies on the geometry and the Hall mobility, which exhibits a significant temperature dependency. The current-related sensitivity (S_I) inversely correlates with the carrier concentration. S_I remains stable across temperature variations for plate doping densities ranging between 10^{15} and 10^{17} cm^3, aligning well with the operating temperatures common in numerous contemporary applications [222].

Typically, a Hall sensor comprises a Hall plate, a Hall spin current bias element, an external magnetic field for appropriately biasing the immobilized magnetic labels, and a readout circuit. The magnetic field induced by the magnetic labels is captured by the embedded Hall-effect sensor. Notably, the magnitude from the B_{MNP} is proportional to the external magnetic field B_{Ext}. Thus the distance between the generator of B_{Ext} and magnetic labels should be minimized. Furthermore, the magnitude of B_{MNP} is asymptotically proportional to the inverse of the cube of the distance between the bead center and the sensor. So, post-processing is required to decrease this distance and enhance sensitivity and biocompatibility. On the other hand, the small magnitude of the magnetic particles causes some undesirable effects such as stray magnetic field, DC offset, and thermal effects, which should be removed. To address his issue, offset-cancellation methods such as spinning-current [223, 224] and X-Hall [225–227] are employed in Hall effect sensors.

Hall Plate Element

The Hall plate is usually a four-terminal device that requires two contacts for the biasing, and two contacts for sensing the Hall voltage. Figure 3.15 illustrates some typical shapes for the Hall plate. The cross shape offers high values of the geometrical correction factor, and in a compact geometry, the square shape exhibits higher sensitivity values [228].

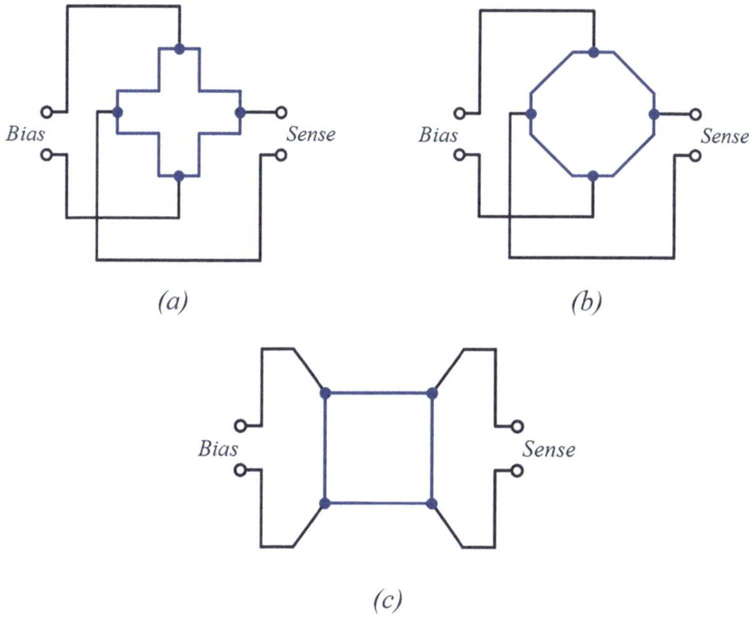

Fig. 3.15 Various shapes of the Hall plate, (**a**) cross (**b**) octagonal (**c**) square with contacts on the angles

Fig. 3.16 Typical planar views of a Hall plate

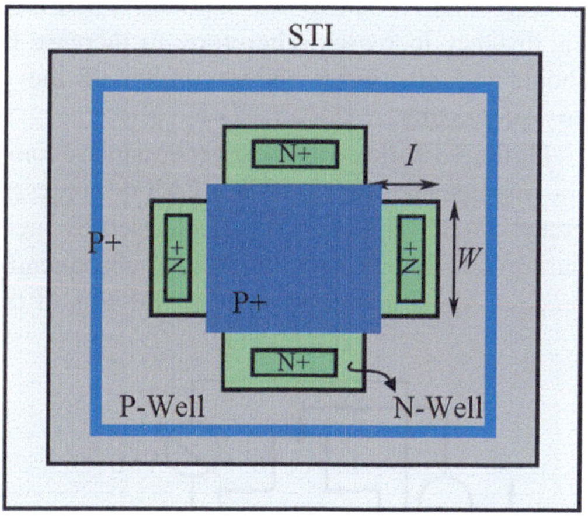

In CMOS technology, a Hall plate can be realized using a diffusion layer or the channel region of a transistor [229]. The N-type well Hall plate is more favorable because of their greater carrier mobility versus p-type wells which leads to higher sensitivity [227, 230–234]. Figure 3.16 shows the typical planar views of a Hall plate [235]. Shallow trench isolation (STI) aims to offer electrical isolation between Hall devices and interface circuits. In this design, an N-well layer with a cross-like shape is implemented on a P-type substrate to create the device's active region.

In this design, to form the device's active region an N-well layer with a cross-like configuration is incorporated into a p-type substrate. For device protection, a guard ring with a layer of a P-well is also established around the N-well. Also, to diminish the resistance of contact, four contact regions with a highly doped N+ implantation layer are formed. To mitigate flicker noise arising from carrier surface recombination, the device's surface is covered with a heavily doped P+ implanting layer [235]. The size of the Hall plate is adjusted for optimal performance according to bead size, signal strength, and physical design guidelines [236].

The Hall plates are operated in either voltage mode or current mode, utilizing four terminals as shown in Figs. 3.17 and 3.18, respectively [237]. In the case of voltage mode, the output signal is voltage-based taken from two non-neighboring output contacts, and the Hall plate is powered by either a current or voltage source through the other two terminals. Usually, Hall plates find application more in voltage-mode circuits. In the current model, the Hall plate is biased by the current and the output of the Hall plate is current [238]. Based on the results reported by Ausserlechner [237], the Hall plate in current mode shows equivalent sensitivity to magnetic field fluctuations and SNR as the conventional Hall plate operating in voltage mode.

Post Processing

In standard multilayer metal processes, the chip surface lies over the active devices, leading to a decrease in the magnetic signal originating from the magnetic bead as the distance increases. Therefore, to increase bead signal strength sensor surface should be positioned in proximity to the embedded Hall-effect sensor by post-processing.

Figure 3.19 shows the post-processing reported by Liu *et. al* [239] for a Hall sensor implemented in a 0.18 μm CMOS process. The sensor area and CMOS integrated circuit (IC) area are safeguarded by metal layers acting as a robust barrier during RIE. The protective mask is subsequently eliminated through a wet etching process. Metal layers serve as hard masks of the sensor area and CMOS IC from

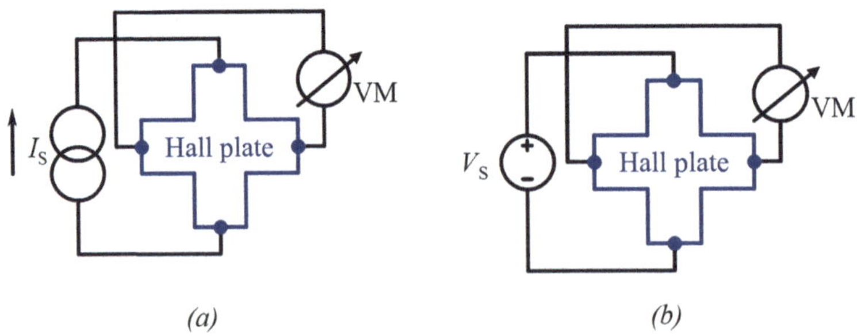

Fig. 3.17 Fundamental circuit concept Hall plate in the voltage mode with (**a**) current source, (**b**) voltage source

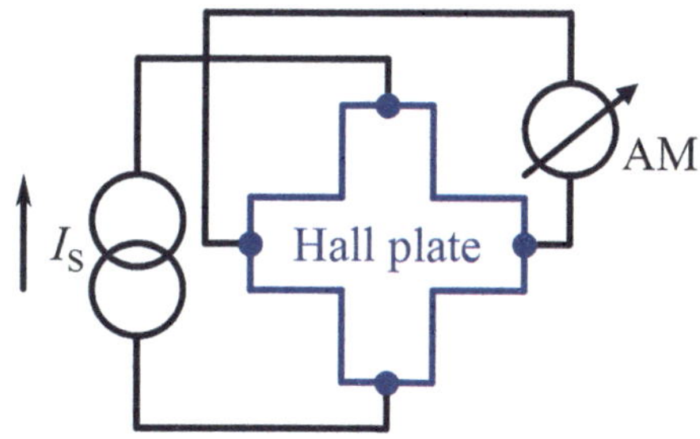

Fig. 3.18 Fundamental circuit concept Hall plate in the current mode

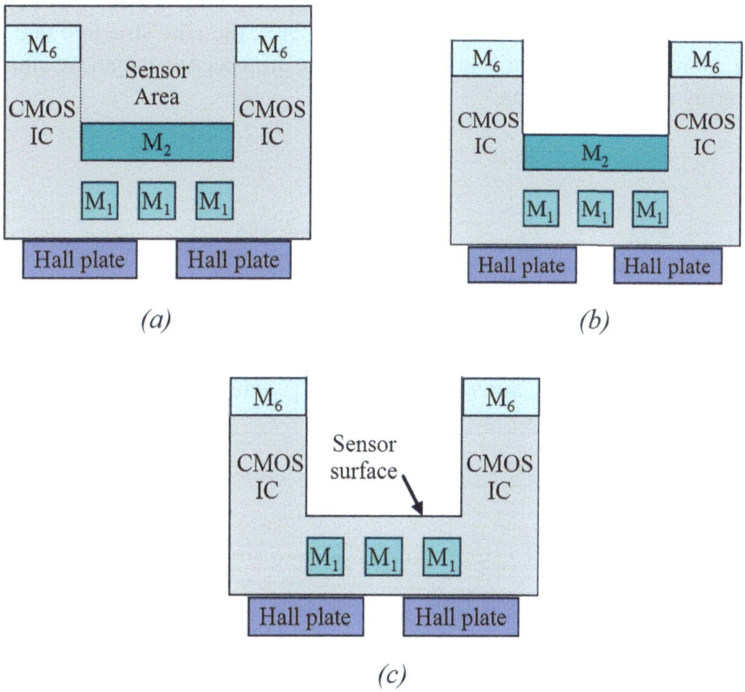

Fig. 3.19 Etching procedures conducted post-CMOS fabrication aimed at minimizing the distance between the beads and the Hall sensor. (**a**) original chip fabricated by CMOS foundry, (**b**) ILDs removed by RIE, (**c**) metal layers removed by wet etching

the RIE. The inter-layer dielectric (ILD) overlying the sensor region is removed by RIE. Then, the hard mask is subsequently eliminated using a wet etching step (optional), which brings the beads nearer to the Hall sensor array. Following the post-processing, only metal and polysilicon remain for interconnects within the sensor region [239]. The photoresist is applied to shield the pad area from etching. Notably, in this study, the post-processing does not require additional masks and can be executed at the wafer level [221].

Magnetic Field

Given that the magnetic moment induced on a bead is directly proportional to the external magnetic field, bringing polarization wires near the bead and increasing the current of magnetic causes a larger magnetic moment and consequently larger signal. To generate the magnetic field integrated wires and micro-coils can be employed (see Fig. 3.20) [240]. The comparison of the average bead signal generated by each structure for the same sensor pitch is reported by Skucha et al. [240]. The achieved results show that the average signals from the various architectures are within 20% of one another for bead sizes ranging from 100 nm to 5 μm. Microcoils perform slightly better for beads smaller than 2 μm in diameter, while wires are more effective for beads larger than 2 μm in diameter. In [240], the wire structure due to the simpler, more compact layout, and smaller voltage drop per row length are employed for the array implementations.

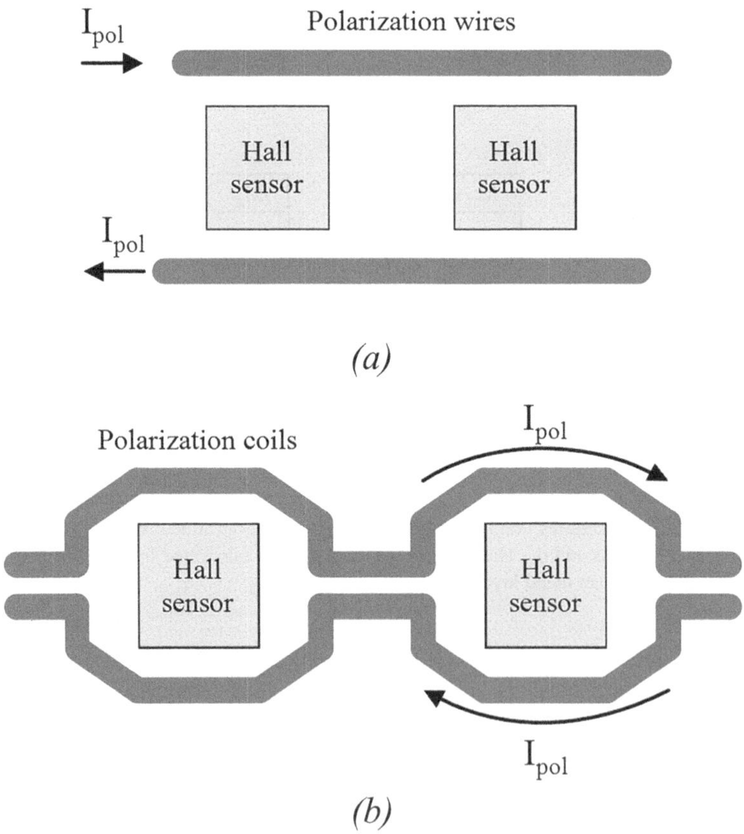

Fig. 3.20 Two polarization field generator architectures based on (**a**) Polarization wires, (**b**) Polarization coils

3.5.2.2 The Operating Principles of Inductive Biosensors

Generally, the core of inductive magnetic sensors consists of a single coil or a couple of coils in which the magnetic particles change the inductance or coupling coefficient, respectively. The most known magnetic sensor based on a single core is known as the frequency-shift magnetic sensor [241], and its principle operation is shown in Fig. 3.21. An alternating current (AC) passing through a single coil induces a magnetic field, leading to the polarization of magnetic particles in its proximity. This augmentation of the total stored magnetic energy within the space consequently elevates the effective inductance of the coil. As a result, the oscillation frequency will be changed.

Figure 3.22 shows the simple model of a magnetic sensor based on coupled coils. It consisted of an excitation (L_1) and pickup coils (L_2). The excitation coil driven by an AC waveform generates a magnetic field and the pickup coil detects the change in magnetic flux due to the presence of a cell decorated with magnetic labels. The presence of magnetic particles modifies the flux coupling between the primary and secondary coils, which produces a voltage at the output of the sensor.

Inductive magnetic sensors seamlessly integrate into the CMOS process without the need for post-processing. Moreover, they operate without the necessity of an external biasing magnetic field, streamlining system implementation and reducing overall costs.

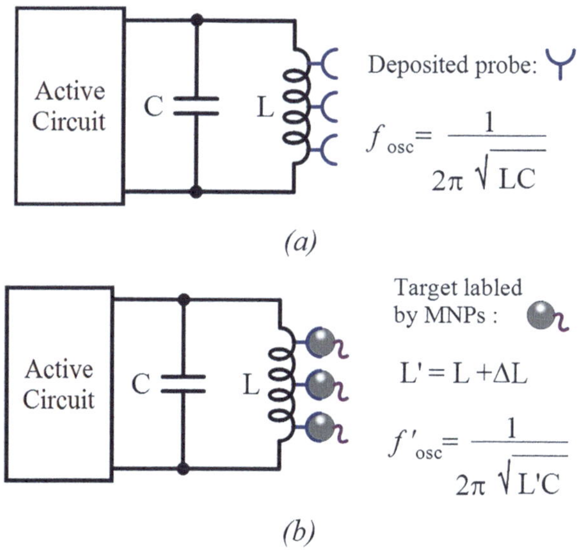

Fig. 3.21 Fundamental principle of the inductive magnetic sensor with frequency-shift structure (**a**) before sensing, (**b**) after sensing

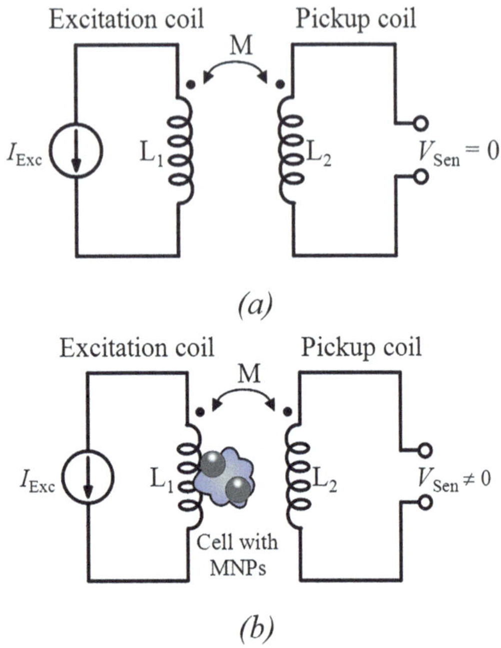

Fig. 3.22 The model of an inductive magnetic sensor with coupled coils structure (**a**) before sensing, (**b**) after sensing

3.5.2.3 The Operating Principles of GMR Biosensors

A material demonstrating magnetoresistance transforms variations in an external magnetic field into alterations in resistance with different mechanisms comprising GMR, anisotropic magnetoresistance (AMR), and tunneling magnetoresistance (TMR). Albert Fert and Peter Grünberg for their discovery of GMR, were honored with the Nobel Prize in Physics in 2007 [242]. The GMR magnetic sensors leverage the giant magnetoresistive effect to detect magnetic fields [243]. The GMR sensors are highly desirable because they are fully compatible with CMOS technology, enabling them to be compact and cost-effective.

The GMR Sensor Film Stack

The focus of this sub-section is examining GMR from a constructed layeries perspective, which can be classified into two major types including multilayer and spin-valve (SV). The multilayer GMR consists of two ferromagnetic layers (free and pinned layer) that are distinct by a thin non-ferromagnetic layer (spacer layer) as shown in Fig. 3.23a [244]. Moreover, a thin biocompatible passivation layer can be applied to form a noncorrosive sensor surface. The magnetic moment of the pinned layer is fixed, as the free layer rotates unrestrictedly within the plane in

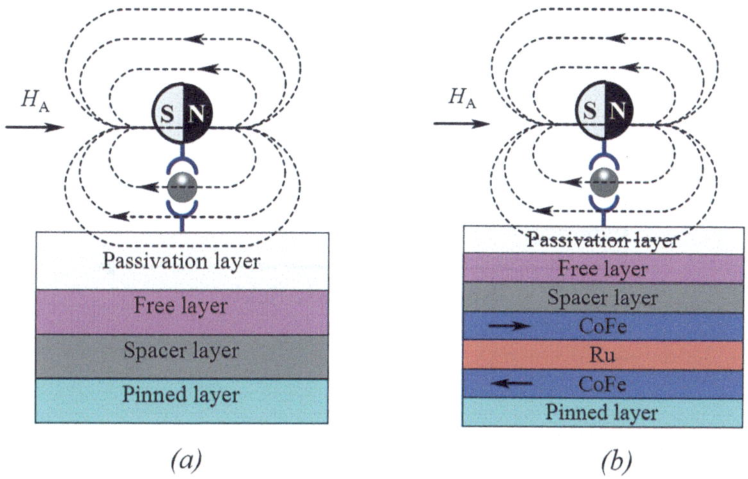

Fig. 3.23 The simplified layer stack of GMR sensor (**a**) multilayer, (**b**) SV

response to the external magnetic field. The resistance of the sensor is determined by the alignment of magnetic moments between the free layer and the pinned layer [242]. When an external magnetic field aligns the free layer parallel to the pinned layer, most carriers in the free layer align with those in the pinned layer. Consequently, electrons can traverse both layers without encountering additional scattering, leading to a decrease in resistance. On the other hand, anti-parallelling the free layer with the pinned layer causes districting the carriers in the free layer from the majority of carriers in the pinned layer. This discrepancy leads to increased electron scattering, resulting in higher resistance.

One constraint of the standard multilayer GMR film stack is the significant magnetic field needed to accomplish a complete magnetization switch from the antiparallel to the parallel state. This tendency compromises the sensors' low-field sensitivity [245]. To address this issue, the GMR SV sensor is introduced (see Fig. 3.23b) that employs a synthetic anti-ferromagnet (CoFe/Ru/CoFe) to the film stack [242, 244, 246–254], which pins the magnetization with exchange coupling. The free layer is capable of rotating freely in response to an external magnetic field, whereas the pinning layer plays a crucial role in determining the magnetization of the synthetic antiferromagnetic structure. Furthermore, the pinning layer serves to regulate the microstructural texture of the subsequent thin films. Consequently, it can be inferred that the strength of the external magnetic field is approximately linearly correlated with the effective resistance of the sensor.

The sensor resistance depends on the angle of the magnetic moments between the layers. As shown in Fig. 3.24 the resistance will be changed according to the applied field. Notably, the sensor's sensitivity is indicated by its magnetoresistive (MR) ratio (see (3.22), representing the maximum resistance change caused by the applied magnetic field.

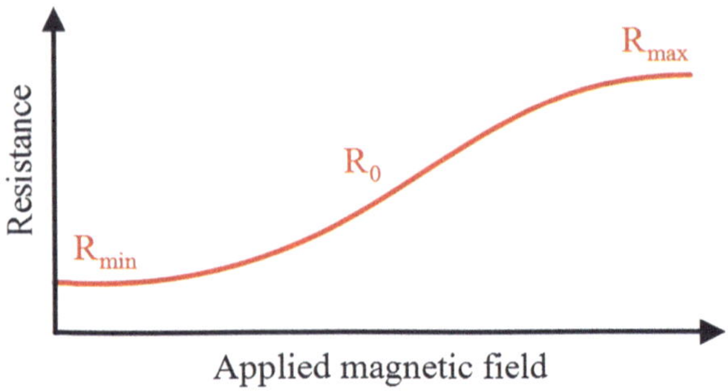

Fig. 3.24 The resistance of sensor vs. applied field

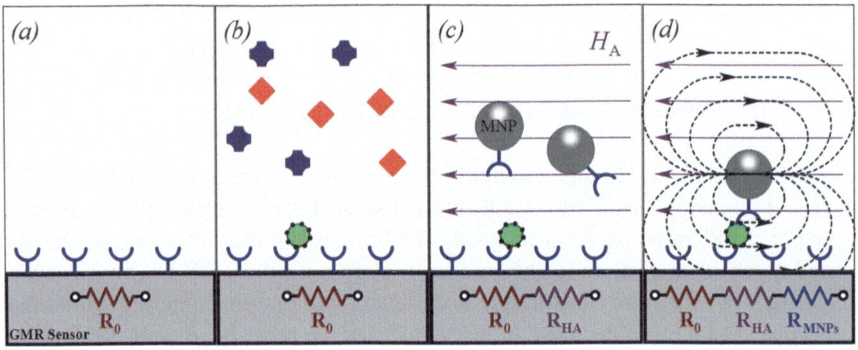

Fig. 3.25 MIA to measure the concentration of target via GMR sensor

$$MR = \frac{R_{max} - R_{min}}{R_{min}} = \frac{\Delta R}{R_{min}} \tag{3.22}$$

where R_{max} and R_{min} are the maximum and minimum resistance of the sensor, respectively.

The Magnetic Immunoassay for GMR Sensors

The GMR sensors detect the levels of specific biomarkers by employing a magnetic immunoassay (MIA). Figure 3.25 shows the sequence of MIA. First, the sensor surface is functionalized with immobilized capture antibodies (Fig. 3.25a). Then, the sample is applied, and the target biomarkers adhere to the immobilized capture antibodies on the sensor surface (Fig. 3.25b). The sensor resistance is R_0, where R_0 represents the nominal resistance of the sensor. In the next step, MNPs labeled detection antibodies are introduced and attached to the target biomarkers, forming a sandwich-like complex (Fig. 3.25c). In this step, the sensor resistance is $R_{HA} + R_0$ (R_{HA} is the magnetoresistance from the applied field, H_A). Lastly, an exter-

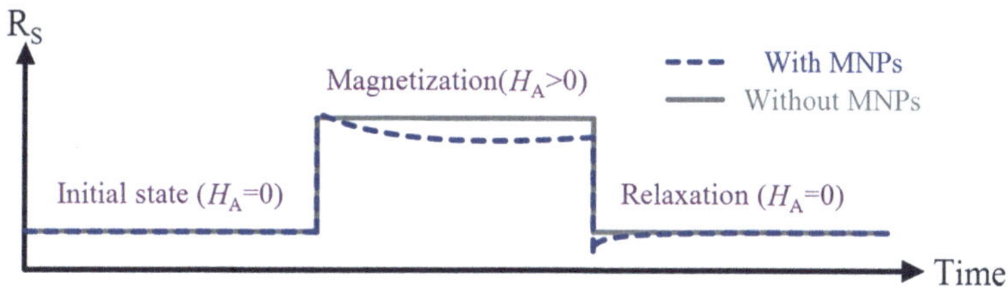

Fig. 3.26 Sensing concept of MRX

nal magnetic field is utilized to align the tethered MNPs, causing them to produce a stray field that opposes the direction of the applied field, H_A (Fig. 3.25d). The magnetoresistance from the MNPs is represented by R_{MNPs} making the the sensor resistance turned to the $R_{MNPs} + R_{HA} + R_0$. The magnetoresistance of R_{MNPs} is directly related to the quantity of tethered MNPs, serving as an indicator of the concentration of the target biomarkers.

Magnetic Sensing Techniques for GMR Sensors

Two common detection techniques that can be employed for GMR sensors are magnetometry and magneto-relaxometry (MRX). Magnetometry quantifies the number of tethered MNPs by measuring the disparity in the magnetic field with and without the presence of MNPs. Conversely, in MRX as illustrated in Fig. 3.26, the applied magnetic field is swiftly eliminated, and the sensors monitor the temporal evolution of the magnetic field as the MNPs gradually randomize, capturing the dynamics.

3.6 NMR

3.6.1 Principles Operation of NMR System

Nuclear magnetic resonance (NMR) is the energy exchange between an RF magnetic field and atomic nuclear spins subjected to static magnetic fields [255], which serves as a powerful means to examine the fundamental physics of atomic nuclei. Because the nuclei of hydrogen atoms (^1H), known as protons, behave like miniature bar magnets owing to their spins, protons are commonly employed in NMR experiments [256].

When no external magnetic field is present, the magnetic moments within the samples exhibit random orientation. As shown in Fig. 3.27a, when an external magnetic field (B_{Ext}, assumed to be along the z-axis) is applied to the nuclei, a fraction of them align with B_{Ext} and have a spin-up state, while others do not align. The interaction between B_{Ext} and magnetic moment, causes the nuclei to proceed around the magnetic field. Subsequently, a radio frequency (RF) magnetic field B_{RF}

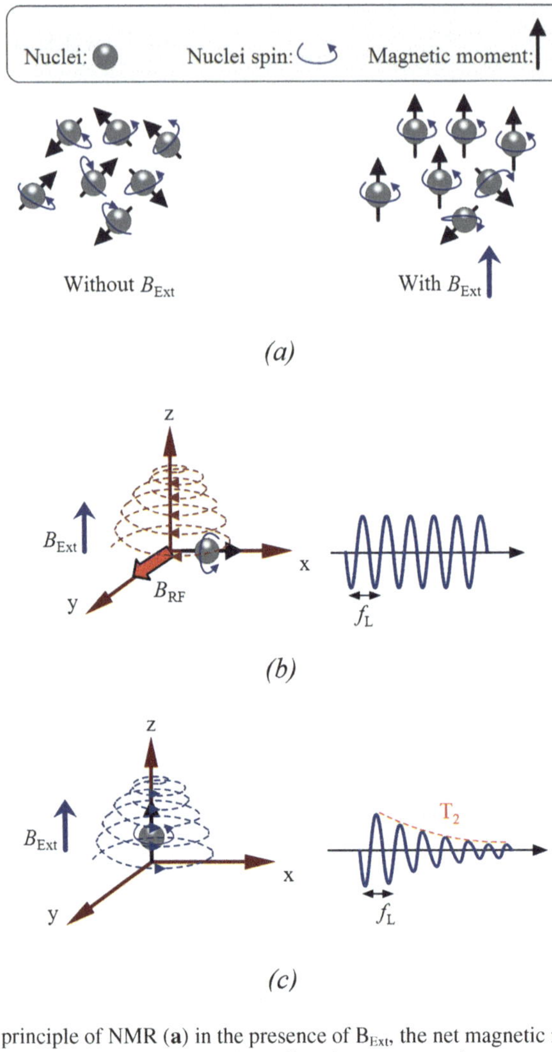

Fig. 3.27 The principle of NMR (**a**) in the presence of B_{Ext}, the net magnetic moment aligns with B_{Ext}, (**b**) applying a magnetic field B_{RF} in the y-direction can cause the magnetization of the nuclei to be deflected away from the z-direction, (**c**) B_{RF} is removed, yet the nuclei continue to resonate and revert to equilibrium, retaining information about the samples within their magnetization

perpendicular to B_{Ext} is applied (see Fig. 3.27b). The nuclei respond by processing around B_{Ext}, engaging in resonant energy exchange between the RF magnetic fields and nuclear spins. Consequently, the bulk magnetization deviates from B_{Ext}. This resonant energy exchange, exclusive to the Larmor frequency (f_L), defines the essence of NMR. It is worth noting that the nuclei only respond to RF excitation at the Larmor frequency that is defined by $f_L = \gamma\ B_{Ext}$, in which γ is the gyromagnetic ratio of the nuclei. After a specific period, the nuclei are deflected away from B_{Ext} at an angle of 90°. At this point, the excitation is terminated and the nuclei continue to resonate at the Larmor frequency and gradually decay with a characteristic decay time known as the spin-spin relaxation time (T_2) (see Fig. 3.27c). Both the T_2 parameter and the resonance frequency rely on material properties, which establishes NMR as an invaluable tool for biomolecule sensing.

3.7 Temperature Sensing Mechanism

3.7.1 The Operating Principles of BJT Temperature Sensor

The PN junction in diodes and bipolar junction transistors (BJTs) exhibit strong thermal dependence characteristics. This makes it a promising option for the design of temperature sensors. Additionally, two types of BJT transistors are available as parasitic devices: lateral and substrate (vertical). These can be utilized as temperature sensors when operated in a diode configuration. It is noteworthy to highlight that while temperature sensors utilizing lateral transistors have been proposed [257–259], the preference for temperature measurement leans towards vertical PNP transistors. This preference is attributed to their heightened sensitivity to process expansion and packaging stress, coupled with the superior exponential relationship between base-emitter voltage and collector current [260–265].

In this type of sensor, the main idea is based on generating a proportional to absolute temperature (PTAT) voltage and a temperature-independent voltage. The ratio of these voltages, which presents a temperature-dependent behavior, can be converted by an ADC to the digital data. Figure 3.28 shows the basic structure of temperature sensors based on BJT [266]. Two diode-connected transistors, which are biased with different currents are used to generate voltages of ΔV_{BE} and V_{BE}. It can be seen from Eq. (3.23) that ΔV_{BE} exhibits a PTAT behavior [267].

$$\Delta V_{BE} = \frac{KT}{q}\ln\left(\frac{NI_{\mathrm{B}}}{I_{\mathrm{S}}}\right) - V_{\mathrm{T}}\ln\left(\frac{I_{\mathrm{B}}}{I_{\mathrm{S}}}\right) = V_{\mathrm{T}}\ln(N) \tag{3.23}$$

Where T represents the absolute temperature, K is Boltzmann's constant, q denotes the electron charge, I_{B} signifies the collector current, I_{S} stands for the saturation current, and N represents the current ratio between two bipolar transistors. For the implementation of a temperature-independent voltage, as illustrated by the equation, a combination of PTAT voltage and a complementary to absolute temperature (CTAT) is required. Generally, this voltage is known as reference voltage (V_{REF}) or band-gap voltage.

$$V_{\mathrm{REF}} = V_{\mathrm{BE}} + \alpha\,\Delta V_{\mathrm{BE}} = V_{\mathrm{T}}\ln\frac{I_{\mathrm{B}}}{I_{\mathrm{S}}} + \alpha V_{\mathrm{T}}\ln(N) \tag{3.24}$$

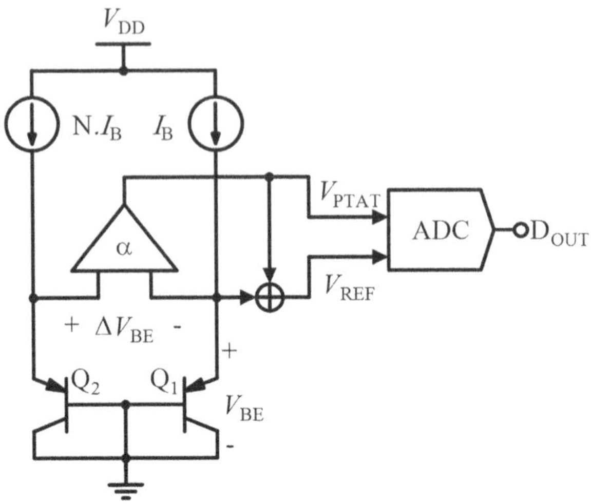

Fig. 3.28 The operational principle of the BJT temperature sensor

3.7.2 *The Operating Principles of MOSFET Temperature Sensor*

To develop a temperature sensor operating below 1 V with low power consumption, instead of the BJT, a metal-oxide-semiconductor field-effect transistor (MOSFET) operated in subthreshold is suggested [268–273]. Generally, compared to BJT temperature sensors, MOSFET temperature sensors have lower accuracy and typically mandate a two-point calibration. Thus applications where the need for high accuracy and resolution can be relaxed are more favorable [271].

3.7.2.1 Subthreshold MOSFET Temperature Sensor

When a MOSFET operates within the subthreshold regime, and the V_{DS} surpasses 0.1 V, the I_{D} of the MOSFET manifests as a temperature-dependent exponential function of the V_{GS}, described by (3.25).

$$I_{\mathrm{D}} = \mu C_{ox} \frac{W}{L}(n-1)V_T^2 \exp\left(\frac{V_{\mathrm{GS}} - V_{\mathrm{th}}}{nV_T}\right) \tag{3.25}$$

Where n represents the subthreshold slope factor, V_{T} (kT/q) signifies the thermal voltage, k denotes Boltzmann's constant, T stands for absolute temperature, and q represents the electron charge [274]. The current of the MOSFET in the subthreshold can be utilized for temperature sensing purposes. Subthreshold MOSFET

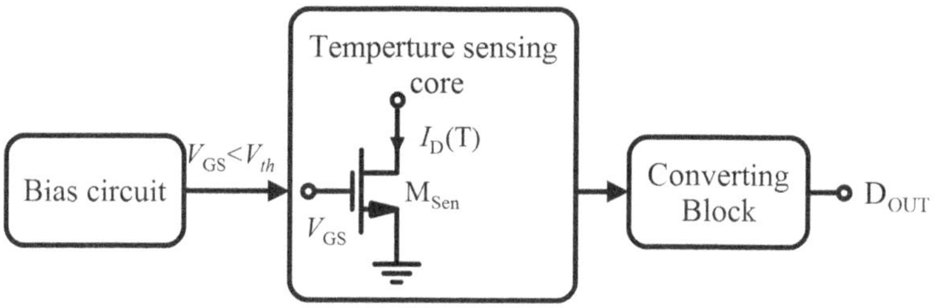

Fig. 3.29 Block diagram of a subthreshold MOSFET temperature sensor

temperature sensors offer the advantages of low voltage operation and low power consumption. While they may have lower accuracy compared to other temperature sensing methods, such as BJT temperature sensors, they can still prove valuable for practical applications where high accuracy and resolution are not critical requirements. It is worth noting that these sensors typically require a two-point calibration to compensate for their lower accuracy.

Figure 3.29 shows the temperature-sensing principle of a subthreshold MOSFET temperature sensor. The main structure of the sensing block is constructed of a single (or couples) MOSFET biased in subthreshold, which turns temperature into current. This current with the help of other circuits can convert to voltage, frequency, or digital data.

3.7.3 The Operating Principles of ETF Temperature Sensor

The principle behind ETF temperature sensors revolves around the thermal diffusivity of silicon, denoted as D, which characterizes the speed of heat dispersion within a silicon substrate from a hot end to a cold end. The relationship between D and temperature follows a power law $D = T^{-1.8}$ [275–277]. In Fig. 3.30, the ETF sensing element consists of a heating element and a temperature sensor created by the junction of two dissimilar materials (thermocouples), placed at a separation distance denoted as S. Applying a signal with a frequency of f_{Drive} to the hot end induces a temperature-dependent phase shift at the cold end, as expressed in (3.26) [278, 279], which can then be converted into digital information to readout.

$$\varnothing_{ETF} \propto \left(S\sqrt{f_{Drive}}\right)T^{0.9} \tag{3.26}$$

where T represents the absolute temperature, with n being approximately 1.8.

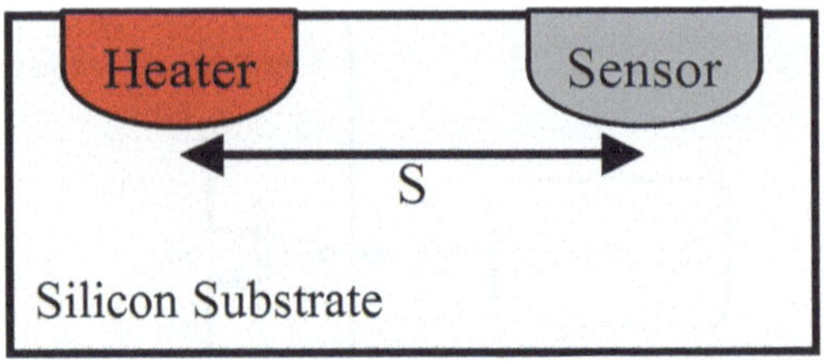

Fig. 3.30 Cross-sectional view of the ETF sensing element

Table 3.1 Characteristics of Different Resistors in CMOS Processes

Resistor type	Metal	Diffusion	N-Well	Poly	Silicided
First-order TC	Large	Medium	Large	Medium or small	Large
Second-order TC	Medium	Medium	Large	Medium	Small
Sheet resistance	Very small	Large	Large	Large	Medium
Supply dependency	Small	Medium	Large	Small	Small
1/f noise	Negligible	Negligible	Negligible	Large	Small
Stress sensitivity	Small	Large	Large	Medium	Small

3.7.4 *The Operating Principles of Resistor Temperature Sensor*

A thermistor (temperature-dependent resistor) can be modeled as (3.27).

$$R(T) = R(T_0)\left(1 + TC_1.\Delta T + TC_2.\Delta T^2\right) \tag{3.27}$$

Where $R(T_0)$ is the resistor at a reference temperature T_0. TC_1 and TC_2 are the first-order and second-order temperature coefficients (TC), respectively, and ΔT is the temperature difference compared to T_0 (the nominal value). Numerous resistors are present in CMOS technology, comprising metal, N-well, diffusion, poly-silicon, and silicide resistors. Their characteristics are outlined in Table 3.1 [280]. To enhance the performance of a resistor temperature sensor, the sensing resistor should meet specific specifications. These include a substantial temperature coefficient (ensuring high linearity) to enhance sensitivity, a significant sheet resistance for reduced spatial requirements and minimal power consumption, low susceptibility to supply variations, stress sensitivity to ensure stable operation, and minimal $1/f$ noise.

Three commonly used thermistor sensors are integrated into the CMOS process, comprising Wheatstone bridge (WhB) [281–288], Wien bridge (WB) [289–294], and polyphase filters (PPFs) [295–299]. The fundamental principle operation of these structures is examined following.

3.7.4.1 Principles of WB Temperature Sensor

The schematic of a WB with the current mode or voltage mode is depicted in Fig. 3.31a, b, respectively. The WB functions as a second-order band-pass filter, where the temperature dependence parameter is determined by the phase shift that is expressed by (3.28) [300].

$$\varnothing(\omega) = -\tan^{-1}\left(\frac{R(T)^2 C^2\omega^2 - 1}{3R(T)C\omega}\right) \tag{3.28}$$

The current and voltage transfer function of this structure is expressed by equations of (3.29) and (3.30), respectively. It is worth mentioning that the current readout schema exhibits a bandpass characteristic in its transfer function, with a phase shift of zero at the center frequency of the filter ($\omega_0 = 1/RC$). Additionally, it maintains a linear behavior around the center frequency. Because the TC of metal-insulator-metal (MIM) capacitors is very low, according to the Eq. (3.28) the phase shift at a constant frequency is primarily influenced by the resistors. This can be inferred from the significantly low TC value of 5.9.

$$\frac{I_{OUT}(\omega)}{V_{IN}(\omega)} = \frac{C\,j\omega}{-R(T)^2 C^2\omega^2 + 3R(T)Cj\omega + 1} \tag{3.29}$$

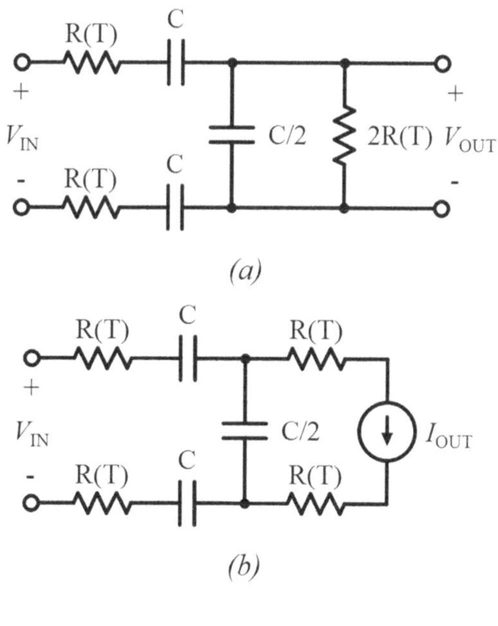

Fig. 3.31 WB sensor with scheme of (**a**) voltage readout, (**b**) current readout

$$\frac{V_{OUT}(\omega)}{V_{IN}(\omega)} = \frac{R(T)C\,j\omega}{1 - R(T)^2 C^2 \omega^2 + 3R(T)Cj\omega} \tag{3.30}$$

3.7.4.2 Principles of WhB Temperature Sensor

Figure 3.32 shows the core structure of the WhB sensor, comprising two resistors with different TCs of positive (R_P(T)) and negative (R_N(T)). Generally, to implement this temperature sensor with high sensitivity and stability, the R_P(T) and R_N(T) are constructed with silicided-p-poly and non-silicided n-poly resistors, respectively [281–285, 287, 288].

3.7.4.3 Principles of Poly-Phase Filter Temperature Sensor

The main architecture of the poly-phase filter (PPF) sensing element comprises two sensing resistors and two reference capacitors that is depicted in Fig. 3.33. Its phase shift and the voltage transfer function are expressed by equations of (3.31) and (3.32), respectively.

$$\frac{V_{OUT}(j\omega)}{V_{IN}(j\omega)} = \frac{1 - R(T)Cj\omega}{1 + R(T)Cj\omega} \tag{3.31}$$

$$\varnothing(\omega) = 2\tan^{-1}\left(-R(T)C\omega\right) \tag{3.32}$$

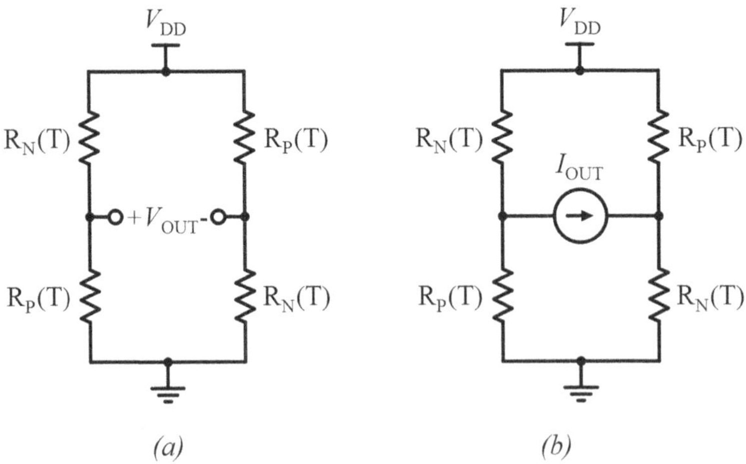

Fig. 3.32 The core structure of the WhB sensor with (**a**) voltage readout, (**b**) current readout

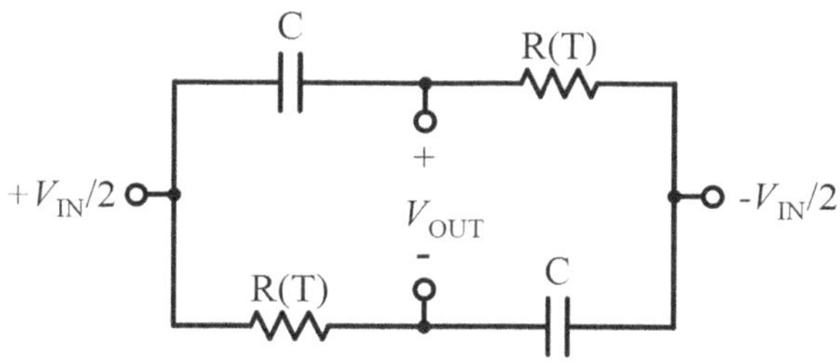

Fig. 3.33 Schematic of PPF sensor

In contrast to the WB structure, the area utilized for the implementation of PPF is beneath. Furthermore, the swing of the PPF output signal is substantially greater (approximately 7 times) than that of the WB [295].

3.7.5 *The Operating Principles of Seebeck Effect Temperature Sensor*

The Seebeck effect refers to a thermoelectric phenomenon that is illustrated in Fig. 3.34. In this effect, the heat energy between thermocouples (A and B) transformed into a voltage potential (ΔV), where the junctions of materials are kept at distinct temperatures. The junction at T and $T + \Delta T$ is known as the cold junction and the hot junction, respectively and the voltage of ΔV is the so-called Seebeck voltage, which can be given by $\Delta V = \alpha_s \Delta T$, where α_s is the Seebeck coefficient expressed in V/K.

In CMOS technology, the thermocouples are constructed from semiconductors and/or metals, where semiconductor layers typically exhibit larger Seebeck coefficients compared to metals [301–303]. Typical reported values for the Seebeck coefficient of CMOS process materials range from 500 to 700 μV/K [304].

Temperature sensors based on the Seebeck effect can be implemented by placing the hot junction on a thermally isolated structure, while the cold junction is strategically positioned on the bulk chip with highly thermally conductive silicon underneath [305]. The fundamental block of this temperature sensor is depicted in Fig. 3.35. Usually, rather than using a single thermocouple, multiple thermocouples connected in series are employed, a configuration known as a thermopile. The generated small voltage by thermopile is amplified by structures such as chopper-based amplifiers [306] and converted to digital data through a digital circuit such as ADC.

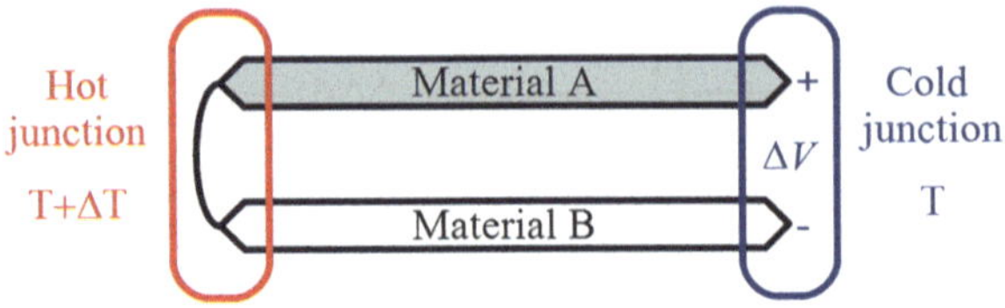

Fig. 3.34 Thermocouples generate voltage in response to temperature differences based on the Seebeck effect

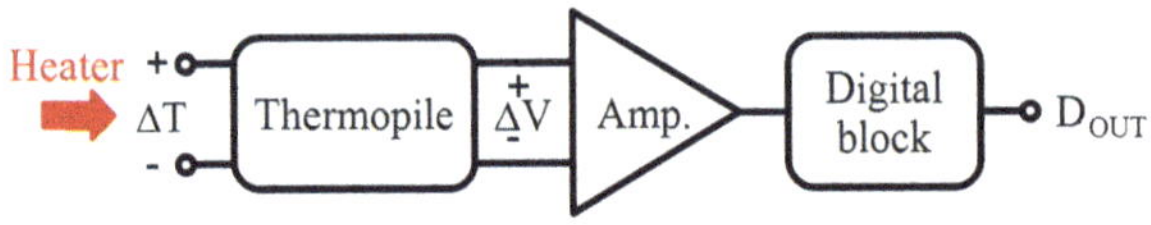

Fig. 3.35 The schematic of the Seebeck-effect temperature sensor

3.8 Summary

This chapter presents a detailed exploration of the various sensing mechanisms and transducer technologies that are central to the functionality of CMOS biosensors. By addressing the design, fabrication, and application of these sensors, the chapter emphasizes their critical role in advancing the detection and measurement of biological and chemical signals. This examination underscores the importance of integrating different sensing approaches to enhance the versatility and effectiveness of CMOS biosensors, paving the way for innovations in medical, environmental, and other applications.

References

1. Harvey D (2010) Analytical chemistry 2.0. LibreTexts
2. Hedayatipour A, Aslanzadeh S, McFarlane N (2019) CMOS based whole cell impedance sensing: challenges and future outlook. Biosens Bioelectron 143:111600
3. Manickam A (2012) Integrated impedance spectroscopy biosensors. The University of Texas at Austin
4. Bard AJ, Faulkner LR, White HS (2022) Electrochemical methods: fundamentals and applications. Wiley
5. Daniels JS, Pourmand N (2007) Label-free impedance biosensors: opportunities and challenges. Electroanalysis 19(12):1239–1257
6. Katz E, Willner I (2003) Probing biomolecular interactions at conductive and semiconductive surfaces by impedance spectroscopy: routes to impedimetric immunosensors, DNA-sensors, and enzyme biosensors. Electroanalysis 15(11):913–947
7. Liu Q, Wang P (2009) Cell-based biosensors: principles and applications. Artech House, Norwood, Massachusetts, United States

8. Prakash SB, Abshire P (2008) Tracking cancer cell proliferation on a CMOS capacitance sensor chip. Biosens Bioelectron 23(10):1449–1457. [Online]. Available: https://www.sciencedirect.com/science/article/abs/pii/S0956566307005064
9. Lu MS-C, Chen Y-C, Huang P-C (2010) 5 × 5 CMOS capacitive sensor array for detection of the neurotransmitter dopamine. Biosens Bioelectron 26(3):1093–1097
10. Nabovati G, Ghafar-Zadeh E, Letourneau A, Sawan M (2018) Smart cell culture monitoring and drug test platform using CMOS capacitive sensor Array. IEEE Trans Biomed Eng 66(4):1094–1104. [Online]. Available: https://ieeexplore.ieee.org/abstract/document/8444751
11. Ghafar-Zadeh E, Sawan M, Chodavarapu VP, Hosseini-Nia T (2010) Bacteria growth monitoring through a differential CMOS capacitive sensor. IEEE Trans Biomed Circuits Syst 4(4):232–238
12. Cornila C et al (1995) Capacitive sensors in CMOS technology with polymer coating. Sensors Actuators B Chem 25(1–3):357–361
13. Hagleitner C, Lange D, Hierlemann A, Brand O, Baltes H (2002) CMOS single-chip gas detection system comprising capacitive, calorimetric and mass-sensitive microsensors. IEEE J Solid State Circuits 37(12):1867–1878
14. Hierlemann A, Weimar U, Baltes H (2002) Hand-held and palm-top chemical microsensor systems for gas analysis. In: Handbook of machine olfaction: electronic nose technology, pp 201–229
15. Kummer AM, Hierlemann A, Baltes H (2004) Tuning sensitivity and selectivity of complementary metal oxide semiconductor-based capacitive chemical microsensors. Anal Chem 76(9):2470–2477
16. Hierlemann A (2005. Digest of technical papers. TRANSDUCERS'05. The 13th international conference on, 2005, vol. 2) Integrated chemical microsensor systems in CMOS-technology. In: Solid-state sensors, actuators and microsystems. IEEE, pp 1134–1137
17. Tashtoush A (2018) Nano-amplification strategy using charge based capacitance measurement for pathogenic bacteria detection, J Biotechnol Strateg Health Res, 2, 2, pp. 87–100
18. Hassibi A, Lee TH (2006) A programmable 0.18-μm CMOS electrochemical sensor microarray for biomolecular detection. IEEE Sensors J 6(6):1380–1388
19. Prakash SB, Abshire P, Urdaneta M, Smela E (2005) A CMOS capacitance sensor for cell adhesion characterization. In: 2005 IEEE international symposium on circuits and systems. IEEE, pp 3495–3498
20. Prakash SB, Abshire P (2007) On-chip capacitance sensing for cell monitoring applications. IEEE Sensors J 7(3):440–447
21. Prakash SB, Abshire P (2005) A CMOS capacitance sensor that monitors cell viability. In: IEEE sensors, 2005. IEEE, p 4
22. Ghafar-Zadeh E, Sawan M, Therriault D (2009) A microfluidic packaging technique for lab-on-chip applications. IEEE Trans Adv Packag 32(2):410–416. [Online]. Available: https://ieeexplore.ieee.org/abstract/document/4476160
23. Ghafar-Zadeh E, Sawan M (2008) Charge-based capacitive sensor array for CMOS-based laboratory-on-chip applications. IEEE Sensors J 8(4):325–332. [Online]. Available: https://ieeexplore.ieee.org/abstract/document/4453910
24. Ghafar-Zadeh E, Sawan M, Therriault D (2009) CMOS based capacitive sensor laboratory-on-chip: a multidisciplinary approach. Analog Integr Circ Sig Process 59(1):1–12
25. Nabovati G, Ghafar-Zadeh E, Mirzaei M, Ayala-Charca G, Awwad F, Sawan M (2015) A new fully differential CMOS capacitance to digital converter for lab-on-Chip applications. IEEE transactions on biomedical circuits and systems 9(3):353–361
26. Moreno-Hagelsieb L et al (2007) Electrical detection of DNA hybridization: three extraction techniques based on interdigitated Al/Al2O3 capacitors. Biosens Bioelectron 22(9–10):2199–2207

27. Nikkhoo N, Man C, Maxwell K, Gulak PG (2008) A 0.18 µm CMOS integrated sensor for the rapid identification of bacteria. In: Solid-state circuits conference, 2008. ISSCC 2008. Digest of Technical Papers. IEEE International. IEEE, pp 336–617
28. Ghafar-Zadeh E, Sawan M (2010) CMOS capacitive sensors for lab-on-chip applications. Springer, New York
29. Couniot N, Francis LA, Flandre D (2016) A 16 ×16 CMOS capacitive biosensor Array towards detection of single bacterial cell. IEEE Trans Biomed Circuits Syst 10(2):364–374. [Online]. Available: https://ieeexplore.ieee.org/abstract/document/7106573
30. Couniot N, Bol D, Poncelet O, Francis LA, Flandre D (2014) A capacitance-to-frequency converter with on-chip passivated microelectrodes for bacteria detection in saline buffers up to 575 MHz. IEEE Trans Circuits Syst II: Express Briefs 62(2):159–163
31. Nabovati G, Ghafar-Zadeh E, Letourneau A, Sawan M (2016) Towards high throughput cell growth screening: a new CMOS 8×8 biosensor Array for life science applications. IEEE Trans Biomed Circuits Syst
32. Thierry B, Winnik FM, Merhi Y, Silver J, Tabrizian M (2003) Bioactive coatings of endovascular stents based on polyelectrolyte multilayers. Biomacromolecules 4(6):1564–1571
33. Chen X, Yan X, Khor KA, Tay BK (2007) Multilayer assembly of positively charged polyelectrolyte and negatively charged glucose oxidase on a 3D Nafion network for detecting glucose. Biosens Bioelectron 22(12):3256–3260
34. Zhang S, Yang W, Niu Y, Li Y, Zhang M, Sun C (2006) Construction of glucose biosensor based on sorption of glucose oxidase onto multilayers of polyelectrolyte/nanoparticles. Anal Bioanal Chem 384(3):736–741
35. Nabovati G, Zhu YW, Sawan M (2015) Capacitive sensor arrays. In: Wiley encyclopedia of electrical and electronics engineering, pp 1–12
36. Hofmann F et al (2002) Passive DNA sensor with gold electrodes fabricated in a CMOS backend process. In: Solid-state device research conference, 2002. Proceeding of the 32nd European. IEEE, pp 487–490
37. Stagni C et al (2006) CMOS DNA sensor array with integrated A/D conversion based on label-free capacitance measurement. IEEE J Solid State Circuits 41(12):2956–2964. [Online]. Available: https://ieeexplore.ieee.org/abstract/document/4014638
38. Guiducci C, Stagni C, Fischetti A, Mastromatteo U, Benini L, Riccoricco B (2006) Microelectrodes on a silicon chip for label-free capacitive DNA sensing. IEEE Sensors J 6(5):1084–1093
39. Sun A, Alvarez-Fontecilla E, Venkatesh A, Aronoff-Spencer E, Hall DA (2017) A 64 × 64 high-density redox amplified coulostatic discharge-based biosensor array in 180nm CMOS. In: ESSCIRC 2017-43rd IEEE European solid state circuits conference. IEEE, pp 368–371. [Online]. Available: https://ieeexplore.ieee.org/abstract/document/8094602
40. Kerman K, Ozkan D, Kara P, Meric B, Gooding JJ, Ozsoz M (2002) Voltammetric determination of DNA hybridization using methylene blue and self-assembled alkanethiol monolayer on gold electrodes. Anal Chim Acta 462(1):39–47
41. Shervedani RK, Mehrjardi AH, Zamiri N (2006) A novel method for glucose determination based on electrochemical impedance spectroscopy using glucose oxidase self-assembled biosensor. Bioelectrochemistry 69(2):201–208
42. Berdondini L, van der Wal PD, de Rooij NF, Koudelka-Hep M (2004) Development of an electroless post-processing technique for depositing gold as electrode material on CMOS devices. Sensors Actuators B Chem 99(2–3):505–510
43. Mallory GO, Hajdu JB (1990) Electroless plating: fundamentals and applications. William Andrew, Orlando
44. Ko JW et al (2010) Electroless gold plating on aluminum patterned chips for CMOS-based sensor applications. J Electrochem Soc 157(1):D46–D49
45. Manickam A, Chevalier A, McDermott M, Ellington AD, Hassibi A (2010) A CMOS electrochemical impedance spectroscopy (EIS) biosensor array. IEEE Trans Biomed Circuits Syst 4(6):379–390

46. Widdershoven F et al (2010) CMOS biosensor platform. In: 2010 IEEE International Electron Devices Meeting (IEDM). IEEE, pp 36.1. 1–36.1. 4. [Online]. Available: https://ieeexplore.ieee.org/abstract/document/5703484.
47. Lemay SG, Laborde C, Renault C, Cossettini A, Selmi L, Widdershoven FP (2016) High-frequency nanocapacitor arrays: concept, recent developments, and outlook. Acc Chem Res 49(10):2355–2362
48. Widdershoven F et al (2018) A CMOS pixelated Nanocapacitor biosensor platform for high-frequency impedance spectroscopy and imaging. IEEE Trans Biomed Circuits Syst
49. Dragas J et al (2017) In vitro multi-functional microelectrode Array featuring 59 760 electrodes, 2048 electrophysiology channels, stimulation, impedance measurement, and neurotransmitter detection channels. IEEE J Solid State Circuits 52(6):1576–1590. [Online]. Available: https://ieeexplore.ieee.org/abstract/document/7913669
50. Ballini M et al (2014) A 1024-channel CMOS microelectrode array with 26,400 electrodes for recording and stimulation of electrogenic cells in vitro. IEEE J Solid State Circuits 49(11):2705–2719. [Online]. Available: https://ieeexplore.ieee.org/abstract/document/6923484
51. Greve F, Lichtenberg J, Kirstein K, Frey U, Perriard J, Hierlemann A (2007) A perforated CMOS microchip for immobilization and activity monitoring of electrogenic cells. J Micromech Microeng 17(3):462
52. Heer F, Hafizovic S, Franks W, Blau A, Ziegler C, Hierlemann A (2006) CMOS microelectrode array for bidirectional interaction with neuronal networks. IEEE J Solid State Circuits 41(7):1620–1629
53. Frey U et al (2010) Switch-matrix-based high-density microelectrode array in CMOS technology. IEEE J Solid State Circuits 45(2):467–482. [Online]. Available: https://ieeexplore.ieee.org/abstract/document/5405139
54. Viswam V et al (2018) Impedance spectroscopy and electrophysiological imaging of cells with a high-density CMOS microelectrode array system. IEEE Trans Biomed Circuits Syst 12:1356–1368
55. Miccoli B et al (2019) High-density electrical recording and impedance imaging with a multi-modal CMOS multi-electrode array chip. Front Neurosci 13:641. [Online]. Available: https://www.frontiersin.org/articles/10.3389/fnins.2019.00641/full
56. Lopez CM et al (2018) A multimodal CMOS MEA for high-throughput intracellular action potential measurements and impedance spectroscopy in drug-screening applications. IEEE J Solid State Circuits 53(11):3076–3086
57. Kandel ER, Schwartz JH, Jessell TM, Siegelbaum S, Hudspeth AJ, Mack S (2000) Principles of neural science. McGraw-hill, New York
58. Mollazadeh M, Murari K, Cauwenberghs G, Thakor N (2009) Wireless micropower instrumentation for multimodal acquisition of electrical and chemical neural activity. IEEE Trans Biomed Circuits Syst 3(6):388–397
59. Patil PG, Turner DA (2008) The development of brain-machine interface neuroprosthetic devices. Neurotherapeutics 5:137–146
60. White JR, Levy T, Bishop W, Beaty JD (2010) Real-time decision fusion for multimodal neural prosthetic devices. PLoS One 5(3):e9493
61. Roham M et al (2008) A wireless IC for wide-range neurochemical monitoring using amperometry and fast-scan cyclic voltammetry. IEEE Trans Biomed Circuits Syst 2(1):3–9
62. Murari K, Stanacevic M, Cauwenberghs G, Thakor NV (2005) Integrated potentiostat for neurotransmitter sensing. IEEE Eng Med Biol Mag 24(6):23–29
63. Johnson M, Franklin R, Scott K, Brown R, Kipke D (2006) Neural probes for concurrent detection of neurochemical and electrophysiological signals in vivo. In: 2005 IEEE engineering in medicine and biology 27th annual conference. IEEE, pp 7325–7328
64. Gosselin B (2011) Recent advances in neural recording microsystems. Sensors 11:4572–4597

65. Yuan X, Emmenegger V, Obien MEJ, Hierlemann A, Frey U (2018) Dual-mode microelectrode array featuring 20k electrodes and high SNR for extracellular recording of neural networks. In: 2018 IEEE Biomedical Circuits and Systems Conference (BioCAS). IEEE, pp 1–4
66. Huys R et al (2012) Single-cell recording and stimulation with a 16k micro-nail electrode array integrated on a 0.18 μm CMOS chip. Lab Chip 12(7):1274–1280
67. Bhatti A, Lee KH, Garmestani H, Lim CP (2017) Emerging trends in neuro engineering and neural computation. Springer
68. Bontorin G (2010) Intelligent multielectrode arrays: improving spatiotemporal performances in hybrid (living-artificial), real-time, closed-loop systems. Université Sciences et Technologies-Bordeaux I
69. Robinson DA (1968) The electrical properties of metal microelectrodes. Proc IEEE 56(6):1065–1071
70. Thomas C Jr, Springer P, Loeb G, Berwald-Netter Y, Okun L (1972) A miniature microelectrode array to monitor the bioelectric activity of cultured cells. Exp Cell Res 74(1):61–66
71. Gross GW, Rieske E, Kreutzberg G, Meyer A (1977) A new fixed-array multi-microelectrode system designed for long-term monitoring of extracellular single unit neuronal activity in vitro. Neurosci Lett 6(2–3):101–105
72. Pine J (1980) Recording action potentials from cultured neurons with extracellular microcircuit electrodes. J Neurosci Methods 2(1):19–31
73. Regehr WG, Pine J, Cohan CS, Mischke MD, Tank DW (1989) Sealing cultured invertebrate neurons to embedded dish electrodes facilitates long-term stimulation and recording. J Neurosci Methods 30(2):91–106
74. Maeda E, Robinson H, Kawana A (1995) The mechanisms of generation and propagation of synchronized bursting in developing networks of cortical neurons. J Neurosci 15(10):6834–6845
75. Oka H, Shimono K, Ogawa R, Sugihara H, Taketani M (1999) A new planar multielectrode array for extracellular recording: application to hippocampal acute slice. J Neurosci Methods 93(1):61–67
76. Müller J et al (2015) High-resolution CMOS MEA platform to study neurons at subcellular, cellular, and network levels. Lab Chip 15(13):2767–2780
77. Bigas M, Cabruja E, Forest J, Salvi J (2006) Review of CMOS image sensors. Microelectron J 37(5):433–451
78. Marblestone AH et al (2013) Physical principles for scalable neural recording. Front Comput Neurosci 7:137
79. Willemin M et al (2001) Optical characterization methods for solid-state image sensors. Opt Lasers Eng 36(2):185–194
80. Hierlemann A, Frey U, Hafizovic S, Heer F (2010) Growing cells atop microelectronic chips: interfacing electrogenic cells in vitro with CMOS-based microelectrode arrays. Proc IEEE 99(2):252–284
81. Shahrokhi F, Abdelhalim K, Serletis D, Carlen PL, Genov R (2010) The 128-channel fully differential digital integrated neural recording and stimulation interface. IEEE Trans Biomed Circuits Syst 4(3):149–161
82. Muller R, Gambini S, Rabaey JM (2011) A 0.013 mm, 5 W, DC-coupled neural signal acquisition IC with 0.5 V supply. IEEE J Solid State Circuits 47(1):232–243
83. Ogi J et al (2017) Twenty-four-micrometer-pitch microelectrode array with 6912-channel readout at 12 kHz via highly scalable implementation for high-spatial-resolution mapping of action potentials. Biointerphases 12(5):05F402
84. Angotzi GN et al (2017) A high temporal resolution multiscale recording system for in vivo neural studies. In: 2017 IEEE International Symposium on Circuits and Systems (ISCAS). IEEE, pp 1–4
85. Berdondini L, Overstolz T, De Rooij N, Koudelka-Hep M, Wany M, Seitz P (2001) High-density microelectrode arrays for electrophysiological activity imaging of neuronal networks. In: ICECS 2001. 8th IEEE international conference on electronics, circuits and systems (Cat. No. 01EX483), vol 3. IEEE, pp 1239–1242

86. Keefer EW, Botterman BR, Romero MI, Rossi AF, Gross GW (2008) Carbon nanotube coating improves neuronal recordings. Nat Nanotechnol 3(7):434–439
87. Livi P, Heer F, Frey U, Bakkum DJ, Hierlemann A (2010) Compact voltage and current stimulation buffer for high-density microelectrode arrays. IEEE Trans Biomed Circuits Syst 4(6):372–378
88. Lopez CM et al (2013) An implantable 455-active-electrode 52-channel CMOS neural probe. IEEE J Solid State Circuits 49(1):248–261
89. Lopez CM et al (2016) 22.7 A 966-electrode neural probe with 384 configurable channels in 0.13 μm SOI CMOS. In: 2016 IEEE International Solid-State Circuits Conference (ISSCC). IEEE, pp 392–393
90. Viswam V et al (2016) 22.8 Multi-functional microelectrode array system featuring 59,760 electrodes, 2048 electrophysiology channels, impedance and neurotransmitter measurement units. In: 2016 IEEE International Solid-State Circuits Conference (ISSCC). IEEE, pp 394–396
91. Bergveld P (1970) Development of an ion-sensitive solid-state device for neurophysiological measurements. IEEE Trans Biomed Eng 1:70–71
92. Kaisti M (2017) Detection principles of biological and chemical FET sensors. Biosens Bioelectron 98:437–448
93. Bausells J, Carrabina J, Errachid A, Merlos A (1999) Ion-sensitive field-effect transistors fabricated in a commercial CMOS technology. Sensors Actuators B Chem 57(1–3):56–62
94. Martinoia S, Grattarola M, Massobrio G (1992) Modelling non-ideal behaviours in H+-sensitive FETs with SPICE. Sensors Actuators B Chem 7(1–3):561–564
95. Massobrio G, Martinoia S, Grattarola M (1994) Use of SPICE for modeling silicon-based chemical sensors. Sens Mater 6:101–101
96. Massobrio G, Martinoia S (1996) Modelling the ISFET behaviour under temperature variations using BIOSPICE. Electron Lett 32(10):936–938
97. Martinoia S, Lorenzelli L, Massobrio G, Conci P, Lui A (1998) Temperature effects on the ISFET behaviour: simulations and measurements. Sensors Actuators B Chem 50(1):60–68
98. Martinoia S, Massobrio G (2000) A behavioral macromodel of the ISFET in SPICE. Sensors Actuators B Chem 62(3):182–189
99. Fernandes PG et al (2012) SPICE macromodel of silicon-on-insulator-field-effect-transistor-based biological sensors. Sensors Actuators B Chem 161(1):163–170
100. Van Hal R, Eijkel J, Bergveld P (1995) A novel description of ISFET sensitivity with the buffer capacity and double-layer capacitance as key parameters. Sensors Actuators B Chem 24(1–3):201–205
101. Sinha S (2014) Modeling and simulation of ISFET microsensor for different sensing films. In: *ISSS international conference on smart materials, Structures and Systems*
102. Yates DE, Levine S, Healy TW (1974) Site-binding model of the electrical double layer at the oxide/water interface. J Chem Soc Faraday Trans 1: Phys Chem Condensed Phases 70:1807–1818
103. Ben-Yaakov D, Andelman D, Podgornik R, Harries D (2011) Ion-specific hydration effects: extending the Poisson-Boltzmann theory. Curr Opin Colloid Interface Sci 16(6):542–550
104. Ozcelik HG, Sozen Y, Sahin H, Barisik M (2020) Parametrizing nonbonded interactions between silica and water from first principles. Appl Surf Sci 504:144359
105. Jiang G, Cheng C, Li D, Liu JZ (2016) Molecular dynamics simulations of the electric double layer capacitance of graphene electrodes in mono-valent aqueous electrolytes. Nano Res 9(1):174–186
106. Shepherd L, Toumazou C (2005) Weak inversion ISFETs for ultra-low power biochemical sensing and real-time analysis. Sensors Actuators B Chem 107(1):468–473
107. Miscourides N, Georgiou P (2016) Linear current-mode ISFET arrays. In: 2016 IEEE International Symposium on Circuits and Systems (ISCAS). IEEE, pp 2827–2830
108. Shoorideh K, Chui CO (2012) Optimization of the sensitivity of FET-based biosensors via biasing and surface charge engineering. IEEE Trans Electron Devices 59(11):3104–3110

109. Syu Y-C, Hsu W-E, Lin C-T (2018) Field-effect transistor biosensing: devices and clinical applications. ECS J Solid State Sci Technol 7(7):Q3196
110. Chen S, Bomer JG, Carlen ET, van den Berg A (2011) Al2O3/silicon nanoISFET with near ideal Nernstian response. Nano Lett 11(6):2334–2341
111. Van Der Wal P et al (2004) High-k dielectrics for use as ISFET gate oxides. In: Sensors, 2004 IEEE. IEEE, pp 677–680
112. Baldacchini C, Montanarella AF, Francioso L, Signore MA, Cannistraro S, Bizzarri AR (2020) A reliable biofet immunosensor for detection of p53 tumour suppressor in physiological-like environment. Sensors 20(21):6364
113. Pullano SA et al (2018) EGFET-based sensors for bioanalytical applications: a review. Sensors 18(11):4042
114. Knopfmacher O et al (2010) Nernst limit in dual-gated Si-nanowire FET sensors. Nano Lett 10(6):2268–2274
115. Spijkman MJ et al (2010) Dual-gate organic field-effect transistors as potentiometric sensors in aqueous solution. Adv Funct Mater 20(6):898–905
116. Khamaisi B, Vaknin O, Shaya O, Ashkenasy N (2010) Electrical performance of silicon-on-insulator field-effect transistors with multiple top-gate organic layers in electrolyte solution. ACS Nano 4(8):4601–4608
117. Duarte-Guevara C et al (2014) Enhanced biosensing resolution with foundry fabricated individually addressable dual-gated ISFETs. Anal Chem 86(16):8359–8367
118. Go J, Nair PR, Alam MA (2012) Theory of signal and noise in double-gated nanoscale electronic pH sensors. J Appl Phys 112(3)
119. Huang Y-J et al (2015) High performance dual-gate ISFET with non-ideal effect reduction schemes in a SOI-CMOS bioelectrical SoC. In: 2015 IEEE International Electron Devices Meeting (IEDM). IEEE, pp 29.2. 1–29.2. 4
120. Cui Y, Lieber CM (2001) Functional nanoscale electronic devices assembled using silicon nanowire building blocks. Science 291(5505):851–853
121. Hahm J-I, Lieber CM (2004) Direct ultrasensitive electrical detection of DNA and DNA sequence variations using nanowire nanosensors. Nano Lett 4(1):51–54
122. Zhang G-J, Chua JH, Chee R-E, Agarwal A, Wong SM (2009) Label-free direct detection of MiRNAs with silicon nanowire biosensors. Biosens Bioelectron 24(8):2504–2508
123. Agarwal A, Buddharaju K, Lao I, Singh N, Balasubramanian N, Kwong D (2008) Silicon nanowire sensor array using top–down CMOS technology. Sensors Actuators A Phys 145:207–213
124. Gao Z et al (2007) Silicon nanowire arrays for label-free detection of DNA. Anal Chem 79(9):3291–3297
125. Gao A et al (2011) Silicon-nanowire-based CMOS-compatible field-effect transistor nanosensors for ultrasensitive electrical detection of nucleic acids. Nano Lett 11(9):3974–3978
126. Zheng G, Patolsky F, Cui Y, Wang WU, Lieber CM (2005) Multiplexed electrical detection of cancer markers with nanowire sensor arrays. Nat Biotechnol 23(10):1294–1301
127. Mishra NN et al (2008) Ultra-sensitive detection of bacterial toxin with silicon nanowire transistor. Lab Chip 8(6):868–871
128. Chua JH, Chee R-E, Agarwal A, Wong SM, Zhang G-J (2009) Label-free electrical detection of cardiac biomarker with complementary metal-oxide semiconductor-compatible silicon nanowire sensor arrays. Anal Chem 81(15):6266–6271
129. Hakim MM et al (2012) Thin film polycrystalline silicon nanowire biosensors. Nano Lett 12(4):1868–1872
130. Patolsky F, Zheng G, Hayden O, Lakadamyali M, Zhuang X, Lieber CM (2004) Electrical detection of single viruses. Proc Natl Acad Sci 101(39):14017–14022
131. Elibol O, Morisette D, Akin D, Denton J, Bashir R (2003) Integrated nanoscale silicon sensors using top-down fabrication. Appl Phys Lett 83(22):4613–4615
132. Torsi L, Magliulo M, Manoli K, Palazzo G (2013) Organic field-effect transistor sensors: a tutorial review. Chem Soc Rev 42(22):8612–8628

133. Yang SY et al (2010) Electrochemical transistors with ionic liquids for enzymatic sensing. Chem Commun 46(42):7972–7974
134. Lai S, Demelas M, Casula G, Cosseddu P, Barbaro M, Bonfiglio A (2012) Ultralow voltage, OTFT-based sensor for label-free DNA detection. Adv Mater 25(1):103–107
135. Mulla MY et al (2015) Capacitance-modulated transistor detects odorant binding protein chiral interactions. Nat Commun 6(1):6010
136. Magliulo M et al (2016) Label-free C-reactive protein electronic detection with an electrolyte-gated organic field-effect transistor-based immunosensor. Anal Bioanal Chem 408:3943–3952
137. Novoselov KS et al (2004) Electric field effect in atomically thin carbon films. Science 306(5696):666–669
138. Wang Z, Jia Y (2018) Graphene solution-gated field effect transistor DNA sensor fabricated by liquid exfoliation and double glutaraldehyde cross-linking. Carbon 130:758–767
139. Zheng C, Huang L, Zhang H, Sun Z, Zhang Z, Zhang G-J (2015) Fabrication of ultrasensitive field-effect transistor DNA biosensors by a directional transfer technique based on CVD-grown graphene. ACS Appl Mater Interfaces 7(31):16953–16959
140. Gao A, Lu N, Wang Y, Li T (2016) Robust ultrasensitive tunneling-FET biosensor for point-of-care diagnostics. Sci Rep 6(1):22554
141. Sarangadharan I et al (2018) High sensitivity cardiac troponin I detection in physiological environment using AlGaN/GaN high electron mobility transistor (HEMT) biosensors. Biosens Bioelectron 100:282–289
142. Borisov SM, Wolfbeis OS (2008) Optical biosensors. Chem Rev 108(2):423–461
143. Li H, Han Y, Zhao H, Jafri H, Tian B (2021) Dyes as labels in biosensing. In: *Dyes and pigments-novel applications and waste treatment*. IntechOpen
144. De Vos K (2010) Label-free silicon photonics biosensor platform withmicroring resonators. Ghent University
145. Hong L, McManus S, Yang H, Sengupta K (2015) A fully integrated CMOS fluorescence biosensor with on-chip nanophotonic filter. In: 2015 Symposium on VLSI Circuits (VLSI Circuits). IEEE, pp C206–C207
146. Jang B, Cao P, Chevalier A, Ellington A, Hassibi A (2009) A CMOS fluorescent-based biosensor microarray. In: 2009 IEEE international solid-state circuits conference-digest of technical papers. IEEE, pp 436–437
147. Khiarak MN, Martel S, De Koninck Y, Gosselin B (2019) High-DR CMOS fluorescence biosensor with extended counting ADC and noise cancellation. IEEE Trans Circuits Syst I: Regular Papers 66(6):2077–2087
148. Manickam A et al (2017) A fully integrated CMOS fluorescence biochip for DNA and RNA testing. IEEE J Solid State Circuits 52(11):2857–2870
149. Steglich P, Bondarenko S, Mai C, Paul M, Weller MG, Mai A (2020) CMOS-compatible silicon photonic sensor for refractive index sensing using local back-side release. IEEE Photon Technol Lett 32(19):1241–1244
150. Strianese M, Staiano M, Ruggiero G, Labella T, Pellecchia C, D'Auria S (2012) Fluorescence-based biosensors. In: Spectroscopic methods of analysis: methods and protocols, pp 193–216
151. Zhu C, Hong L, Yang H, Sengupta K (2022) A packaged multiplexed fluorescent biomolecular sensor array and ultralow-power wireless interface in CMOS for ingestible electronic applications. IEEE Sensors J 22(24):24060–24074
152. Zhu C, Wen Y, Liu T, Yang H, Sengupta K (2023) An ingestible pill with CMOS fluorescence sensor Array, bi-directional wireless Interface and packaged optics for in-vivo bio-molecular sensing. IEEE Trans Biomed Circuits Syst
153. Simpson ML et al (2001) An integrated CMOS microluminometer for low-level luminescence sensing in the bioluminescent bioreporter integrated circuit. Sensors Actuators B Chem 72(2):134–140
154. Eltoukhy H, Salama K, Gamal AE (2006) A 0.18 um CMOS bioluminescence detection lab-on-chip. IEEE J Solid State Circuits 41(3):651–662

155. Liu Q et al (2022) A threshold-based bioluminescence detector with a CMOS-integrated photodiode Array in 65 nm for a multi-diagnostic ingestible capsule. IEEE J Solid State Circuits
156. Chang Y-W, Yu P-C, Huang Y-T, Yang Y-S (2007) A CMOS-compatible optical biosensing system based on visible absorption spectroscopy. In: 2007 IEEE conference on electron devices and solid-state circuits. IEEE, pp 1099–1102
157. Chang Y-W, Yu P-C, Huang Y-T, Yang Y-S (2009) A high-sensitivity CMOS-compatible biosensing system based on absorption photometry. IEEE Sensors J 9(2):120–127
158. Hofmann A, Meister M, Rolapp A, Reich P, Scholz F, Schäfer E (2021) Light absorption measurement with a CMOS biochip for quantitative immunoassay based point-of-care applications. IEEE Trans Biomed Circuits Syst 15(3):369–379
159. Yan R, Mestas SP, Yuan G, Safaisini R, Dandy DS, Lear KL (2009) Label-free silicon photonic biosensor system with integrated detector array. Lab Chip 9(15):2163–2168
160. K. De Vos, "Label-free silicon photonics biosensor platform with microring resonators," 2010
161. Luan E, Shoman H, Ratner DM, Cheung KC, Chrostowski L (2018) Silicon photonic biosensors using label-free detection. Sensors 18(10):3519
162. Adamopoulos C et al (2021) Lab-on-Chip for everyone: introducing an electronic-photonic platform for multiparametric biosensing using standard CMOS processes. IEEE Open J Solid-State Circuits Soc 1:198–208
163. Mai A, Mai C, Steglich P (2022) From lab-on-chip to lab-in-app: challenges towards silicon photonic biosensors product developments. Results Opt 9:100317
164. Ning S et al (2023) Silicon photonic chip-based biosensor for COVID-19 and flu detection with high sensitivity and specificity. In: Ultra-high-definition imaging systems VI, vol 12444. SPIE, pp 26–28
165. Sajan SC, Singh A, Sharma PK, Kumar S (2023) Silicon photonics biosensors for cancer cells detection-a review. IEEE Sensors J
166. Suarasan S et al (2020) Superhydrophobic bowl-like SERS substrates patterned from CMOS sensors for extracellular vesicle characterization. J Mater Chem B 8(38):8845–8852
167. Ehrlich K et al (2017) pH sensing through a single optical fibre using SERS and CMOS SPAD line arrays. Opt Express 25(25):30976–30986
168. Wang L, Wang G, Yang K, Liu W (2023) Plasmonic biosensor with annular aperture array integrated on a resonant cavity LED. Opt Commun 535:129336
169. Singh AK, Anwar M, Pradhan R, Ashar MS, Rai N, Dey S (2023) Surface Plasmon resonance based-optical biosensor: emerging diagnostic tool for early detection of diseases. J Biophotonics:e202200380
170. Shakoor A et al (2016) Plasmonic sensor monolithically integrated with a CMOS photodiode. ACS Photonics 3:1926–1933
171. Salazar A, Camacho-Leon S, Martínez-Chapa SO, Rossetto O (2013) Towards a SPR-based biosensing platform incorporating a CMOS active column sensor. Analog Integr Circ Sig Process 77:365–372
172. Koppa S, Joo Y (2013) Compact, low cost CMOS integrated SPR biosensor system. In: SENSORS, 2013 IEEE. IEEE, pp 1–4
173. J. R. Lakowicz, "Principles of fluorescence spectroscopy," 2006
174. Hwang R-B (2021) A theoretical design of evanescent wave biosensors based on gate-controlled graphene surface plasmon resonance. Sci Rep 11:1–10
175. Wang J, Sanchez MM, Yin Y, Herzer R, Ma L, Schmidt OG (2020) Silicon-based integrated label-free optofluidic biosensors: latest advances and roadmap. Adv Mater Technol 5:1901138
176. Huertas CS, Calvo-Lozano O, Mitchell A, Lechuga LM (2019) Advanced evanescent-wave optical biosensors for the detection of nucleic acids: an analytic perspective. Front Chem:724
177. Xiao-Hong Z et al (2014) A reusable evanescent wave immunosensor for highly sensitive detection of bisphenol a in water samples. Sci Rep 4:1–7
178. Wangüemert-Pérez JG et al (2014) Evanescent field waveguide sensing with subwavelength grating structures in silicon-on-insulator. Opt Lett 39:4442–4445
179. Taitt CR, Anderson GP, Ligler FS (2005) Evanescent wave fluorescence biosensors. Biosens Bioelectron 20:2470–2487

180. Hutchinson AM (1995) Evanescent wave biosensors. Mol Biotechnol 3:47–54
181. C. Adamopoulos and V. Stojanovic, "A fully integrated electronic-photonic platform for label-free biosensing," 2020
182. Gowri A, Kumar NA, Anand BS (2021) Recent advances in nanomaterials based biosensors for point of care (PoC) diagnosis of COVID-19–a minireview. TrAC Trends Anal Chem 137:116205
183. Strianese M, Staiano M, Ruggiero G, Labella T, Pellecchia C, D'Auria S (2012) Fluorescence-based biosensors. In: Spectroscopic methods of analysis. Springer, pp 193–216
184. M. C. Morris, "Fluorescence-based biosensors: from concepts to applications," 2012
185. Mader H, Li X, Saleh S, Link M, Kele P, Wolfbeis O (2008) Fluorescence methods and applications: spectroscopy, imaging, and probes. Ann N Y Acad Sci 1130:218
186. Hassibi A et al (2018) Multiplexed identification, quantification and genotyping of infectious agents using a semiconductor biochip. Nat Biotechnol 36:738–745
187. Manickam A et al (2017) A fully integrated CMOS fluorescence biochip for DNA and RNA testing. IEEE J Solid State Circuits 52:2857–2870
188. Singh RR, Ho D, Nilchi A, Gulak G, Yau P, Genov R (2010) A CMOS/thin-film fluorescence contact imaging microsystem for DNA analysis. IEEE Trans Circuits Syst I: Regular Papers 57:1029–1038
189. Jang B, Cao P, Chevalier A, Ellington A, Hassibi A. A CMOS fluorescent-based biosensor microarray
190. Hong L, McManus S, Yang H, Sengupta K. A fully integrated CMOS fluorescence biosensor with on-chip nanophotonic filter
191. Hong L, Li H, Yang H, Sengupta K (2017) Fully integrated fluorescence biosensors on-chip employing multi-functional nanoplasmonic optical structures in CMOS. IEEE J Solid State Circuits 52:2388–2406
192. Barnes WL, Dereux A, Ebbesen TW (2003) Surface plasmon subwavelength optics. Nature 424(6950):824–830
193. Jiang Y et al (2018) A nano-filter-integrated CMOS image sensor for fluorescent biomedical imaging. In: 2018 IEEE Biomedical Circuits and Systems Conference (BioCAS). IEEE, pp 1–4
194. Tang S, Saeedkia D (2016) Advances in imaging and sensing. CRC Press
195. DeHennis A, Getzlaff S, Grice D, Mailand M (2015) An NFC-enabled CMOS IC for a wireless fully implantable glucose sensor. IEEE Journal of Biomedical and Health Informatics 20:18–28
196. Tyndall D, Rae B, Li D, Richardson J, Arlt J, Henderson R (2012) A 100Mphoton/s time-resolved mini-silicon photomultiplier with on-chip fluorescence lifetime estimation in 0.13 μm CMOS imaging technology. IEEE
197. Ta-chien DH et al (2011) Gene expression analysis with an integrated CMOS microarray by time-resolved fluorescence detection. Biosens Bioelectron 26:2660–2665
198. Yoon H-J, Itoh S, Kawahito S (2009) A CMOS image sensor with in-pixel two-stage charge transfer for fluorescence lifetime imaging. IEEE Transactions on Electron Devices 56:214–221
199. Ta-chien DH, Sorgenfrei S, Gong P, Levicky R, Shepard KL (2009) A 0.18-$\mu $ m CMOS array sensor for integrated time-resolved fluorescence detection. IEEE J Solid State Circuits 44:1644–1654
200. Stoppa D, Mosconi D, Pancheri L, Gonzo L (2009) Single-photon avalanche diode CMOS sensor for time-resolved fluorescence measurements. IEEE Sensors J 9:1084–1090
201. Patounakis G, Shepard KL, Levicky R (2006) Active CMOS array sensor for time-resolved fluorescence detection. IEEE J Solid State Circuits 41:2521–2530
202. Zhang L, Niknejad AM (2019) Design and analysis of a microwave-optical dual modality biomolecular sensing platform. IEEE J Solid State Circuits 55:639–649
203. Khiarak MN et al (2018) A 17-bit 104-dB-DR high-precision low-power CMOS fluorescence biosensor with extended counting ADC and noise cancellation. In: 2018 16th IEEE International New Circuits and Systems Conference (NEWCAS). IEEE, pp 100–103

204. Gradišnik V, Gumbarević D (2018) a-Si: H pin Photodiode as a Biosensor. In: Advances in Photodetectors-Research and Applications. IntechOpen
205. Titus AH, Cheung MC, Chodavarapu VP (2011) CMOS photodetectors. Photodiodes-world activities in 2011. IntechOpen
206. Ghione G (2009) Semiconductor devices for high-speed optoelectronics
207. Mosconi D, Stoppa D, Pancheri L, Gonzo L, Simoni A (2006) CMOS single-photon avalanche diode array for time-resolved fluorescence detection. In: 2006 Proceedings of the 32nd European solid-state circuits conference. IEEE, pp 564–567
208. Baselt DR, Lee GU, Natesan M, Metzger SW, Sheehan PE, Colton RJ (1998) A biosensor based on magnetoresistance technology. Biosens Bioelectron 13(7–8):731–739
209. Morrish AH (2001) The physical principles of magnetism
210. Ida N (2015) Engineering electromagnetics
211. Wohlfarth EP, Buschow KHJ (1989) Ferromagnetic Mater 4
212. Wolf WP (1961) Ferrimagnetism. Rep Prog Phys 24:212
213. Marshall W (1955) Antiferromagnetism. Proc R Soc Lond Series A Math Phys Sci 232(1188):48–68
214. Akbarzadeh A, Samiei M, Davaran S (2012) Magnetic nanoparticles: preparation, physical properties, and applications in biomedicine. Nanoscale Res Lett 7:1–13
215. Issadore D et al (2014) Magnetic sensing technology for molecular analyses. Lab Chip 14:2385–2397
216. Lee H, Yoon T-J, Figueiredo J-L, Swirski FK, Weissleder R (2009) Rapid detection and profiling of cancer cells in fine-needle aspirates. Proc Natl Acad Sci 106(30):12459–12464
217. Lee H, Yoon TJ, Weissleder R (2009) Ultrasensitive detection of bacteria using Core–Shell nanoparticles and an NMR-Filter system. Angew Chem 121(31):5767–5770
218. Liong M, Tassa C, Shaw SY, Lee H, Weissleder R (2011) Multiplexed magnetic labeling amplification using oligonucleotide hybridization. Adv Mater 23:H254–H257
219. Peterson VM, Castro CM, Lee H, Weissleder R (2012) Orthogonal amplification of nanoparticles for improved diagnostic sensing. ACS Nano 6:3506–3513
220. Hall EH (1879) On a new action of the magnet on electric currents. Am J Math 2(3):287–292
221. Skucha K, Liu P, Megens M, Kim J, Boser B (2011) A compact Hall-effect sensor array for the detection and imaging of single magnetic beads in biomedical assays. In: 2011 16th international solid-state sensors, actuators and microsystems conference. IEEE, pp 1833–1836
222. Sze SM (2008) Semiconductor devices: physics and technology. Wiley
223. Mosser V, Matringe N, Haddab Y (2017) A spinning current circuit for Hall measurements down to the nanotesla range. IEEE Trans Instrum Meas 66(4):637–650
224. Crescentini M, Marchesi M, Romani A, Tartagni M, Traverso PA (2018) A broadband, on-chip sensor based on Hall effect for current measurements in smart power circuits. IEEE Trans Instrum Meas 67(6):1470–1485
225. Crescentini M et al (2020) Experimental assessment of a broadband current sensor based on the X-Hall architecture. In: 2020 IEEE International Instrumentation and Measurement Technology Conference (I2MTC). IEEE, pp 1–6
226. Crescentini M et al (2020) The X-Hall sensor: toward integrated broadband current sensing. IEEE Trans Instrum Meas 70:1–12
227. Syeda SF, Crescentini M, Marchesi M, Traverso PA, Romani A (2023) A wideband and low-noise CMOS-integrated X-Hall current sensor operating in current mode. IEEE Trans Instrum Meas
228. Crescentini M, Syeda SF, Gibiino GP (2021) Hall-effect current sensors: principles of operation and implementation techniques. IEEE Sensors J 22(11):10137–10151
229. Liu PP et al (2012) Magnetic relaxation detector for microbead labels. IEEE J Solid State Circuits 47(4):1056–1064
230. Popovic RS (2003) Hall effect devices. CRC Press

231. Gambini S, Skucha K, Liu PP, Kim J, Krigel R (2012) A 10 kPixel CMOS hall sensor array with baseline suppression and parallel readout for immunoassays. IEEE J Solid State Circuits 48(1):302–317
232. Skucha K, Gambini S, Liu P, Megens M, Kim J, Boser B (2013) Design considerations for CMOS-integrated Hall-effect magnetic bead detectors for biosensor applications. J Microelectromech Syst 22(6):1327–1338
233. Fan H, Yue H, Bonizzoni E, Feng Q, Wei Q (2023) Modelling of three-axis hall effect sensor based on CMOS process. IEEE Sensors J
234. Zou H, Lei K-M, Martins RP, Mak P-I (2023) A CMOS hall sensors array with integrated readout circuit resilient to local magnetic interference from current-carrying traces. IEEE Sensors J
235. Xu Y, Wang B, Hu X, Jiang L (2022) A CMOS front-end Hall sensor microsystem for linear magnetic field measurement with best tradeoff between sensitivity and SNR. IEEE Trans Instrum Meas 71:1–8
236. Liu PP et al (2012) Magnetic relaxation detector for microbead labels. IEEE J Solid State Circuits 47:1056–1064
237. Ausserlechner U (2023) Comments on "a CMOS front-end hall sensor microsystem for linear magnetic field measurement with best tradeoff between sensitivity and SNR". IEEE Trans Instrum Meas 72:1–3
238. Heidari H, Gatti U, Maloberti F (2015) Sensitivity characteristics of horizontal and vertical Hall sensors in the voltage-and current-mode. In: 2015 11th Conference on Ph. D. Research in Microelectronics and Electronics (PRIME). IEEE, pp 330–333
239. Liu P (2012) A CMOS magnetic sensor chip for biomedical applications
240. Skucha K, Gambini S, Liu P, Megens M, Kim J, Boser BE (2013) Design considerations for CMOS-integrated Hall-effect magnetic bead detectors for biosensor applications. J Microelectromech Syst 22:1327–1338
241. Wang H, Chen Y, Hassibi A, Scherer A, Hajimiri A (2009) A frequency-shift CMOS magnetic biosensor array with single-bead sensitivity and no external magnet. IEEE
242. Fullerton EE, Schuller IK (2007) The 2007 Nobel prize in physics: magnetism and transport at the nanoscale. ACS Nano 1:384–389
243. Hardman U (1996) Magnetic thin film and multilayer systems: physics, analysis and industrial applications, Series in material science. Springer
244. Zhou X (2020) Magnetoresistive biosensor circuits and systems for ultrasensitive point-of-care diagnostics
245. Cubells-Beltrán M-D et al (2014) Monolithic integration of Giant magnetoresistance (GMR) devices onto standard processed CMOS dies. Microelectron J 45:702–707
246. Adem S, Jain S, Sveiven M, Zhou X, O'Donoghue AJ, Hall DA (2020) Giant magnetoresistive biosensors for real-time quantitative detection of protease activity. Sci Rep 10:1–10
247. De Boer BM, Kahlman J, Jansen T, Duric H, Veen J (2007) An integrated and sensitive detection platform for magneto-resistive biosensors. Biosens Bioelectron 22:2366–2370
248. Hall DA et al (2010) GMR biosensor arrays: a system perspective. Biosens Bioelectron 25:2051–2057
249. Hall DA, Gaster RS, Makinwa KAA, Wang SX, Murmann B (2013) A 256 pixel magnetoresistive biosensor microarray in 0.18 μm CMOS. IEEE J Solid State Circuits 48:1290–1301
250. Hall DA, Gaster RS, Osterfeld SJ, Makinwa K, Wang SX, Murmann B (2011) A 256 channel magnetoresistive biosensor microarray for quantitative proteomics. IEEE
251. Hall DA, Gaster RS, Osterfeld SJ, Murmann B, Wang SX (2010) GMR biosensor arrays: correction techniques for reproducibility and enhanced sensitivity. Biosens Bioelectron 25:2177–2181
252. Zhou X, Huang C-C, Hall DA (2017) Giant magnetoresistive biosensor array for detecting magnetorelaxation. IEEE Trans Biomed Circuits Syst 11:755–764
253. Zhou X et al (2021) A 9.7-nTrms, 704-ms magnetic biosensor front-end for detecting magneto-relaxation. IEEE J Solid State Circuits 56:2171–2181

254. Zhou X, Sveiven M, Hall DA (2019) 11.4 a fast-readout mismatch-insensitive magnetoresistive biosensor front-end achieving sub-ppm sensitivity. IEEE
255. Rabi II, Zacharias JR, Millman S, Kusch P (1938) A new method of measuring nuclear magnetic moment. Phys Rev 53(4):318
256. Sun N, Liu Y, Lee H, Weissleder R, Ham D (2009) CMOS RF biosensor utilizing nuclear magnetic resonance. IEEE J Solid State Circuits 44(5):1629–1643
257. Krummenacher P, Oguey H (1990) Smart temperature sensor in CMOS technology. Sensors Actuators A Phys 22(1–3):636–638
258. Bianchi R, Dos Santos FV, Karam J, Courtois B, Pressecq F, Sifflet S (1998) CMOS compatible temperature sensor based on the lateral bipolar transistor for very wide temperature range applications. Sensors Actuators A Phys 71(1–2):3–9
259. Bianchi R, Karam J, Courtois B, Nadal R, Pressecq F, Sifflet S (2000) CMOS-compatible temperature sensor with digital output for wide temperature range applications. Microelectron J 31(9–10):803–810
260. Bakker A, Huijsing JH (1996) Micropower CMOS temperature sensor with digital output. IEEE J Solid State Circuits 31(7):933–937
261. Meijer GC (1996) Concepts for bandgap references and voltage measurement systems. In: Analog circuit design: low-noise, low-power, low-voltage; mixed-mode design with CAD tools; voltage, current and time references, pp 243–268
262. Fruett F, Wang G, Meijer GC (2000) The piezojunction effect in NPN and PNP vertical transistors and its influence on silicon temperature sensors. Sensors Actuators A Phys 85(1–3):70–74
263. Meijer GC, Wang G, Fruett F (2001) Temperature sensors and voltage references implemented in CMOS technology. IEEE Sensors J 1(3):225–234
264. Pertijs MA, Meijer GC, Huijsing JH (2004) Precision temperature measurement using CMOS substrate PNP transistors. IEEE Sensors J 4(3):294–300
265. Aita AL, Makinwa KA (2007) Low-power operation of a precision CMOS temperature sensor based on substrate PNPs. In: SENSORS, 2007 IEEE. IEEE, pp 856–859
266. Pertijs MA, Huijsing J (2006) Precision temperature sensors in CMOS technology. Springer Science & Business Media
267. Meijer GC (1986) Thermal sensors based on transistors. Sensors Actuators 10(1–2):103–125
268. Zhao W, Pan R, Ha Y, Yang Z (2014) A 0.4 V 280-nW frequency reference-less nearly all-digital hybrid domain temperature sensor. In: 2014 IEEE Asian Solid-State Circuits Conference (A-SSCC). IEEE, pp 301–304
269. Azcona C, Calvo B, Medrano N, Celma S (2015) 1.2 V–0.18μm CMOS temperature sensors with quasi-digital output for portable systems. IEEE Trans Instrum Meas 64(9):2565–2573
270. Bashir M, Sreehari Rao P (2019) A low power, miniature temperature sensor with one-point calibrated accuracy of±0.25 C from− 55 to 125 C in 65 nm CMOS process. Analog Integr Circ Sig Process 99(2):311–323
271. Someya T, Islam AM, Sakurai T, Takamiya M (2019) An 11-nW CMOS temperature-to-digital converter utilizing sub-threshold current at sub-thermal drain voltage. IEEE J Solid State Circuits 54(3):613–622
272. Krishna R, Mal AK, Mahapatra R (2020) Time-domain smart temperature sensor using current starved inverters and switched ring oscillator-based time-to-digital converter. Circuits, Syst Signal Process 39(4):1751–1769
273. Moisello E, Ippolito CM, Bruno G, Malcovati P, Bonizzoni E (2023) A MOS-based temperature sensor with inherent inaccuracy reduction enabled by time-domain operation. IEEE Trans Instrum Meas
274. Wang A, Calhoun BH, Chandrakasan AP (2006) Sub-threshold design for ultra low-power systems. Springer
275. Touloukian Y, Powell R, Ho C, Nicolaou M (1974) Thermophysical properties of matter-the TPRC data series. Volume 10. Thermal diffusivity. DTIC Document

276. Makinwa KA, Snoeij MF (2006) A CMOS temperature-to-frequency converter with an inaccuracy of less than ±0.5°C from (3σ) from −40°C to 105°C. IEEE J Solid State Circuits 41(12):2992–2997
277. Kashmiri S, Makinwa K (2009) Measuring the thermal diffusivity of CMOS chips. In: SENSORS, 2009 IEEE. IEEE, pp 45–48
278. Makinwa KA, Snoeij MF (2006) A CMOS temperature-to-frequency converter with an inaccuracy of less than ±0.5°C (3σ) from −40°C to 105°C. IEEE J Solid State Circuits 41(12):2992–2997
279. van Vroonhoven CP, Makinwa KA (2008) A CMOS Temperature-to-Digital Converter with an Inaccuracy of±0.5°C (3σ) from-55 to 125°C. In: 2008 IEEE international solid-state circuits conference-digest of technical papers. IEEE, pp 576–637
280. Pan S, Makinwa KA (2018) Energy-efficient high-resolution resistor-based temperature sensors. In: Hybrid ADCs, smart sensors for the IoT, and sub-1V & advanced node analog circuit design: Advances in analog circuit design 2017, pp 183–200
281. Pan S, Jiang H, Makinwa KA (2017) A CMOS temperature sensor with a 49fJK 2 resolution FoM. In: *2017 Symposium on VLSI Circuits*. IEEE, pp C82–C83
282. Pan S, Makinwa KA (2018) A 0.25 mm 2-resistor-based temperature sensor with an inaccuracy of 0.12° C (3 σ) from– 55° C to 125° C. IEEE J Solid State Circuits 53(12):3347–3355
283. Park H, Kim J (2018) A 0.8-V resistor-based temperature sensor in 65-nm CMOS with supply sensitivity of 0.28 C/V. IEEE J Solid State Circuits 53(3):906–912
284. Xin H, Andraud M, Baltus P, Cantatore E, Harpe P (2018) A 174 pW–488.3 nW 1 S/s–100 kS/s all-dynamic resistive temperature sensor with speed/resolution/resistance adaptability. IEEE Solid-State Circuits Letters 1(3):70–73
285. Pan S, Makinwa KA (2019) 10.4 A Wheatstone Bridge Temperature Sensor with a Resolution FoM of 20fJ. K 2. In: 2019 IEEE International Solid-State Circuits Conference-(ISSCC). IEEE, pp 186–188
286. Jiang H, Huang C-C, Chan MR, Hall DA (2020) A 2-in-1 temperature and humidity sensor with a single FLL wheatstone-bridge front-end. IEEE J Solid State Circuits 55(8):2174–2185
287. Pan S, Makinwa KA (2020) A 10 fJ·K 2 Wheatstone bridge temperature sensor with a tail-resistor-linearized OTA. IEEE J Solid State Circuits 56(2):501–510
288. Pan S, Makinwa KA (2020) A 6.6-μW wheatstone-bridge temperature sensor for biomedical applications. IEEE Solid-State Circuits Letters 3:334–337
289. Shahmohammadi M, Souri K, Makinwa KA (2013) A resistor-based temperature sensor for MEMS frequency references. In: 2013 Proceedings of the ESSCIRC (ESSCIRC). IEEE, pp 225–228
290. Park P, Ruffieux D, Makinwa KA (2015) A thermistor-based temperature sensor for a real-time clock with ± 2 ppm frequency stability. IEEE J Solid State Circuits 50(7):1571–1580
291. Weng C-H, Wu C-K, Lin T-H (2015) A CMOS thermistor-embedded continuous-time delta-sigma temperature sensor with a resolution FoM of 0.65 pJ °C^2. IEEE J Solid State Circuits 50(11):2491–2500
292. Pan S, Luo Y, Shalmany SH, Makinwa KA (2017) A resistor-based temperature sensor with a 0.13 pJ·K2 resolution FoM. IEEE J Solid State Circuits 53(1):164–173
293. Angevare J, Makinwa KA (2018) A 6800-μm 2 resistor-based temperature sensor in 180-nm CMOS. In: 2018 IEEE Asian Solid-State Circuits Conference (A-SSCC). IEEE, pp 43–46
294. Pan S, Gürleyük Ç, Pimenta MF, Makinwa KA (2019) 10.3 A 0.12 mm 2 Wien-bridge temperature sensor with 0.1° C (3σ) inaccuracy from −40° C to 180° C. In: 2019 IEEE International Solid-State Circuits Conference-(ISSCC). IEEE, pp 184–186
295. Choi W et al (2018) A compact resistor-based CMOS temperature sensor with an inaccuracy of 0.12° C (3σ) and a resolution FoM of 0.43 pJ·K 2 in 65-nm CMOS. IEEE J Solid State Circuits 53(12):3356–3367
296. Lee Y, Choi W, Kim T, Song S, Makinwa KA, Chae Y (2019) A 5800-μm 2 resistor-based temperature sensor with a one-point trimmed inaccuracy of±1.2 C (3σ) from– 50 C to 105 C

in 65-nm CMOS. In: ESSCIRC 2019-IEEE 45th European Solid State Circuits Conference (ESSCIRC). IEEE, pp 68–71
297. Khashaba A, Zhu J, Elmallah A, Ahmed M, Hanumolu PK (2020) 3.2 A 0.0088 mm 2 Resistor-Based Temperature Sensor Achieving 92fJ·K 2 FoM in 65nm CMOS. In: 2020 IEEE International Solid-State Circuits Conference-(ISSCC). IEEE, pp 60–62
298. Angevare JA, Chae Y, Makinwa KA (2021) 5.3 a highly digital 2210μm 2 resistor-based temperature sensor with a 1-point trimmed inaccuracy of±1.3° C (3 σ) from-55° C to 125° C in 65nm CMOS. In: 2021 IEEE International Solid-State Circuits Conference (ISSCC), vol 64. IEEE, pp 76–78
299. Lee Y, Kim T, Chae Y (2023) A 0.9 V 6,400-μm2 resistor-based temperature sensor with a one-point trimmed 3σ inaccuracy of 10.64° C from. 50 to 125° C. IEEE Trans Circuits Syst II: Express Briefs
300. Pan S, Makinwa KA (2022) Resistor-based temperature sensors in CMOS technology. Springer
301. Sze SM (1994) Semicondutor sensors. In: *Semicondutor sensors*, pp 550–550
302. Middelhoek S et al (1995) Silicon sensors. Meas Sci Technol 6(12):1641
303. Akin T (2005) CMOS-based thermal sensors. CMOS—MEMS, pp 479–512
304. Van Herwaarden A, Sarro P (1986) Thermal sensors based on the Seebeck effect. Sensors Actuators 10(3–4):321–346
305. Hierlemann A, Baltes H (2003) CMOS-based chemical microsensors. Analyst 128(1):15–28
306. Moisello E, Vaiana M, Castagna ME, Bruno G, Bonizzoni E, Malcovati P (2019) A chopper interface circuit for thermopile-based thermal sensors. In: 2019 IEEE International Symposium on Circuits and Systems (ISCAS). IEEE, pp 1–5

Chapter 4
Interface Circuits

This chapter provides an in-depth exploration of the interface circuits designed for a variety of CMOS biosensors including voltammetric, impedimetric, capacitive, field-effect transistor (FET)-based, optical, magnetic, nuclear magnetic resonance (NMR), and temperature sensors as well as neural stimulation/recording systems. Each section of the chapter is designed to provide a comprehensive understanding of the circuits that drive these various CMOS biosensors, illustrating their significance in modern biochemical technologies.

4.1 CMOS Interface Circuits for Voltammetric and Impedimetric Sensing

As discussed earlier, voltammetric and impedimetric sensors function by utilizing electron transfer, producing either current or voltage output via electrochemical cell reactions. Simple basic electrochemical cells can be configured with two [1–7] or three [8, 9] electrodes. In a two-electrode setup, consisting of a working electrode (WE) and a reference electrode (RE), maintaining a constant reference voltage during current flow is challenging, prompting the preference for a three-electrode configuration with an additional counter electrode (CE) to address this issue and enhance measurement accuracy. As seen in Fig. 4.1, the electrochemical instrumentation for these electron transfer-based sensors comprises (1) a signal generator, (2) a potentiostat, (3) a readout circuit, and (4) a communication block. The signal generator shapes stimulus signals, and designing a low-noise signal generator is essential for high-resolution applications. The potentiostat controls the cell and acquires current. The readout circuit amplifies and processes sensor responses. Finally, the signal processing and communication block is responsible for transmitting the output signal to external devices or systems for further analysis or display.

E. Ghafar-Zadeh et al., *Advanced CMOS Biochips*, Analog Circuits and Signal Processing, https://doi.org/10.1007/978-94-007-0099-4_4

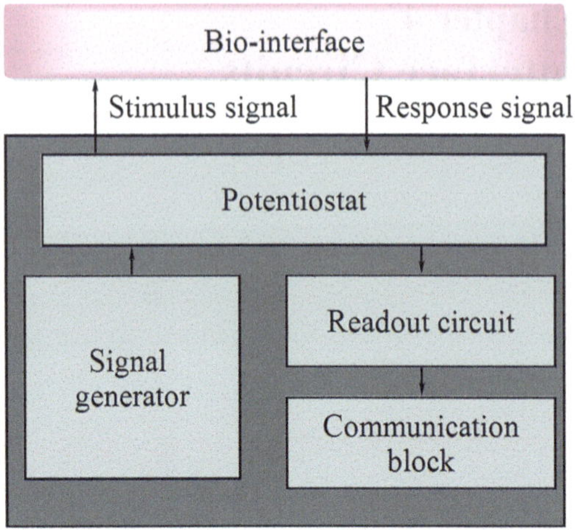

Fig. 4.1 Block diagram of an electron transfer-based sensor comprising a signal generator, a potentiostat, a readout circuit, and a communication block

The excitation signals of voltammetric and impedimetric sensors can be externally generated or integrated into the sensor's components. For example, Ghoreishizadeh et al. [10] developed a direct digital synthesizer (DDS) for generating sub-Hertz triangular waveforms, while Li et al. [11] designed a digital-controlled, programmable multi-mode voltage waveform generator to support various voltammetric techniques. For electrochemical impedance spectroscopy (EIS), precise sinusoidal signals with low noise and stability are necessary, achievable through frequency synthesizers. Crystal oscillators offer higher precision compared to nonlinear oscillators, with techniques like DDS and phase-locked loop (PLL) commonly used for signal generation in EIS applications [12].

Potentiostats facilitate connections to the electrode-electrolyte interface and the circuits designed for measuring direct currents (DC currents) and alternating currents (AC currents), essential for voltammetric and impedimetric measurements, respectively. After acquiring and processing the signal using the potentiostat and readout circuit, the transmission of processed sensor data to external devices or systems for analysis, storage, or display can be facilitated through various interfaces, including wired or wireless connections. Depending on the specific application and system setup, these connections may utilize serial communication protocols like UART, SPI, or I2C, as well as Ethernet, Wi-Fi, or Bluetooth. The implementation of this communication block may vary, with options for on-chip or off-chip integration, tailored to the requirements of applications such as handheld, wearable, or implantable devices, and the desired signal-to-noise ratios (SNRs).

This section will cover CMOS potentiostats, and readout circuits for voltammetric and impedimetric sensors.

4.1.1 Potentiostats

A potentiostat, an electronic device essential for managing the electrochemical cell's potential and acquiring current, is particularly vital in setups employing constant voltage amperometry, impedance spectroscopy, and cyclic voltammetry (CV) within a three-electrode configuration.

Three-electrode setups provide three configurations [13]: a WE-grounded setup, widely used; a RE-grounded setup, primarily found in multi-electrode arrangements [10]; and a CE-grounded setup, less common but potentially advantageous for reducing external electromagnetic interference [14]. Usually, the output current is measured through either the WE or CE. In situations where a direct link between the WE and the actual ground is lacking, environmental noise and interference may arise, underscoring the significance of connecting the WE directly to the ground and measuring the current via the CE. Two main types of circuits for acquiring current in potentiostats are a transimpedance amplifier (TIA) and a current conveyor (CC). These circuits will be explored further in subsequent sections.

4.1.1.1 Current Acquisition via Transimpedance Amplifiers (TIA)

In many scenarios, the ability to both source and sink reaction currents, such as those in redox reactions, is essential. One common method involves converting bidirectional currents into voltages using capacitive or resistive feedback through an operational transconductance amplifier (OTA), configured as a TIA [1] (see Fig. 4.2a). To ensure that the voltages of the WE and RE change correspondingly, it is crucial to maintain a consistent voltage difference between them, typically equal to the stimulating voltage (V_{st}). To achieve this, TIA-based potentiostats often employ a buffer to prevent current flow through the RE and establish a specific voltage difference between the WE and RE [11].

The functionality of single-ended potentiostats is constrained by the CMOS process's low power supply trend, as biosensors' redox potentials may surpass the supply voltage, leading to a compromised dynamic range and vulnerability to common mode noise and interference. To overcome these limitations, fully differential potentiostats were introduced [15–22], aiming to mitigate the challenges associated with single-ended designs. Figure 4.2b and c illustrate the block diagrams of a conventional single-ended potentiostat and the fully differential potentiostat introduced by Martin et al. [23], respectively. The fully differential potentiostat developed by this group enhances the V_{cell} output range of the single-ended counterpart, facilitating the detection of various analytes by chemical micro-transducers, even in low-voltage and high-performance processes. Nonetheless, it still exhibits deficiencies in sensitivity and accuracy. In an effort, Ghodsevali et al. [8] implemented a method utilizing high gain and rejection ratio amplifiers to mitigate voltage drop across the sense resistor, R_{Sense}, enabling the use of elevated resistance values for low current sensing, thereby enhancing the circuit's sensitivity without compromising its dynamic range.

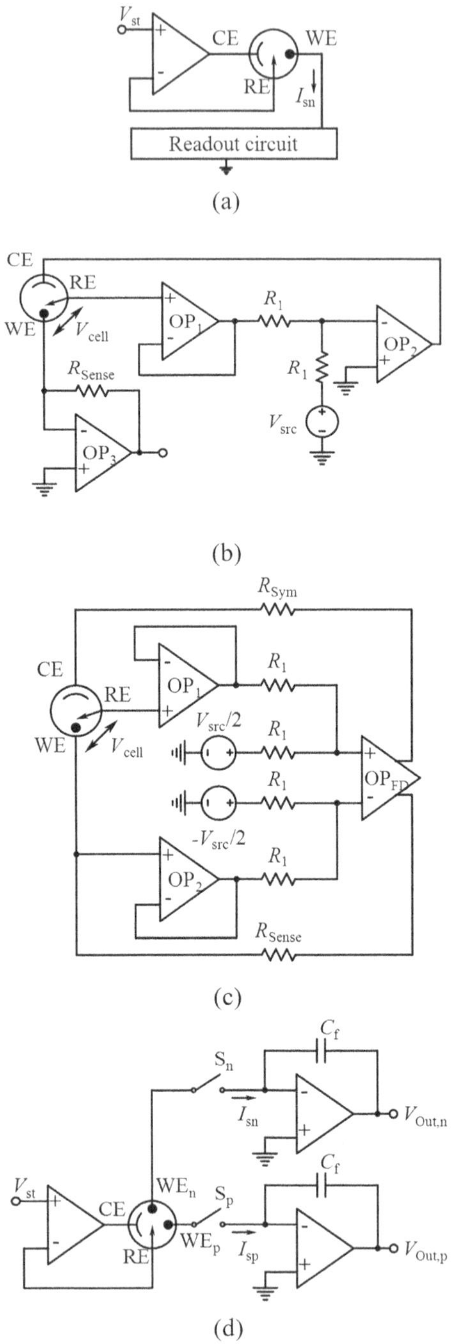

Fig. 4.2 (**a**) Basic structure of a three-electrode TIA-based system, (**b**) Single-ended potentiostat diagram, (**c**) A fully differential potentiostat, (**d**) A pseudo-differential amperometry system

To address the effects of charging currents and undesired analyte-related currents, alternative amperometric readout circuits were devised [24–26]. Demonstrated in Fig. 4.2d, the diagram portrays a pseudo-differential readout design, incorporating switches S_n and S_p to control the reading process. Through the subtraction of currents from WE_n and WE_p, most parasitic currents can be canceled out, preserving the desired analytical signal. However, this approach involves the utilization of two WEs instead of one [25].

4.1.1.2 Current Acquisition via Current Conveyor (CC)

Another prevalent approach for monitoring the reaction current involves the use of a current conveyor (CC), serving as a buffer to insulate the sensor from subsequent stages [2, 27–31]. In this technique, the reaction current originating from the WE is conveyed to a high-impedance output node while maintaining a virtual potential, before undergoing conversion into voltage, frequency, or time [1]. This strategy is frequently adopted in two-electrode configurations for one-way current measurement, particularly advantageous for densely packed on-chip arrays due to their compactness and minimal power demands. CCs can be designed relatively simply, sometimes consisting of only an OTA and an additional transistor, as illustrated in Fig. 4.3a, removing the necessity for large resistors or capacitors and resulting in negligible power consumption and footprint. Furthermore, since the OTA in this setup is directly linked to the transistor gate, it operates with exceedingly low power usage [32].

The literature also explores bidirectional current measurement techniques, either through symmetrical circuits [33, 34] or by introducing offset current to the CC [1]. However, the latter method poses challenges, including increased risk of error due to bias current noise and the need for high-resolution analog-to-digital converters (ADCs). To address this, Jafari et al. [1] devised a bidirectional CC-based circuit employing both P-channel metal-oxide semiconductor (PMOS) and N-channel metal-oxide semiconductor (NMOS) transistors, M_p and M_n, respectively, linked to an OTA feedback. This setup, illustrated in Fig. 4.3b, mirrors the currents of M_p and M_n at the CC output, integrating them on the load capacitor for sampling. Additionally, OTA chopping helps mitigate flicker noise effects.

In high-density array recordings, using amplifiers presents challenges due to their size and power requirements. To tackle this, certain array setups adopt a method where half of the amplifier circuit serves multiple recording electrodes within a row, cutting down on size and power needs [32, 35–38]. White et al. [36, 39] implemented such a strategy by employing a half-shared OpAmp design, allowing for the integration of a 32 × 32 amplifier and electrode array on a single chip with reduced power consumption and area. In their approach (shown in Fig. 4.3c), the non-inverting input transistor is part of the shared half OpAmp, while the inverting transistor is specific to each TIA (see Fig. 4.3d). Negative feedback is utilized to regulate the voltage at electrode N in order to match V_{ref} at the non-inverting input.

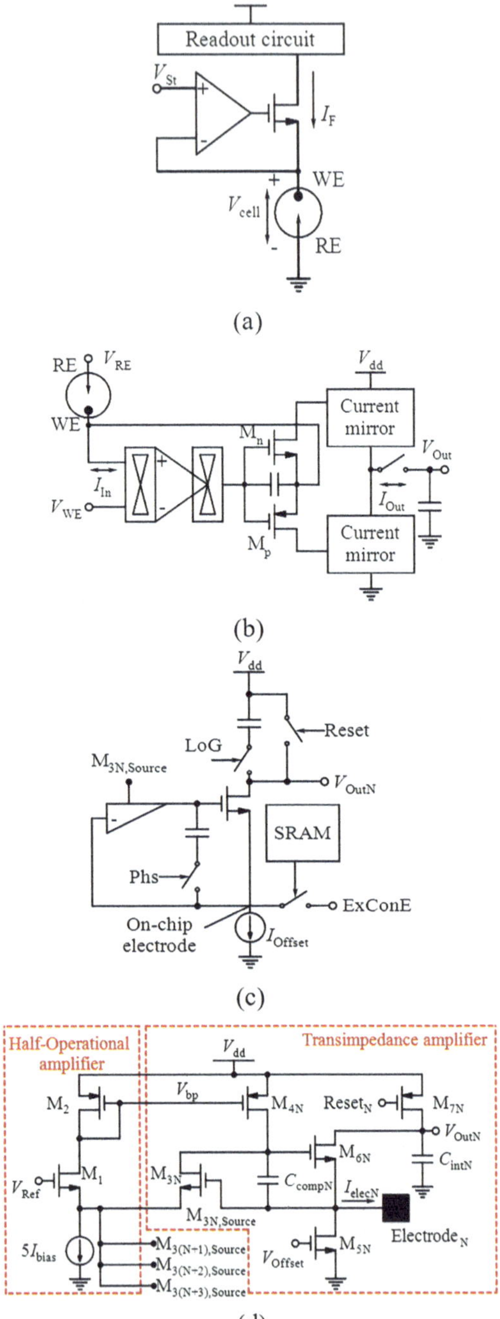

Fig. 4.3 (**a**) Basic structure of a two-electrode CC-based system, (**b**) A two-electrode chopper-stabilized bidirectional CC, (**c**) Each pixel of a CC-based array architecture including a half TIA, (**d**) The half-shared OpAmp and half TIA designs for the array architecture mentioned in (**c**)

Each TIA incorporates a 1-bit static random-access memory (SRAM), as shown in Fig. 4.3c, addressable by decoders, ensuring efficient operation within the array structure.

Differential techniques were also explored, as demonstrated by Wang et al. [15], who presented both single-ended and fully differential potentiostats to address linearity and dynamic range limitations. The fully differential configuration outperformed the single-ended counterpart, providing a wider output voltage swing and improved linearity for enhanced dynamic range in the detection of low-level sensor currents.

4.1.2 *Readout Techniques for Potentiostats' Output Current*

In this section, various kinds of readout circuits are examined alongside the potentiostats utilized to measure DC or AC output currents in voltammetric and impedimetric sensors.

4.1.2.1 DC Current Readout

In voltammetric sensors, the usual output is DC. There are several methods for converting this current into a voltage signal using a TIA. One way is by configuring the TIA with feedback components like resistors or capacitors, or by using a switch-capacitor circuit. Another method involves integrating the output current from current-controlled potentiostats with capacitors. Additionally, techniques like digitization or current-to-frequency conversion can also be employed to translate the current into a digital signal.

Capacitive and/or Resistive Readout Circuits

Ghoreishizadeh and colleagues [10] designed a combined chronoamperometry (CA) and CV sensor integrated onto a single chip, along with a signal generator and five WEs. The entire setup is illustrated in Fig. 4.4a. During CV operation, a triangular waveform is routed to the WE using a TIA, while a constant voltage is delivered to the RE via a potentiostat. This setup enables the exploration of both positive and negative voltage ranges between V_{WE} and V_{RE} (V_{WE}-V_{RE}). Moreover, the TIA reads the bidirectional current in the CV mode readout circuit. The resulting current passes through a resistor, R_M, converting into a voltage, that is then buffered by two OpAmps, OP_2 and OP_3. Following this, a differential amplifier enhances the buffered voltage across R_M. Additionally, the ultimate amplifier introduces a DC voltage to the signal to ensure it remains within the supply voltage limits.

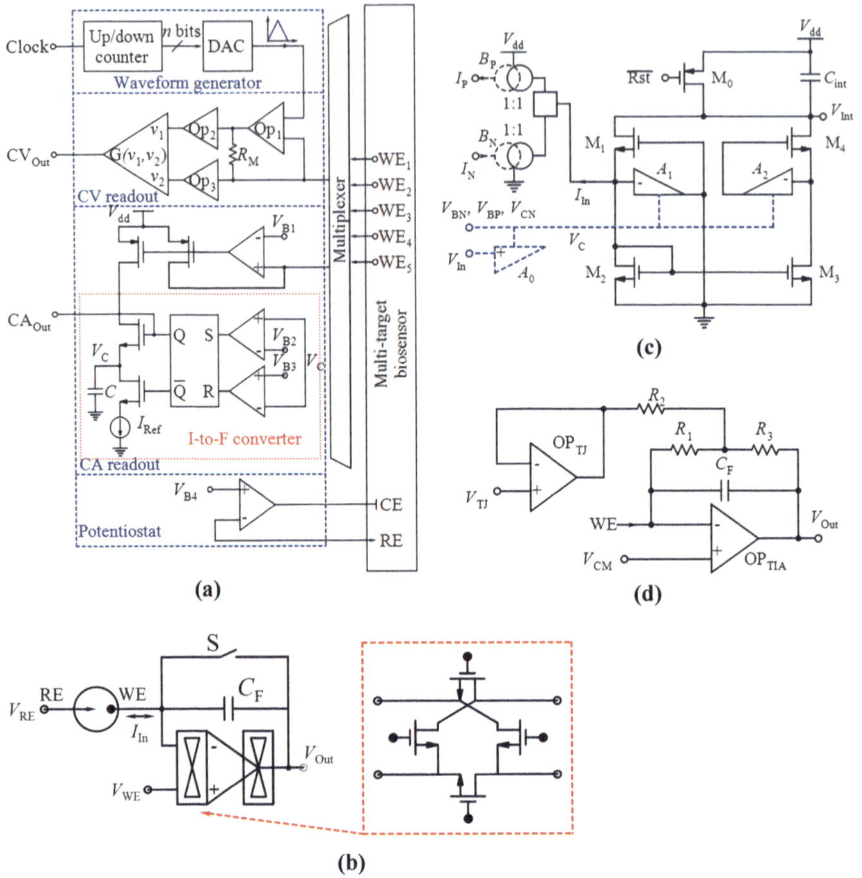

Fig. 4.4 (**a**) Schematic of an electrochemical sensor driver/readout interface including a potentiostat, a waveform generator, and two readout circuits for CA and CV, (**b**) A TIA with a chopper-stabilized bidirectional-input along with a capacitive feedback, (**c**) Bidirectional-current potentiostat unit along with an integrating capacitor, (**d**) A read channel equipped with a T-network of resistors for high amplification, in conjunction with a system based on TIA

Thermal noise can be introduced into the biosensor by resistors [1]. To achieve high SNR and gain, large resistors may be utilized, occupying significant area. Despite efforts [40, 41] to reduce the area by employing an active feedback structure instead of resistive feedback, the total area remains substantial, allowing only eight channels to occupy approximately 9 mm^2. Additionally, in multi-channel readout circuits employing resistive feedback TIAs, gain calibration is necessary due to significant gain variations resulting from resistance mismatch caused by process variations [32].

One approach to transform the current resulting from the reaction into voltage is by employing a TIA along with capacitive feedback and switch capacitor methods. A switch capacitor feedback TIA acts as an integrator, ideal for measuring small currents, and the capacitive feedback, functions as an low-path filter (LPF), effectively eliminating high-frequency noise [1]. For instance, Jafari and colleagues [1] devised a readout circuit based on TIA in a setup with two electrodes, employing a chopper-stabilized OTA and capacitive feedback (C_F). As depicted in Fig. 4.4b, this circuit functions in two phases depending on the switch, S, whether it is in an activated or deactivated state. During activation, the input current integrates over C_F, while the deactivated switch discharges the feedback capacitor, ensuring any remaining charge on C_F is cleared at the cycle's conclusion.

As previously mentioned in Sect. 4.1.1.2, a specific type of potentiostats utilizes CC structures, which can easily work in conjunction with an integrator to convert the reaction current into voltage. As an example, in the 32 × 32-array outlined by White and colleagues [36, 39] shown in Fig. 4.3c, d, the output current, I_{elecN}, is integrated using a capacitor for integration, denoted as C_{intN}. Similarly, Dorta-Quiñones et al. [42] utilized a shared amplifier arrangement alongside an integrating capacitor, as depicted in Fig. 4.4c. This circuit comprises inverting half amplifiers, A_1 and A_2, cascade transistors M_1 and M_4, mirror transistors M_2 and M_3, an integrating capacitor C_{int} and switch M_0. This configuration was utilized in a 64-channel array for fast-scan cyclic voltammetry (FSCV) detection, where each unit integrates 14 transistors in addition to an integrating capacitor.

An alternative method for converting current to voltage involves combining capacitors and resistors. As an example, Martin and colleagues [24] implemented a circuit combining capacitive and resistive elements with a pseudo-differential potentiostat. In a separate investigation, Tedjo and co-authors [43] utilized a TIA incorporating T-network resistive feedback in conjunction with capacitors to achieve I-to-V conversion across 16,064 channels. Illustrated in Fig. 4.4d, each TIA read channel comprises the OP_{TIA} with R_{1-3}. The resultant voltage from this setup is determined by:

$$V_{out} = -I_{in} R_1 \left(1 + \frac{R_3}{R_2}\right) \tag{4.1}$$

Remarkably, the T-network setup increases both amplification and noise in contrast to the TIA with a single resistor.

Readout Circuits with Digital and Pseudo-Digital Outputs

Various circuits are capable of transforming DC output currents into pseudo-digital outputs, like frequency-modulated signals, or digital outputs [4, 7, 10, 13, 44–48]. Considering that electrochemical sensors commonly produce signals in the current domain and emphasize compatibility with low voltage, resistance to noise, and efficient use of space, circuits operating in the current mode such as current-controlled oscillators (CCOs) and quantizers based on CCOs are appropriate for incorporation into sensor arrays. For instance, Nazari et al. [4] implemented a potentiostat based on CC alongside an ADC, incorporating an current-to-frequency converter and a single-slope ADC. Figure 4.5a displays a single pathway from the 8 × 12-array constructed by this group, capable of measuring bidirectional currents. Moreover, Ghoreishizadeh and team [10] introduced a sensor tailored for multiple targets, engineered for both CV and CA assessments utilizing five WEs, employing a three-electrode configuration alongside an current-to-frequency mechanism for the CA mode (refer to Fig. 4.4a). In this operational mode, a stable voltage is administered to the designated WE, and a one-way current is replicated via a current mirror. Following this, a conversion from current to pulse width generates a width of pulse inversely proportional to this resultant current. The resultant sensor readings can be conveniently transmitted off the chip without necessitating an ADC.

Sutula et al. [13] proposed an innovative approach that utilizes the prolonged time constant of an electrochemical cell to develop a compact and energy-efficient interface circuit for electrochemical ΔΣ modulation, eliminating the need for large capacitors on the chip. Shown in Fig. 4.5b, the time constant of the electrochemical cell is repurposed within a loop to create a continuous-time noise shaper of the first-order. The remaining components of the system, including a sample-and-hold unit, a single-bit quantizer, and a feedback digital-to-analog converter (DAC), can be entirely implemented in the electronic domain. Maintained at the desired potential V_{ref} through the modulator's closed loop, V_{rsw} enables the output current I_{sens} to be digitally modulated to q_{mod}, available at the input of the DAC. The conversion of analog to digital is accomplished using an LPF, adjusting the sampling frequency to meet the Nyquist criterion.

4.1.2.2 AC Current Readout

Circuits for reading impedance evaluate sensing impedance by contrasting excitation and response signals, often utilizing methods such as auto-balanced bridge (ABB), discrete Fourier transform (DFT) multiply-sum (MAc) units, DDS coupled with an ADC, or lock-in techniques. Auto-balanced bridges suit frequencies up to 100 kHz, whereas lock-in techniques, popular in CMOS technology, enable impedance measurement within the same frequency range without rapid sampling requirements. CMOS impedimetric biosensors are categorized into three groups: lock-in detection, phase/amplitude technique, and silicon cochlea-based sensors, with lock-in detection being the predominantly reported method, particularly validated experimentally with on-chip electrodes [12].

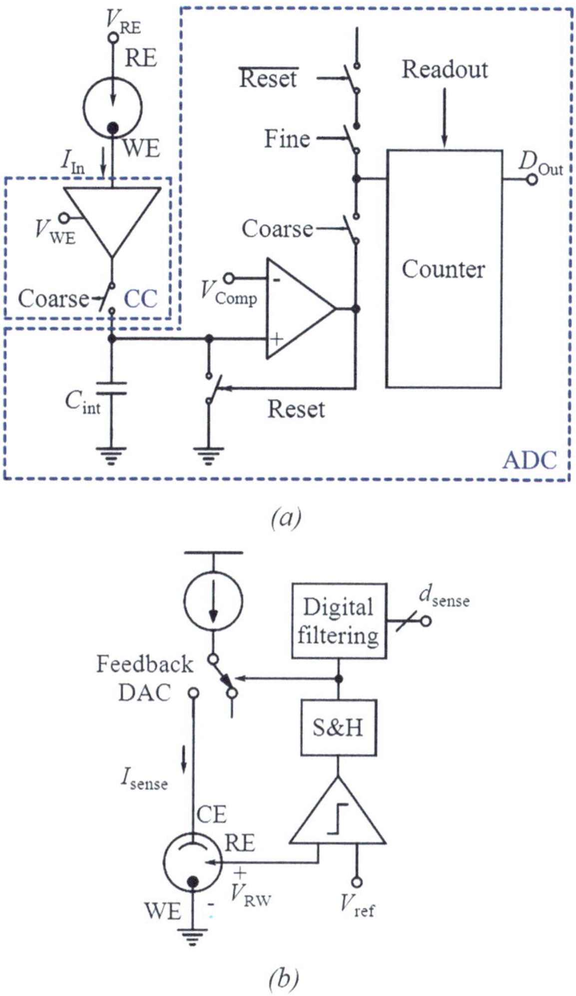

Fig. 4.5 (**a**) One channel of a two-electrode CC-based system with digitized output, (**b**) A potentiostat including a delta-sigma (ΔΣ) modulation loop

Lock-in Technique

Figure 4.6a demonstrates the functioning of the lock-in method, where the sensing impedance, offset, and low-frequency noise undergo modulation to a higher frequency through a designated signal. Whether it operates in the voltage or current mode, the process necessitates a voltage-to-current (V-to-I) or I-to-V conversion and subsequent amplification before down-conversion. The original signal is then recovered through synchronous demodulation aided by LPFs. By utilizing a quadrature demodulator, it is possible to extract both the actual and imaginary parts of the

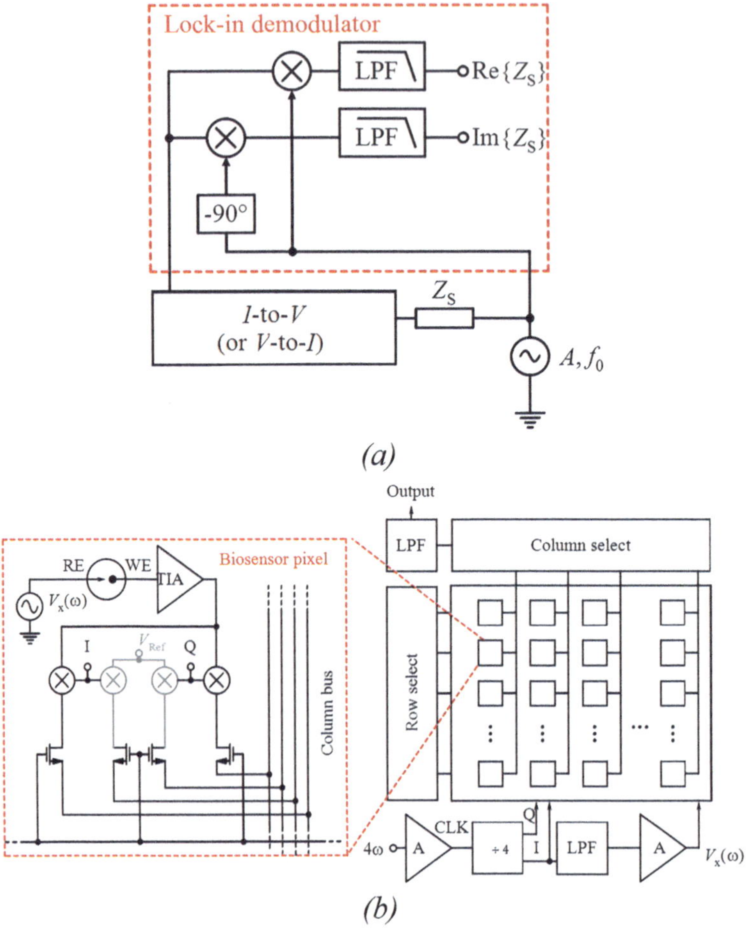

Fig. 4.6 (**a**) Simple block diagram of the lock-in technique, (**b**) An array of EIS biosensors based on a lock-in technique

sensing impedance (Z_S) by multiplying the signal with the (Q) and in-phase (I) signals. Although commonly employed in impedance spectroscopy applications [5–7, 49–51], there are cases where this method has been modified for ultra-wideband dielectric spectroscopy and sensing of complex permittivity [52–54].

Manickam et al. [6, 7] introduced the pioneering fully integrated CMOS impedimetric biosensor featuring a 10 × 10 on-chip electrode array (Fig. 4.6b). Each pixel of this array incorporates a coherent demodulator comprising a low-noise TIA and two mixers. The TIA boosts the current from the sensing impedance, Z_S, which is subsequently multiplied by sinusoidal signals (Q and I that are orthogonal to each other) at the angular frequency ω. The DC values of the mixer outputs, V_I and V_Q, yield the amplitude and phase of the sensing admittance, $Y_S(\omega) = Z_S(\omega)^{-1}$, as expressed in Eqs. (4.2) and (4.3), respectively:

$$\left|Y_{\mathrm{S}}(\omega)\right| = \frac{\sqrt{V_{\mathrm{I}}^2 + V_{\mathrm{Q}}^2}}{A_{\mathrm{TIA}} \cdot \left|V_{\mathrm{x}}(\omega)\right|} \tag{4.2}$$

$$\angle Y_{\mathrm{S}}(\omega) = \tan^{-1}\left(\frac{V_{\mathrm{Q}}}{V_{\mathrm{I}}}\right) \tag{4.3}$$

$V_x(\omega)$ and the quadrature signals (I and Q) are produced externally by a reference clock functioning at 4ω. Following input into a digital counter divided by 4, which is powered by this clock, the quadrature signals are generated, while $V_x(\omega)$ is obtained from the processed I signal through an LPF and an amplifier in Fig. 4.6b.

While the lock-in detection technique, despite its synchronous nature, faces issues concerning alignment, built-in DC offsets, and synchronization discrepancies, obtaining simultaneous measurements of real and imaginary components in systems with multiple channels or frequencies presents alignment challenges. This requires accurate synchronization between the injection and measurement phases. Additionally, offset cancellation techniques like chopping are necessary to eliminate DC offsets, potentially increasing circuit complexity [55]. Moreover, this method requires signal filtration through an LPF, leading to extended measurement times, particularly at low frequencies. Furthermore, the application of each frequency individually restricts measurement speed, particularly for achieving high-frequency resolution [56].

Phase/Amplitude Technique

An alternative to the lock-in method involves measuring the phase and magnitude of the sensing impedance using a modulator, comparator, XOR, and integrator circuitries, as depicted in Fig. 4.7a. This technique is scarcely documented alongside on-chip electrodes, according to current knowledge.

The phase/amplitude circuit devised by Kassanos et al. [55] exemplifies this method, employing a single frequency at a time with off-chip electrodes. Through multiplication, the magnitude is determined, with instrumentation amplifiers (IAs) measuring voltage differences across a known current sensing resistor (R_{Isense}) and the sensing impedance (see Fig. 4.7b). Subsequently, clockless comparators transform amplifier outputs into square waves, generating a pulse signal via an XOR gate that signifies the phase delay induced by the sensing impedance at the specified frequency. This pulse, processed by a g_m-C integrator, produces a sawtooth wave proportional to the phase. The phase detector's output is calculated using $\theta = 360f\Delta t$, where θ signifies the phase, Δt is the pulse width, and f stands for the signal frequency. The square wave also serves as a clock signal for synchronous rectification. Following low-pass filtering, the magnitude (M) of the sensing impedance is equal to:

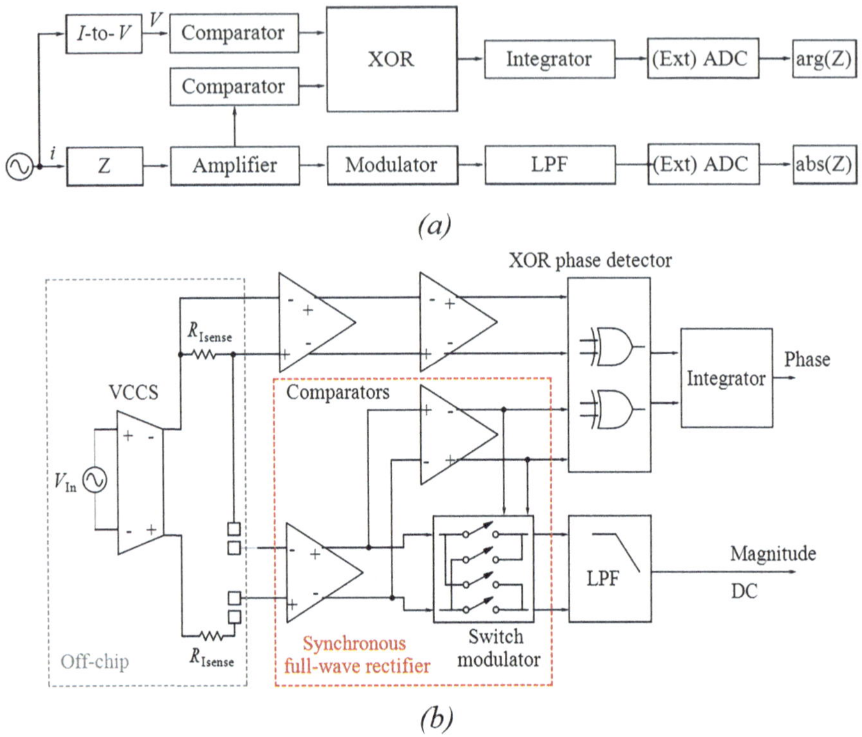

Fig. 4.7 (**a**) Simple block diagram of the phase/magnitude technique, (**b**) Schematic of the integrated phase/amplitude circuit for impedance measurement using square wave analysis

$$M = \frac{\pi V_{DC}}{2.A_v.I_{inj}} \tag{4.4}$$

where Av denotes amplifier gain, I_{inj} is the injected current amplitude, and V_{DC} represents the filter output.

Silicon Cochlea-Based Technique

Employing a multi-frequency signal to stimulate the electrodes enhances measurement efficiency compared to the lock-in technique. Utilizing silicon cochlea, sinusoidal stimuli are generated at periodically spaced frequencies. Following the summation of these stimuli, the analyzer segregates the output based on frequency to establish a relationship between impedance and frequency [56].

In an effort, Hamilton et al. [57] introduced an impedance sensor illustrated in Fig. 4.8a, utilizing silicon cochleae in place of a conventional band-pass filter bank due to their sharper and more precise high-frequency cut-offs. This adaptation allows for the rejection of out-of-band frequencies without necessitating higher-order filters with increased complexity, power consumption, and area. In the illustrated setup, the stimulus cochlea, as shown in Fig. 4.8b, produces sinusoidal signals at frequencies spaced logarithmically. These signals are then summed and introduced into the test structure. Subsequently, the analyzer cochlea segregates the test structure's output based on frequency to establish the relationship between impedance and frequency, as depicted in Fig. 4.8a. In this representation, $Z(i)$ is determined by the ratio of the ith current from the analyzer cochlea ($I_{out}(i)$) to the ith current from the stimulus cochlea ($I_{ref}(i)$), adjusted by a constant established by the V-to-I converter (*Scale*):

$$Z(i) = \frac{I_{out}(i)}{I_{ref}(i)} \times scale \tag{4.5}$$

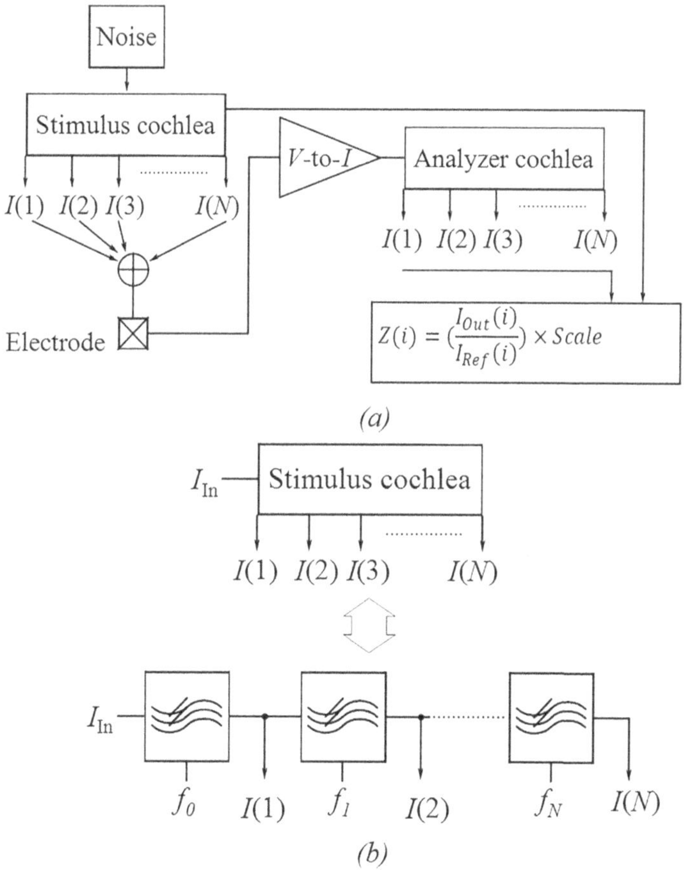

Fig. 4.8 (**a**) An impedance measurement system based on silicon cochlea, (**b**) The silicon cochlea cascade structure

4.2 CMOS Interface Circuits for Capacitive Sensing

Capacitive sensors necessitate an interface circuit to translate biochemical capacitance into readable signals such as current, voltage, frequency, or digital outputs. These signals can be transmitted to users via wired or wireless methods, which can be integrated on-chip or off-chip depending on the sensor's application, whether handheld, wearable, or implantable. This section primarily concentrates on the interface circuitry, excluding discussions on communication techniques.

Various categories of CMOS capacitive interface circuits are utilized for biosensing applications, including (1) oscillator-based capacitive sensors, (2) lock-in detection, (2) charge redistribution techniques, (4) charge-based capacitance measurement (CBCM), and (5) triangular voltage analysis.

4.2.1 Oscillator-Based Capacitive Sensors

Capacitive sensor readout circuits can be realized through various oscillator structures, including comparator-based relaxation oscillators, voltage-controlled oscillators (VCOs), and ring oscillators (ROs).

4.2.1.1 Comparator-Based Capacitance-to-Frequency Converters (CFCs)

Certain kinds of sensors utilize relaxation oscillators to modulate the frequency output based on variations in the sensing capacitance [58–60]. Fig. 4.9a illustrates a CFC as an example of this mechanism. A reference current (I_B) charges and discharges the sensing capacitor, C_S. Subsequently, a comparator assesses the capacitor voltage against a threshold voltage (V_{th}), triggering a switch to reset the voltage to zero upon reaching V_{th}. The output pulse frequency (f_{Out}) is inversely related to C_S [58], as depicted by:

$$f_{Out} = \left(\frac{C_S . V_{th}}{I_B} + \tau_d \right)^{-1} \tag{4.6}$$

The delay resulting from the comparator, denoted as τ_d, is considered negligible.

A different setup for managing the sensing capacitor charging and discharging involves employing two identical source and sink reference currents [60]. Switching between these currents is achieved using a comparator with hysteresis, like a Schmitt trigger. This configuration offers an alternative method to control the discharging and charging processes of the capacitor, enabling versatile operation in various sensing applications.

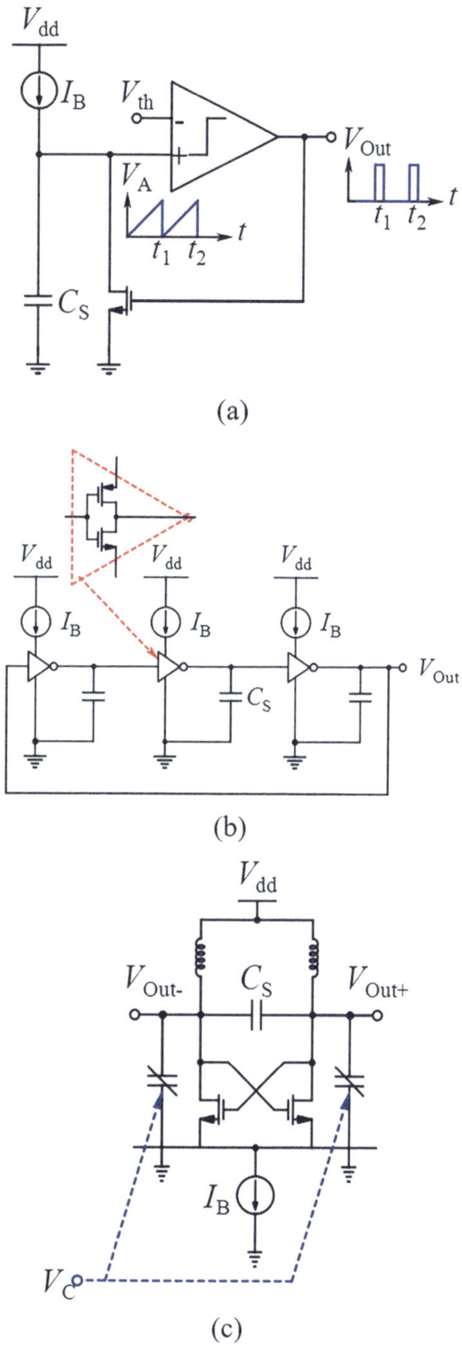

Fig. 4.9 A basic structure of: (**a**) A comparator-based CFC, (**b**) A 3-stage ring *RO-based CFC,* (**c**) *An LC VCO-based sensor.*

When developing relaxation oscillators with comparators, ensuring accurate current references and comparator precision is vital. Various elements, such as parasitic capacitances and process-related parameters like resistors, as well as temperature-related factors like transistor transconductance, can influence the output frequency. Accounting for these factors is key to enhancing performance and precision, especially in applications where precise frequency control is essential.

4.2.1.2 Ring Oscillator (RO)-Based Capacitance-to-Frequency Converters (CFCs)

ROs can also be employed to convert sensing capacitance into frequency [59, 61–68]. Illustrated in Fig. 4.9b is a CFC featuring three delay cells, where the delays are contingent upon the charge of their load capacitors driven by the current I_B to a designated voltage V_{osc}. Within these cells, one is designated as the sensing capacitor, C_S, described by $C_S=C_R+\Delta C$, with C_R representing the reference capacitance and ΔC denoting capacitance changes. The period of an M-stage RO can be calculated by [65]:

$$T_{osc} = 2\left[\frac{C_S.V_{osc}}{I_B} + (M-1)\frac{C_R.V_{osc}}{I_B}\right] \tag{4.7}$$

This technique is also reported in a differential structure by Mohammad et al. [63] using two ROs, where one is linked to the sensing electrode. A pulse-width modulated signal is generated by detecting the frequency difference between the ROs.

Despite being susceptible to factors such as fluctuations in process, supply voltage, and temperature, CFCs provide the benefit of a semi-digital output, streamlining the conversion to digital representation utilizing a counter without necessitating additional ADCs, thereby lessening system complexity and power consumption.

4.2.1.3 Voltage-Controlled Oscillator (VCO)-Based Capacitive Sensors

Capacitive sensors based on VCOs are frequently employed in dielectric spectroscopy and measuring complex permittivity over a wide spectrum of frequencies ranging from mega- to giga-Hertz [69–77]. These sensors typically consist of a sensing VCO paired with a frequency detector. An instance of an LC VCO-based sensor is illustrated in Fig. 4.9c, where C_S contributes to the LC tank [69, 72]. When an analyte is present, electric field alterations induce a frequency change in the VCO. The relative frequency variation concerning the pre-exposure frequency f_0 of the LC oscillator can be calculated by [77]:

$$\frac{\Delta f}{f_0} = \frac{1}{\sqrt{1+\Delta C_{tot}(f_0)/C_{tot}}} - 1 \tag{4.8}$$

where C_{tot} identifies the total capacitance, encompassing C_S, varactors, and parasitic capacitors, and $\Delta C_{tot}(f_0)/C_{tot}$ denotes the relative change in total capacitance concerning C_{tot}.

Single VCO-based sensors are prone to environmental influences and low-frequency temperature variations, driving the adoption of a differential approach employing two VCOs, a reference and a sensing VCO, with differentiated output frequencies to mitigate sensitivity to external effects. Ensuring similarity between the VCOs is critical for optimal performance, necessitating periodic activation to prevent frequency pulling and noise filtering [72]. Closed-loop frequency detectors, such as PLL architectures, expedite capacitance measurement at specific frequencies, facilitating faster measurement times by tuning and stabilizing frequency shifts [69, 70, 77]. Additionally, studies [74–76] advocate for quadrature voltage-controlled oscillators (QVCOs) to enhance SNR, and precision incorporating LC tank-based injection-locked oscillators (ILOs) in various applications.

4.2.2 Lock-in Detection

Lock-in detection, commonly utilized in impedance spectroscopy, extends its application to capacitive sensors as well [6, 7, 49, 50]. For example, Ciccarella et al. [78, 79] achieved a resolution surpassing 100 zF for counting single μm-sized airborne particles. Despite its effectiveness, this method poses challenges like increased complexity, synchronization issues, and sensor mismatch. Each channel's setup consists of a charge preamplifier with adaptable high-pass filtering, a square-wave mixer, a tunable LPF, and a digital network, as illustrated in Fig. 4.10. Utilizing rail-to-rail square waveforms maximizes charge injection into the preamplifier. The lock-in demodulation employs a low-pass g_m-C filter and a non-return-to-zero (NRZ) passive mixer. A voltage amplifier is inserted between the charge preamplifier and the lock-in demodulator to mitigate g_m-C filter noise. Furthermore, to ensure a balanced condition in the differential input capacitance and address saturation of the front-end amplifier, a digital-to-capacitance converter (DCC) is utilized.

4.2.3 Charge Redistribution Techniques

These techniques can be divided into three subcategories including methods relying on (1) the principle of charge sharing, (2) charge-sensitive amplifiers (CSAs), and (3) switch-capacitor circuits.

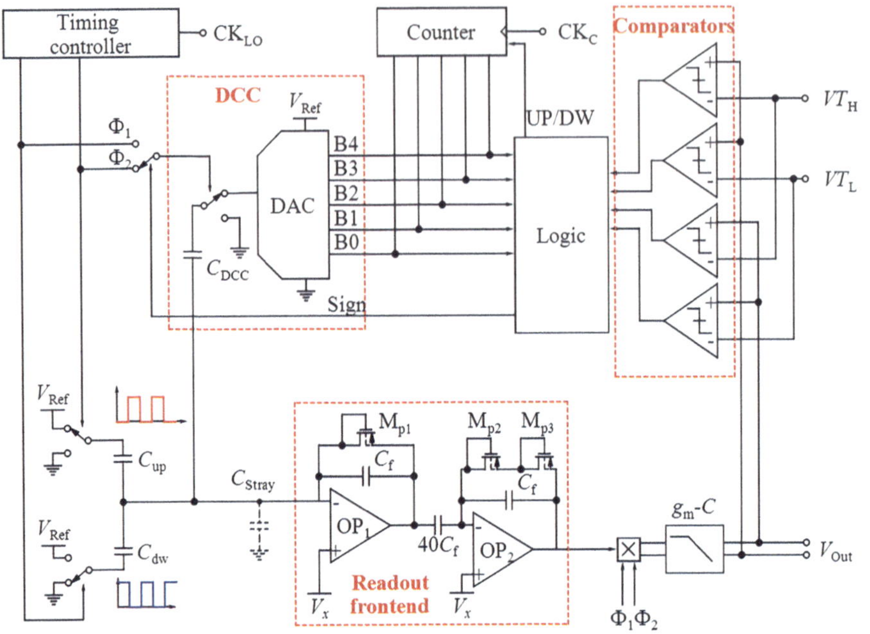

Fig. 4.10 One channel of a multi-channel CMOS capacitive sensor based on Lock-in detection method

4.2.3.1 Charge Sharing Principle

The operational principle of this method relies on manipulating the charge and discharge cycles of multiple capacitors [80–82]. An example is depicted in Fig. 4.11a [80, 81]. In this system, switches M_{1-3} govern the discharging and charging processes of capacitors N_1 and N_2. The circuit operates in two phases: the reset phase and the evaluation phase, controlled by clock pulses. During the reset phase, nodes N_1 and N_2 are charged with V_{dd} and V_{ss}, respectively, while in the evaluation phase, charge redistribution occurs between their capacitances. The output voltage, determined by C_S, is mathematically expressed as:

$$V_{Out} = \frac{\left(C_{p1} + C_S\right).V_{dd} + C_{p2}.V_{ss}}{C_{p1} + C_{p2} + C_S} \tag{4.9}$$

The notations C_{p1} and C_{p2} stand for the parasitic capacitances of the nodes N_1 and N_2, respectively.

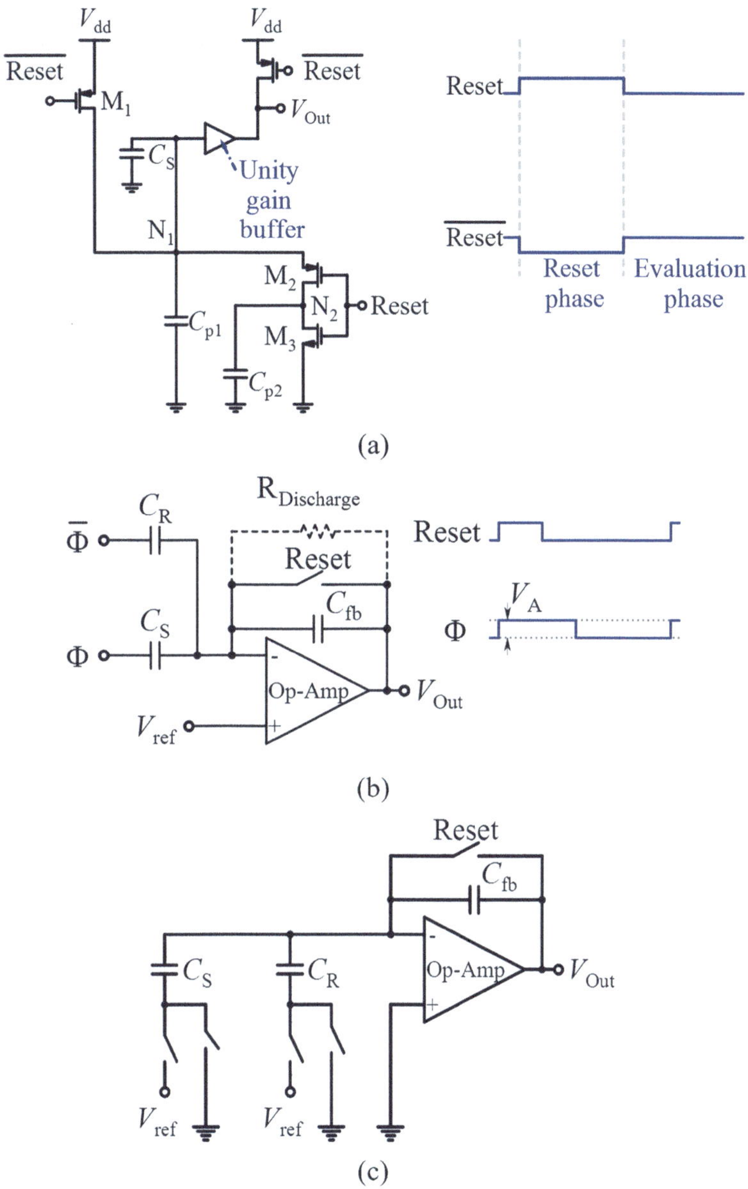

Fig. 4.11 A simple example of charge redistribution techniques using: (**a**) Charge sharing principle, (**b**) CSA, (**c**) Switch-capacitor method

4.2.3.2 Charge-Sensitive Amplifier (CSA)-Based Techniques

An alternative approach, known as the CSA technique, serves to redistribute charges [83–85]. The CSA technique, depicted in Fig. 4.11b, involves applying a voltage pulse, Φ, to C_S, followed by the transfer of charge from C_S to a reference capacitor, C_R. The voltage across C_R is then integrated using a capacitive feedback amplifier, with a reset switch included in the feedback path to prevent amplifier saturation. By comparing the charges on C_R and C_S and completing the integration, the output voltage of the integrator is directly proportional to the difference between C_S and C_R [84]:

$$V_{\mathrm{Out}} = V_{\mathrm{A}} \frac{C_{\mathrm{S}} - C_{\mathrm{R}}}{C_{\mathrm{fb}}} \tag{4.10}$$

where V_A denotes the Φ signal's amplitude. De Venuto et al. [83] employed the CSA technique for output voltage measurement, opting to use a resistor instead of a reset switch to discharge the feedback capacitor.

4.2.3.3 Switch-Capacitor Circuits

Switch-capacitor circuits, akin to CSAs in function, differ in that they accept DC voltage inputs instead of voltage pulses. Illustrated in Fig. 4.11c, these configurations utilize several switches to charge and discharge the reference and sensing capacitors, effectively mitigating parallel parasitic capacitances while sustaining minimal input impedance [84].

Sawtooth waveform output frequency modulation involves an amplifier and counter, while conversion of level output voltage to digital necessitates an ADC [86, 87]. Various ADC types, such as successive-approximation register (SAR), pipeline ADCs, and $\Delta\Sigma$ ADCs are applicable, with switch-capacitor circuits enabling direct or voltage conversion-based digital signal conversion [88–90]. Nevertheless, switch-capacitor systems face challenges such as offsets induced by switches and injected charge, often addressed through methods like auto-correction and dual sampling, though this leads to elevated power usage and circuit intricacy. These challenges are pervasive in fields utilizing switch-capacitor circuits, prompting the need for advanced techniques balancing power efficiency and circuit performance.

4.2.4 Charge-Based Capacitance Measurement (CBCM)

The CBCM method employs a sensing capacitor (C_S) and a reference capacitor (C_R) as well as pseudo-inverters with pull-down and pull-up switches for controlled charging and discharging of capacitors (see the green rectangle in Fig. 4.12a, b). Clock pulses Φ_1 and Φ_2 control these switches, preventing short-circuit currents by

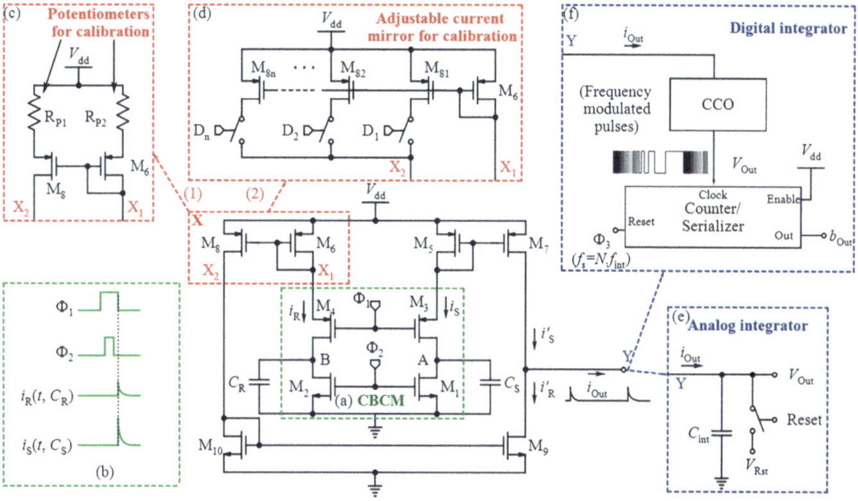

Fig. 4.12 (**a**) A differential Core-CBCM capacitance-to-current converter (The CBCM core is shown in the green rectangle), (**b**) The waveforms of the CBCM core shown in (**a**), (**c**, **d**) The components within rectangle X in (**a**) can be substituted with either (**c**) potentiometers, or (**d**) an adjustable current mirror, for calibration, (**e**, **f**) The output differential current at node Y, i_{Out}, can be integrated in either the analog domain using the integrator shown in (**e**), or in the digital domain employing the integrator shown in (**f**)

charging capacitors through pull-up switches (M_3 and M_4) and discharging them via pull-down switches (M_1 and M_2). Instantaneous currents $i_R(C_R,t)$ and $i_S(C_S,t)$ exhibit sharp, time-dependent exponential profiles, with the capacitance difference $\Delta C=C_S-C_R$ indicating analyte changes. Average currents I_R and I_S over one clock pulse period, T_S, are proportional to each branch's capacitance, allowing ΔC determination by subtracting the average reference branch current from the sensing branch:

$$I_S - I_R = \frac{1}{T_s}\int_0^{T_s}\left(C_S\frac{dv_s(t)}{dt} - C_R\frac{dv_R(t)}{dt}\right)dt$$

$$= f_S\left(V_{dd} - V_{Am}\right).\Delta C \tag{4.11}$$

This technique enables precise ΔC extraction from C_S using the frequency of Φ_1 and Φ_2 ($f_S = 1/T_S$). While implementable with half the circuit using one electrode and one pseudo-inverter, recent advances include integrated readout circuits for processing CBCM currents instead of relying on external elements like ammeters [91–104].

Differential voltage-based techniques involve integrating core-CBCM currents, i_S and i_R, before or after subtraction. In one approach, two distinct integrating capacitors are employed to average i_S and i_R currents. Subsequently, these averages are amplified and subtracted using a differential amplifier, balancing resolution and dynamic range to enhance sensitivity [94, 95]. To address the challenge of limited dynamic range in differential voltage mode, the latter approach can be used as illustrated in Fig. 4.12a [97, 98]. This approach entails the utilization of current mirrors to subtract and amplify the currents i_S and i_R, followed by the injection of the resulting differential current ($\Delta i = i_S - i_R$) into an integrating capacitor (Fig. 4.12e). To calibrate the offset voltage (V_{off}), potentiometers, R_{P1} and R_{P2} (Fig. 4.12c), are employed alongside adjustable current gain and current mirrors, as depicted in Fig. 4.12d. Another approach described in articles referenced in [100, 101] outlines a fully differential rail-to-rail capacitance-to-voltage converter (CVC) for on-chip cell monitoring, doubling the capacitance measurement's dynamic range by addressing issues like parasitic capacitances and common-mode noise.

Previous versions of core-CBCM sensors faced dynamic range constraints, as they converted output current to voltage before digitization, limiting the integrating capacitor's voltage swing due to supply voltage limitations. To address this, a current-mode approach can be used (see Fig. 4.12f), employing a core-CBCM CFC, where amplified currents from the CBCM core are directed to a CCO, converting them into pulse frequency to track fluctuations, with the resultant output frequency averaged using a counter, correlating with ΔC [104–106].

CBCM offers a blend of high precision and minimal power consumption, which is highly desirable for life science applications. CBCM showcases exceptional accuracy down to the atto-Farad range while consuming mere micro-watts of power.

4.2.5 *Triangular Voltage Analysis*

A method utilizing a triangular voltage signal can measure capacitance and resistance individually. This signal is either an output generated by a pulse current stimulator, as shown in Fig. 4.13a, or it is applied to stimulate the analyte, as depicted in Fig. 4.13b. The calculation for obtaining C_S in the first scenario involves using a CCO, relying on the slope of each rising or falling segment of the output voltage, as per research by Druart et al. [107]. In the second scenario, the triangular voltage waveform stimulates the analyte, generating a square current through C_S. The capacitance is determined only in the "valley" and "peak" regions of the triangular voltage input, where the second derivative is not equal to zero. Lee et al. [108] utilized a switch-capacitor circuit to process the output current, enabling direct impedance measurement with triangular voltage analysis, achieving a resolution of roughly 1 pF.

4.3 Interface Circuits for Neural Stimulation/Recording

CMOS interface circuits are crucial in neural interface technology, facilitating both neural stimulation and recording processes. They serve as a crucial link between biological systems and electronic devices, enabling researchers to interact with the complex signals of the nervous system. Neural stimulation circuits deliver precise

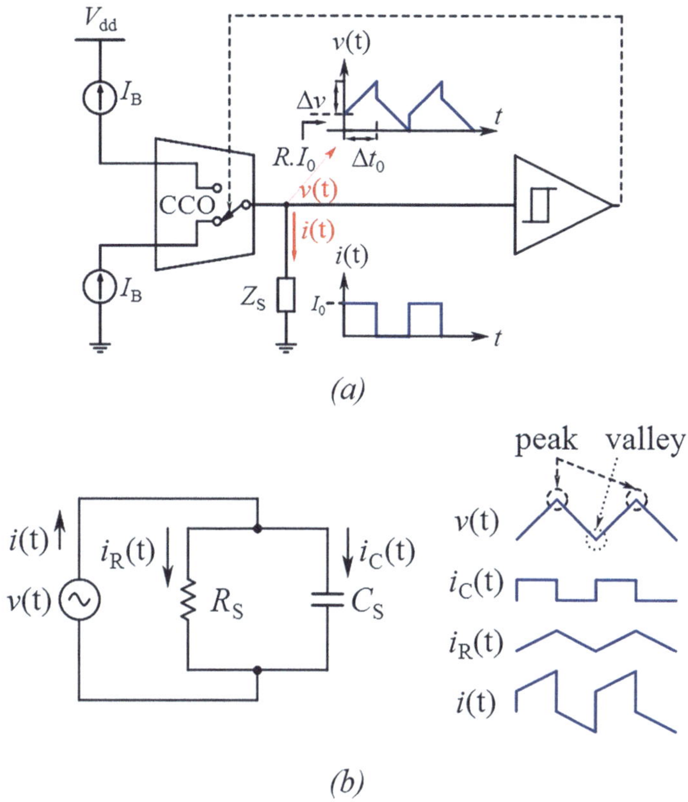

Fig. 4.13 The triangular voltage analysis method with: (**a**) An output triangular voltage waveform, (**b**) An input triangular voltage waveform

electrical impulses to targeted areas of the nervous system, aiding in research and potentially treating neurological disorders. Conversely, neural recording circuits capture and analyze neural signals, enabling the monitoring of brain activity and the study of neural networks. With advancements in CMOS technology, these circuits have evolved to offer high precision, low power consumption, and enhanced scalability to meet the diverse needs of neuroscience research and clinical applications. This section briefly discusses the circuits employed for neural stimulation and recording, excluding discussions on communication methodologies.

4.3.1 Neural Stimulation

Neural stimulation relies on delivering controlled electrical charges to initiate action potentials (APs), primarily achieved through current-controlled stimulation (CCS) [109–111]. This method ensures precise charge delivery and mitigates potential tissue damage by utilizing bidirectional current sources and an electrode interface

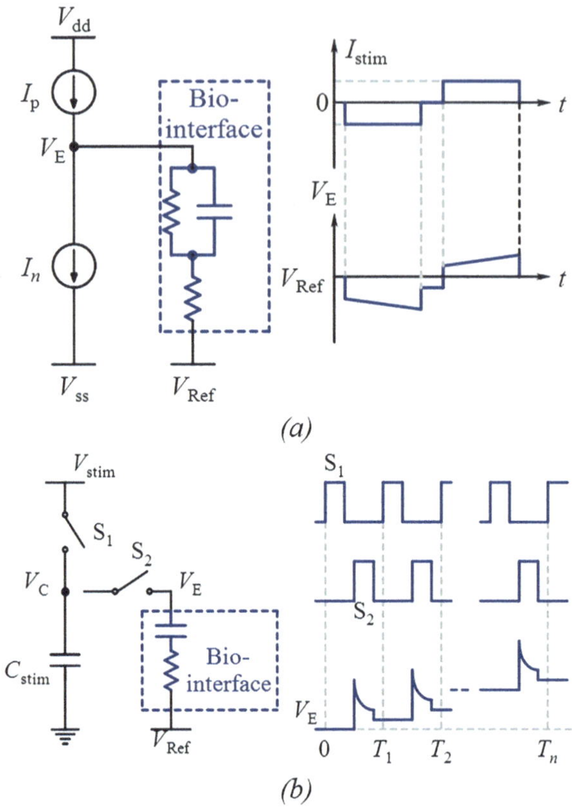

Fig. 4.14 (**a**) The standard setup of a bidirectional current stimulator and illustrations showing the current and voltage waveforms of the bidirectional current stimulator, (**b**) The setup of a high-frequency switch-capacitor and voltage pattern on the electrode with control signals from the stimulator's switch

model comprising capacitance and resistance (Fig. 4.14a) [112, 113] . Voltage/current-controlled stimulation (V/CCS) offers concurrent regulation of output voltage and current, enhancing precision and safety in stimulation protocols [50, 114]. Integration of buffer circuits, like those described in prior studies, further refines control over stimulation parameters, considering electrode impedance and voltage-only control strategies. Additionally, techniques such as high-frequency stimulation methods and switched capacitor stimulation (SCS) are explored for improved power efficiency and charge control, albeit with challenges in on-chip integration and large capacitor integration [115–117].

Figure 4.14b demonstrates a high-frequency switching method for stimulation, allowing for a significant reduction in the required capacitance (C_{stim}) and enabling efficient on-chip integration. It also shows the timing and voltage waveform of the electrode (V_E), where a phase difference between S_1 and S_2 prevents a dead zone, and V_E rises with successive switches until the charge accumulation triggers an action potential [113].

Efficient neural stimulation circuitry design emphasizes safety and power efficiency. Techniques like adiabatic CCS architecture enhance energy-saving performance by tracking electrode voltage changes and recovering electric charge from nerve tissue [157]. The predominant use of CCS in neural stimulators necessitates considerations for wireless power supplies in implantable devices and battery operation in wearable units [110]. Ensuring stimulation safety involves voltage detection circuits and pulse injection systems to monitor and remove the residual charge from tissues promptly [112, 118, 119]. Peak efficiency, often reaching 80%, is crucial in evaluating performance, alongside considerations for maximum stimulation current to determine the effectiveness of neural or muscular stimulation [113].

4.3.2 Neural Recording

In a closed-loop neural setup, the integration of neural recording and stimulation allows for real-time feedback and control based on recorded neural signals. Unlike the robust stimulator signals, neural recordings entail the sampling of low-amplitude and low-frequency local field potential (LFPs), necessitating specialized analog frontends to amplify, filter, and digitize these signals from extracellular electrodes for compatibility with computing systems. These analog frontends are meticulously designed to execute these tasks efficiently, ensuring seamless processing and analysis of neural recordings within the closed-loop architecture [113, 120].

LFPs, occupying the lower frequency spectrum of 1–200 Hz, and APs, with higher frequencies ranging from 200 Hz to 10 kHz, demand stringent measures to maintain signal fidelity and improve SNR. To achieve this, the neural recording circuit must exhibit high input impedance (Z_{in}) compared to electrode impedance (Z_{in} > 1 GΩ), while also limiting the electrode's DC current to 100 pA [113]. Employing a high-gain low-noise amplifier (LNA) (>40 dB) at the recording front end, coupled with digital quantization circuits, enables precise quantization of microvolt-level nerve signals, ensuring accurate signal capture and conversion [114, 121–123]. Additionally, the integration of a high-pass filter (HPF) with a low cutoff frequency helps eliminate DC offsets in neural signals, preventing recording saturation and facilitating reliable data acquisition and analysis within the closed-loop system [113].

4.3.2.1 Amplification

The cornerstone of frontends employed in neural signal recording is the LNA, also referred to as a neural amplifier. Its primary function revolves around amplifying and filtering neural waveforms while effectively eliminating any observed DC offset across a pair of differential electrodes [114, 124]. A robust LNA design necessitates sufficient gain, appropriate bandwidth, high SNR, excellent linearity, and high rejection ratios for common mode and power supply (CMRR and PSRR), all crucial for ensuring desired signal quality [125, 126]. In multi-channel configurations, where each electrode requires its own sensory circuit, LNAs must exhibit low power consumption, compact size, and scalability for multiple parallel channels [120].

Various OTA configurations, notably the two-stage OpAmp [121, 127, 128] and the current mirror OTA [129–132], are favored for their low noise characteristics. Alternative methodologies have been explored to minimize power overhead and reduce noise from the second stage, including folded cascode OpAmps and fully-differential self-biased OTAs. A capacitive network-based topology proposed in [133] enhances noise efficiency factor (NEF) by leveraging source degeneration resistors within the active load of a differential pair, significantly reducing noise contribution from this branch compared to that of the differential pair (Fig. 4.15a). Efforts by Shen et al. [134] introduced innovative approaches for closed-loop amplifiers, resulting in enhanced transconductance and noise reduction without additional current consumption. Meanwhile, alternative designs like that proposed in [135] feature active feedback loops, offering competitive noise performance and remarkably small chip area compared to traditional configurations [120].

Adapted versions of neural amplifier configurations have found widespread application in capturing lower-frequency signal types like LFPs and electroencephalography (EEG) signals [125]. Employing dynamic methods such as chopper stabilization, these setups effectively counteract $1/f$ noise within CMOS-integrated systems across a spectrum of frequency ranges [136, 137]. Demonstrating flexibility, these configurations support different frequency spectrums [128, 129, 133, 138, 139], utilizing various approaches to achieve specific bandwidth adjustments, such as tuning resistance values in filtration or modifying operational parameters. In particular setups, the higher cutoff is adapted by adjusting the gate voltage of a weakly inverted MOSFET [140, 141] or a pseudo-resistor [133, 142], whereas the lower cutoff is altered by directly modifying the operational state of the low-noise OTA [125] or by altering its capacitive loading through the selection of distinct output capacitors [143]. However, many of these setups face significant distortion and fluctuations in the higher cutoff due to the voltage-sensitive resistance of MOS elements, requiring strategies to linearize these constituents [129, 144]. These strategies, further refined in [145], achieve exceptional linearity exceeding 74 dB within ±200 mV and frequency cutoff values independent of process variations. Additionally, a configurable switch-capacitor neural amplifier, as reported in [182], presents adaptability for multimodal measurements, accommodating various low- and high-frequency cutoffs while sustaining minimal noise and satisfactory amplification [120].

4.3.2.2 DC Offset Suppression

Creating compact devices that balance low noise and power consumption while preserving neural signals across a broad frequency spectrum presents a significant design obstacle. This challenge stems from the need to incorporate an ultra-low

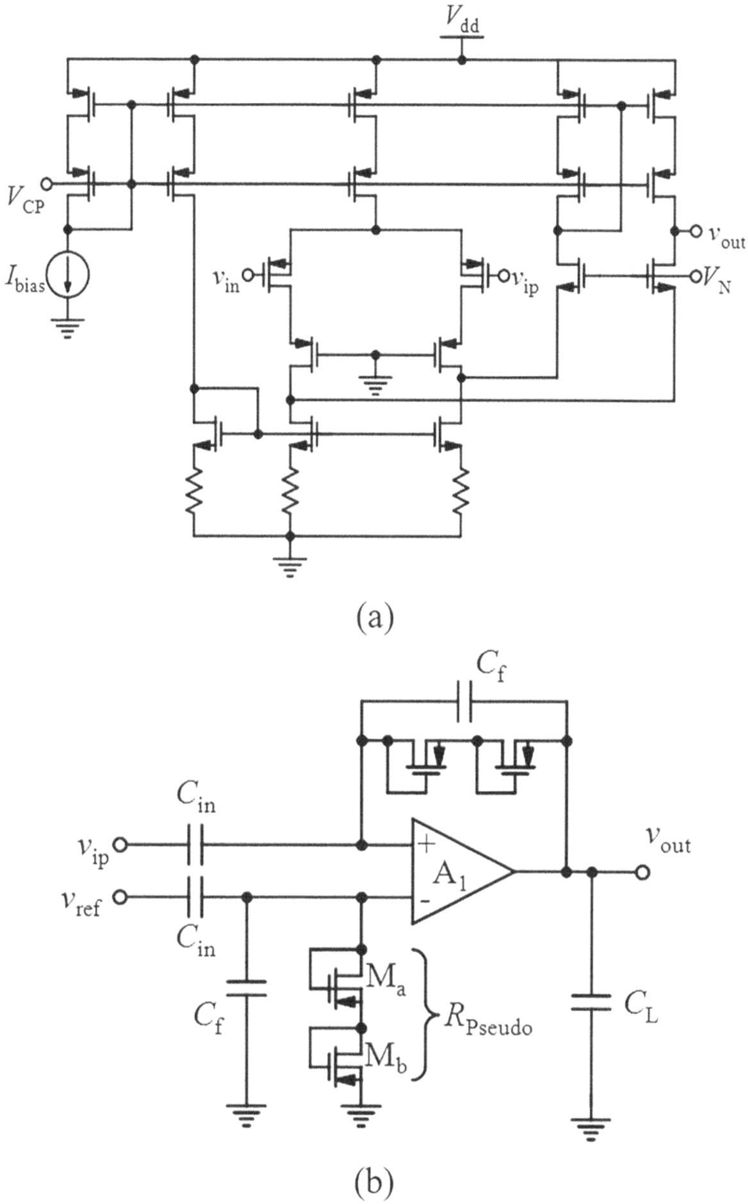

Fig. 4.15 (**a**) The folded OTA with source degeneration, (**b**) The schematic of a neural amplifiers showcasing a capacitive feedback combined with an ADC

cutoff frequency. While some approaches prioritize achieving minimal noise levels [146] or ultra-low power consumption [147], the evolution of integrated neural amplifiers has shifted towards closed-loop configurations. Initially, techniques involved loading the recording site with a high-value resistor, achieved through methods like employing a reverse-biased diode [148] or utilizing subthreshold transistors to construct an HPF in conjunction with electrode capacitance [140].

Recent advancements have seen closed-loop DC suppression methods replacing open-loop approaches, with one common strategy, depicted in Fig. 4.15b, involving the integration of a capacitive feedback network alongside a highly resistive metal-oxide-semiconductor (MOS)-bipolar element to establish closed-loop gain with a low-frequency pole [125]. MOS-bipolar elements can feature equivalent resistors in the several-thousand giga-Ohms range for small voltages, enabling the use of small integrated capacitors in the feedback network to achieve a low-frequency cut off in the mHz range. The feedback loop typically integrates a low-noise OTA with varied implementations [120].

4.3.2.3 Signal Quantization

Proposing an innovative neural-recording integrated circuit (IC) design, Jeon et al. [149] introduced a VCO-based approach for direct signal quantization, achieving a remarkable improvement in input dynamic range (IDR). The circuit incorporates an AC-coupled input transconductance mechanism, converting voltage signals into differential currents, subsequently processed by two CCOs. Utilizing negative feedback controlled by a DAC, the input resistance is adjusted to ensure a wide linear input range, enhancing recording stability by directly connecting the circuit input to the MOSFET gate, leveraging its substantial input impedance [113]. Meanwhile, the selection of an ADC in neural-recording front-ends commonly favors the power-efficient SAR-ADC [50, 150–153]. Nevertheless, challenges arise when dealing with large input swings, potentially leading to IA saturation at the front end, thus necessitating a balance between input range and voltage gain. Despite limitations posed by capacitor matching in modern CMOS processes, efforts are underway to address this trade-off in the voltage domain through various methods explored in recent studies [124, 154–156].

Exploring innovative architectures and signal processing techniques, these approaches aim to mitigate the input range/gain trade-off while enhancing resolution and dynamic range. For instance, frequency-shaping amplifier architectures and oversampled ADCs offer potential solutions, albeit with varying trade-offs in input-referred noise and dynamic range. Alternative strategies, such as direct conversion from voltage to frequency domain using VCO-based ADCs [155], and novel architectures like the continuous-time delta-sigma modulator (CTΔΣM) [156], present promising directions for future development, offering high input impedance, low power consumption, and compact form factors [113].

4.4 CMOS Interface Circuits for Bio/ChemFET-Based Sensing

This section delves into interface circuits designed for Bio/ChemFET sensors, with a particular emphasis on handheld devices, while omitting discussions related to communication components.

Bio/ChemFETs parameters can be evaluated using external tools like a semiconductor parameter analyzer and a potentiostat [157–160], or through on-chip circuits [161–166]. In the linear region, ISFET's output current is expressed by Eq. (3.11), while its threshold voltage is determined by Eq. (3.13) in Chap. 3. However, the actual gate-source voltage and drain-source voltage of ISFET are, $V_{GS,ISFET} = V_{GS}-R_sI_D$ and $V_{DS,ISFET} = V_{DS}-(R_s + R_d)I_D$, respectively, influenced by internal resistances, R_s and R_d, leading to reduced sensitivity. To tackle this, shortening drain and source diffusions becomes imperative, whilst devising readout circuits that show insensitivity to series resistances. Counterbalancing pH-induced threshold voltage changes can be accomplished by adjusting the gate-source voltage, V_{GS}, in the presence of a constant I_D under a set drain-source voltage, V_{DS} [167].

Current-mode readout circuits typically operate in linear mode, particularly in triode ISFETs with low V_{DS}, where the output current can be approximated by [168]:

$$I_D = \mu C_{ox} \frac{W}{L}\left[\left(V_{GS} - V_{th(ISFET)}\right)V_{DS}\right] \tag{4.12}$$

exhibiting linear sensitivity to pH [168]:

$$\frac{dI_D}{dpH} = g_m\left(pH\right) = -2.3\alpha\mu C_{ox}\frac{W}{L}V_T V_{DS} \tag{4.13}$$

The width of the channel (W) is determined by gain requirements, with a trade-off between occupied area and gain, crucial in array structures aiming for suitable array density. The transistor length (L) should be sufficient to mitigate short-channel effects as well as second-order non-linearity sources like mobility degradation.

The method to evaluate the threshold voltage of saturated ISFETs is akin to that of triode variants. Furthermore, ISFETs operating in weak inversion are ideal for crafting energy-efficient, low-voltage circuits, frequently utilized as translinear components.

Velocity saturation, a characteristic of short-channel devices, operates linearly, making it suitable for current-mode readout circuits. It exhibits little sensitivity to mobility (μ), length (L) mismatches, and V_{DS}, particularly in configurations with minimum length:

$$\frac{dI_D}{dpH} = g_m\left(pH\right) = -2.3\alpha V_T v_{sat} C_{ox} W \tag{4.14}$$

In velocity saturation, transistors are typically designed as short-channel devices, with a narrow width advisable to limit the biasing current [168].

Bio/ChemFETs face non-idealities, and several techniques are employed to address these challenges. Trapped charges, causing unpredictable threshold voltage variations, are tackled through methods such as ultraviolet (UV) radiation and hot-electron injection. UV radiation, using a small aperture on ISFETs, stimulates charge migration, aiding in matching electrical characteristics in arrays [169]. Hot-electron injection involves adding electrons to the floating gate, calibrating the threshold voltage [170]. Temperature sensitivity is mitigated using circuit compensation techniques, including differential OpAmp configurations to match ISFETs with MOSFETs [171]. Tuning bias conditions, empirical thermal operating points, and periodic gate resets further cancel temperature coefficients [172, 173] . Flicker noise, a dominant low-frequency noise in ISFETs, is reduced by opting for p-MOSFET-based ISFETs due to their lower noise characteristics [174]. These strategies collectively enhance the reliability of Bio/ChemFETs [170–174].

Here, the readout circuits are classified into seven groups: (1) variable voltage reference in feedback mode, (2) constant-voltage constant-current (CVCC), (3) current-mode readout circuits, (4) Bio/ChemFET logic, (5) Time/frequency modulation, (6) Bio/ChemFET-based active pixel sensors (APSs), and (7) differential measurement.

4.4.1 *Variable Voltage Reference in Feedback Mode*

Fluctuations in I_D are managed via a feedback loop, and adjusting the reference electrode potential with respect to drain and source voltage. So, V_{th} variations can be compensated by modifying V_{gs} using a reference voltage [175–177]. An example is an automatically balanced bridge circuit that compensates for V_{th} variations by adjusting V_{gs} via the RE [175]. However, this method may impose a specific voltage on the analyte, particularly problematic if it lacks grounding, rendering the system sensitive to static electricity and electric fields [167]. Additionally, it is not suitable for measuring multiple ISFETs with a single RE [178]. Figure 4.16 illustrates a readout circuit featuring a programmable gate (PG)-ISFET, featuring a feedback loop enabling comparison and adjustment of the ISFET's current with a reference current, I_{Ref} [176]. This configuration, while effective, may prove unsuitable for array structures due to the need for distinct REs for each pixel, increasing sensor complexity [179].

4.4.2 *Constant-Voltage Constant-Current (CVCC)*

The preferred method for readout circuits of Bio/ChemFET sensors, proposed by Bergveld [167], involves maintaining constant drain voltage and current while allowing the source voltage to vary with pH. This setup automatically adjusts

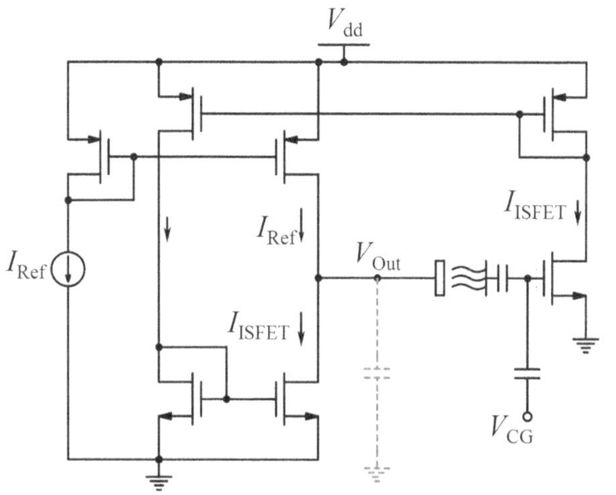

Fig. 4.16 The circuit utilized to evaluate ISFET drift operating in feedback mode

source/drain potentials relative to a constant liquid potential, with grounding the liquid being the optimal choice. Various groups have used this technique for the readout of BioChemFETs [162, 167, 178, 180, 181]. A widely used circuit for achieving these conditions and monitoring ISFET threshold voltage changes is the source/drain follower circuit [167]. In this configuration, the ISFET's floating gate remains unaffected by pH-induced capacitive scaling. Additionally, array sensors utilizing the CVCC technique are compact, requiring only a switch and an ISFET for each pixel [179].

Figure 4.17a depicts a straightforward source/drain follower, as an example, utilizing unsaturated ISFET [178]. With the OpAmp's input voltages equal and V_{R1} and V_{R2} forming part of constant V_{ref}, maintaining constant $V_{R1} = V_{R3}$, and $V_{R2} = V_{ds}$. Consequently, $I_d = V_{R3}/R_3$ remains constant. This setup enables V_{gs} to automatically adjust the source voltage, compensating for variations in ISFET threshold voltage (V_{Th}), ensuring the output voltage accurately represents the change in oxide surface potential. In cases of a system exceeding its limits, indicator diodes illuminate, indicating a restriction on V_{Out} and consequently the source voltage.

These circuits ensure high linearity by maintaining stable biasing and effectively mitigating parasitic capacitance from various nodes to the floating gate, aligning output and input voltages closely [182]. However, using OpAmps leads to increased area occupation and power consumption, particularly critical for arrays with multiple pixels, where sharing readout circuits among pixels in the same row or column serves as an alternative [161, 183–187]. In an effort, Duan et al. [181] introduced a floating CMOS ISFET array featuring cost-effective auto-compensation and enhanced offset distribution tolerance. Their readout circuit employs a P-N complementary source follower to extend the input range and ensure high offset distribution tolerance (see Fig. 4.17b). Digital common-mode voltage adjustment effectively compensates for signal offsets across a wide range before amplification and quantization.

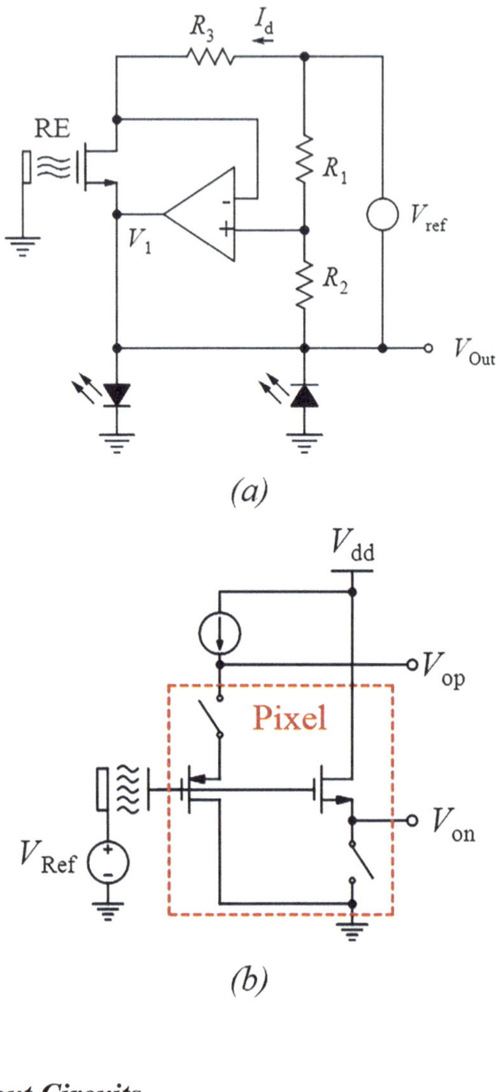

Fig. 4.17 (**a**) A simple source/drain follower structure, (**b**) An ISFET front-end system utilizing a complementary source follower

4.4.3 Current-Mode Readout Circuits

Several circuits for reading ISFET output current have been documented [168, 188–201], utilizing current-mode techniques compatible with linear region, velocity saturation, and weak inversion states [179]. Additionally, many of these circuits employ CCs, serving as buffers within voltage-mode setups.

The drain current range provided by FETs in the weak inversion region typically falls within the nano-ampere range or lower, making them ideal for low-power sensor designs. Moreover, this region offers the highest transconductance-to-current ratio, maximizing intrinsic voltage gain [189]. Additional advantages include minimal requirements for V_{ds} and gate voltage, as well as reduced gate capacitance [202]. The exponential correlation between V_{gs} and I_d facilitates novel design possibilities, including log-domain filters, through translinear and bipolar circuit techniques, such as log-domain filters.

Shepherd et al. [189, 203] introduced a hydrogen cell (Hcell) employing translinear operation, producing an output current directly correlated to pH, as depicted in Fig. 4.18a. Another innovation by Georgiou et al. [190, 204] involved a log-domain filter integrating an ISFET biased in weak inversion at its input. Figure 4.18b illustrates a first-order log-domain filter showcasing this feature. Additionally, Fig. 4.18c presents an alternative setup where the drain current of the MOSFET, functioning in weak inversion, is substituted by a chemically modulated signal, allowing filter parameters such as gain and cutoff frequency to depend on the ion concentration of the analyte. To maintain DC stability, certain current-mode circuits utilize feedback mechanisms [191, 200, 201].

4.4.4 Bio/ChemFET Logic

Wong et al. [205] introduced discrete ISFET logic for chemical reaction threshold detection, negating the need for precise pH measurement. Using components like comparators such as a NAND gate [40], a Schmitt trigger [206], or a switch [207, 208], an inverter's switching threshold can yield a binary response to pH changes. Various configurations of ISFET inverters, depicted in Fig. 4.19a-c, utilize either single p-type or n-type ISFETs or a combination of both, with sensitivity to threshold voltage varying based on the ratio of PMOS and NMOS aspect ratios (β_p/β_n) [209]. For example, Al-Ahdal et al. [207, 208] proposed a complementary pair of n-type and p-type ISFETs sharing the same ion-sensitive membrane, acting as an ISFET-based chemical switch (Fig. 4.19a). Nabovati et al. [209] expanded upon these switches in an 8 × 8 array, achieving a sensitivity of 50 mV/pH across a wide pH range from 1 to 14.

4.4.5 Time/Frequency Modulation

A method discussed for interpreting ISFET outputs involves translating pH values into time and pulse-width modulation (PWM) signals [163, 182, 210–221]. This process can be accomplished using complementary ISFET-based inverters, forming the foundation of a pH-to-time converter, which interacts capacitively with a triangular wave. The switching point of this wave, and consequently the resulting pulse width, adapts to pH fluctuations. Adopting a purely time-based readout offers the advantage of a compact layout and addresses speed limitations, as highlighted by [210, 222].

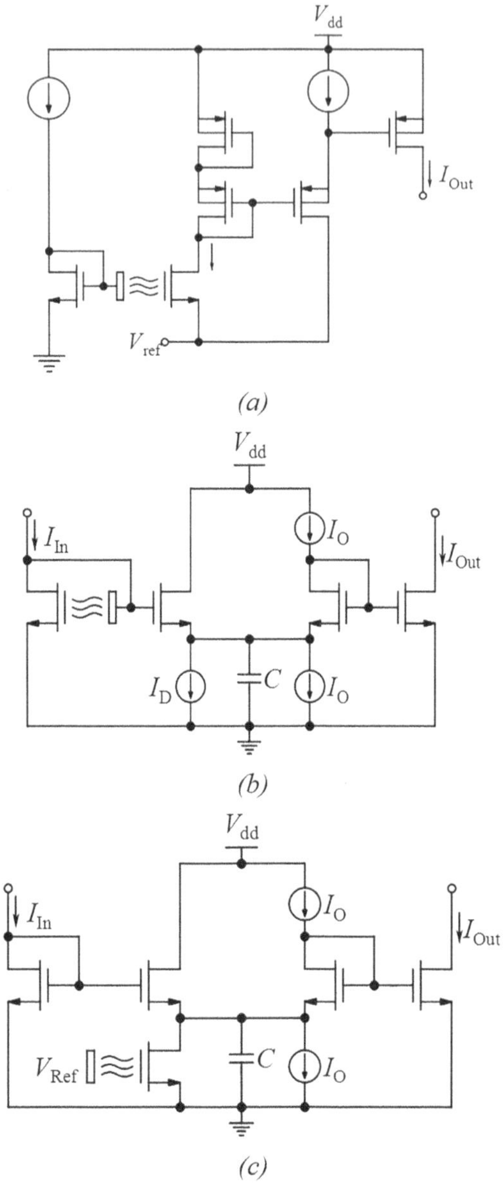

Fig. 4.18 (**a**) An HCell operating in a translinear mode, (**b**) A first-order filter in a log-domain configuration utilizing an ISFET at its input, (**c**) A log-domain filter chemically adjustable

PWM-based methods show potential in improving the SNR through in-pixel quantization, as emphasized in [179], yet caution is warranted regarding readout synchronization and parasitic effects in extensive arrays, as acknowledged in [182]. Illustrated in Fig. 4.20a, Liu et al. [210] presented a PWM-based interface requiring additional amplification to ensure accurate data conversion without introducing noise into the chemical signal. In another effort, Moser et al. [211–213] introduced

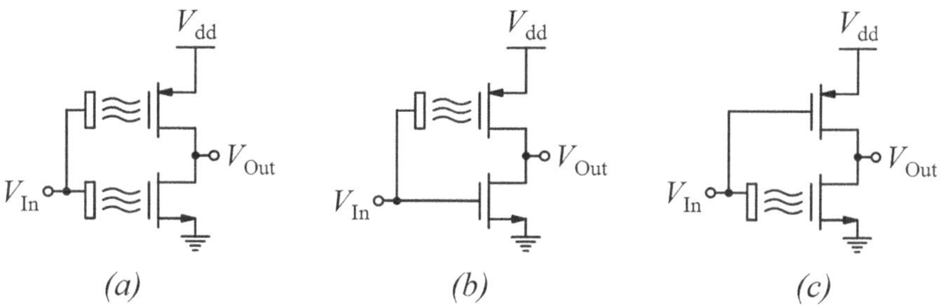

Fig. 4.19 Three variations of ISFET inverters where: (**a**) both n-type and p-type ISFETs utilize a common membrane, (**b**) an n-type MOSFET and a p-type ISFET sharing a membrane, and (**c**) a p-type MOSFET paired with an n-type ISFET, both with a membrane

an APS-driven pH-to-time conversion system, illustrated in Fig. 4.20b, utilizing current discharging output points and a cyclic reset strategy coupled with capacitor discharging via the ISFET to translate pH into pulse duration.

4.4.6 Bio/ChemFET-Based Active Pixel Sensors (APSs)

Integrated APS sensors utilizing ISFETs either replace photodiodes using charge transfer [223, 224] or function as standard buffers [225, 226]. These sensors typically employ common source circuits to convert chemical voltage to current or voltage output, either via current output using CCs [227] or discharging load capacitors [213]. However, managing constant biasing and capacitor ratios in floating gates is crucial to mitigate non-linearity and signal reduction, necessitating calibration and pH-to-voltage mapping due to insufficient linearity in open-loop methods.

In certain sensor arrays [227, 228], a traditional pixel readout, akin to the CVCC method shown in Fig. 4.21a, is utilized, integrating an ISFET and two switches. Huang et al. [225] introduced a dual-mode sensor merging a CMOS image sensor with an ISFET acting as standard buffers, as illustrated in Fig. 4.21b, incorporating additional circuitry in one pixel for optical sensing alongside pH measurement. Sawada et al. [223, 224, 229, 230] proposed a charge transfer-based accumulation technique for ion sensing utilizing a four-transistor APS, depicted in Fig. 4.21c, transforming surface potential variations into electrical charge packets and converting them into voltage through and the source follower and the floating diffusion (FD) amplifier. To enhance spatial resolution and reduce pixel size, a simplified three-transistor APS was introduced (Fig. 4.21d), charging electrons into the FD and selectively discharging them based on the sensing area's potential level, followed by readout via a source follower circuit [231].

Fig. 4.20 (**a**) A PWM-based interface providing time output, (**b**), an APS-based pH-to-time converter with current discharging output nodes

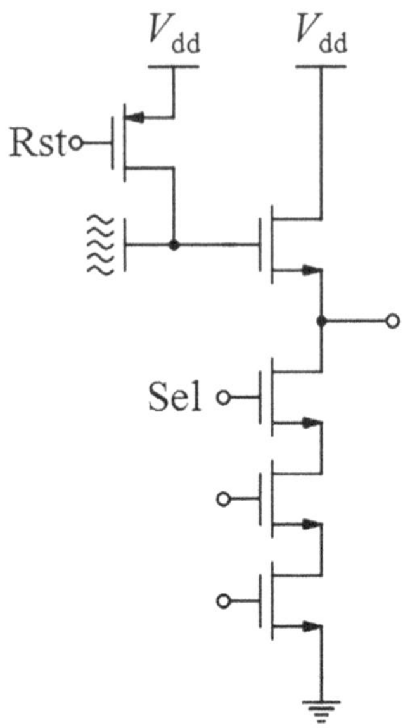

(a)

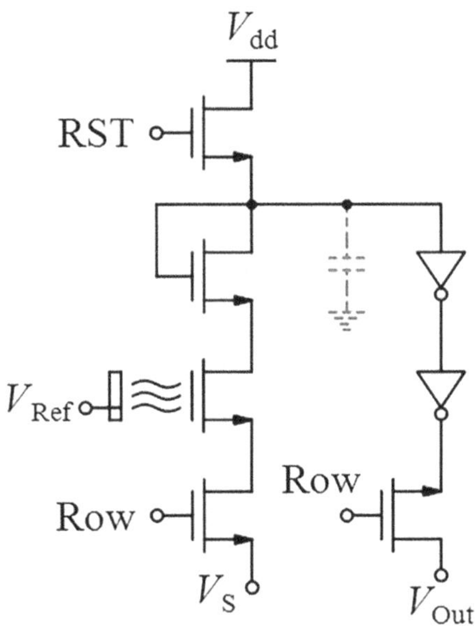

(b)

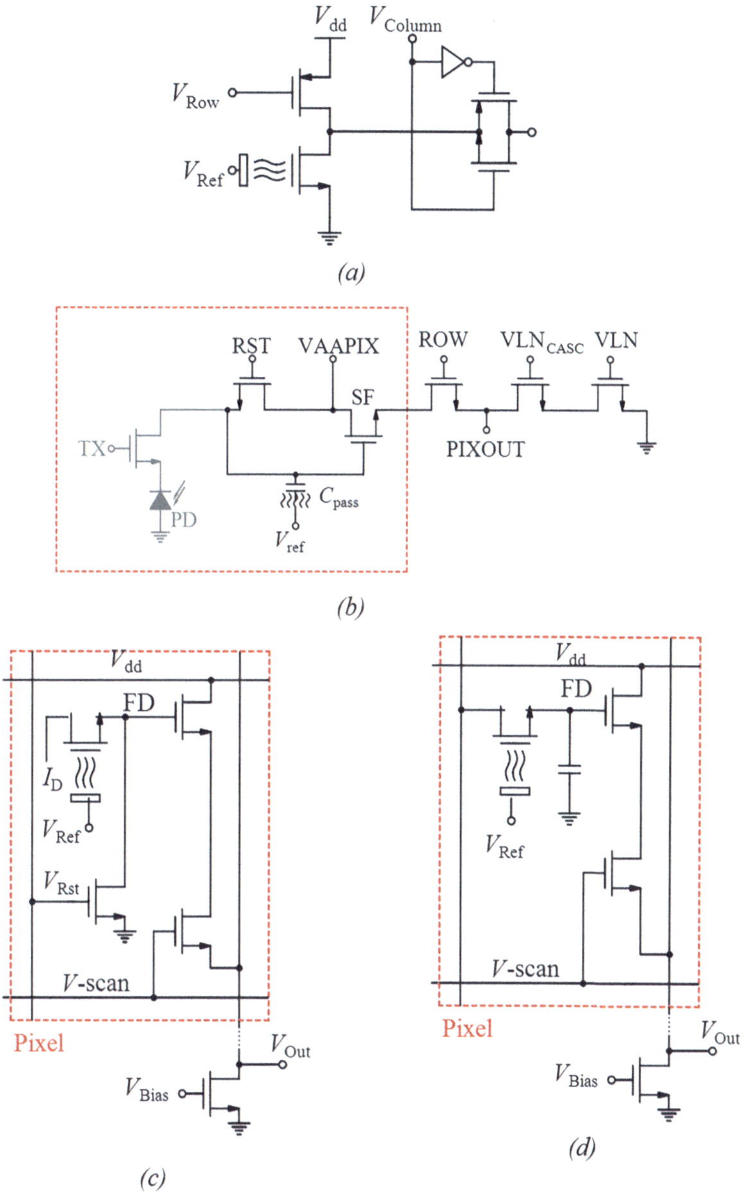

Fig. 4.21 (**a**) A typical ISFET pixel readout, (**b**) a dual-function circuit combining a source follower with a CMOS image sensor, (**c**) A four-transistor APS topology, (**d**) A three-transistor APS topology

4.4.7 Differential Measurements

These approaches rely on contrasting the output signals from two ISFETs with identical REs, termed differential measurement, aiming to alleviate temperature fluctuations, common-mode noise, and long-term drift. An inherent challenge with Bio/ChemFET-based sensors lies in the limited lifespan of liquid-filled REs, often requiring a sizable RE alongside a small sensor probe, restricting measurement volumes [165, 171, 186, 232–239]. Consequently, the interest in differential measurement techniques between ISFETs and identical reference FETs (REFETs) has surged due to their minimal sensitivity to sample ion concentration. In this method, a metal wire grounds the sample solution, enabling the biasing of a differential structure comprising an ISFET and REFET using a common counter-electrode, termed the pseudo-reference electrode (PRE) [178]. Typically crafted from noble metals like platinum or gold, the PRE facilitates determining the electrolyte voltage without external REs.

Creating low-sensitive REFETs usually involves applying an extra ion-insensitive membrane to the ISFET's gate oxide, achieved through methods such as surface site chemical [240] or polymer use [232, 241], with source and bulk connections often short-circuited [232].

Hammond et al. [186] introduced a digital pH meter designed for wireless diagnostic capsules, featuring multiplexers and on-chip programmable voltage references controlled by a microcontroller. The analog segment of this differential pH measurement system is portrayed in Fig. 4.22, where two source/drain followers for REFET and ISFET as well as a common PRE are integrated, with their outputs directed to an IA.

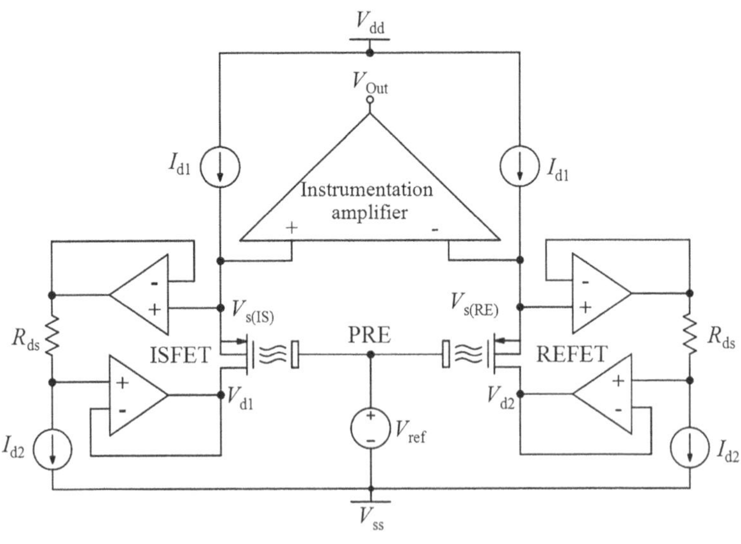

Fig. 4.22 A pixel configuration for differential pH measurement featuring ISFET and REFET, designed for an array structure.

4.5 CMOS Optical Biosensors

Fluorescent and luminescent biosensors are typically the widespread and preferred options for producing a detectable signal in the optical spectrum. In such sensors, the light signals generated by biochemical reactions convert into a measurable current signal through a photo-sensor element. The need for bulky laboratory setups to detect weak generated optical signals severely hampers the widespread application of optical biosensors. Fortunately, CMOS technology, through its integration capabilities, stands out as the ideal solution to overcome this obstacle. On the other hand, precise current measurement at the input stage of the readout circuit holds significant importance in CMOS optical biosensors. Also, a data converter is crucial to generate the output data in a digital format. According to the researcher's reports, the most commonly used current conveyors for optical sensing are the negative-feedback transimpedance amplifier (NF-TIA), and direct current integration (DCI), which will be examined following.

4.5.1 Current Conveyor Circuits

In this section, two widely used structures of current conveyor circuits including NF-TIA and DCI will be described.

4.5.1.1 Negative-Feedback Transimpedance Amplifier (NF-TIA)

The basic NF-TIA topology shown in Fig. 4.23, uses a voltage amplifier with a feedback network of resistor or capacitor to convert the photodiode current to the detectable voltage [242–248]. By utilizing a resistive feedback TIA (RF-TIA) structure with a high resistance, there is the potential for achieving high gain and low noise performance in CMOS optical biosensors. However, the trade-off lies in the fact that a large resistor can limit the bandwidth and require more physical space [249]. To address this issue capacitive feedback TIA (CF-TIA) is more favorable structures in optical biosensors [242–248]. Alternatively, CF-TIA can be utilized

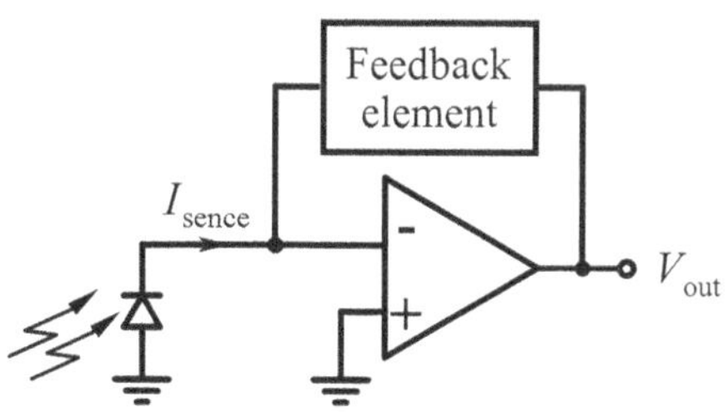

Fig. 4.23 Schematic of the NF-TIA

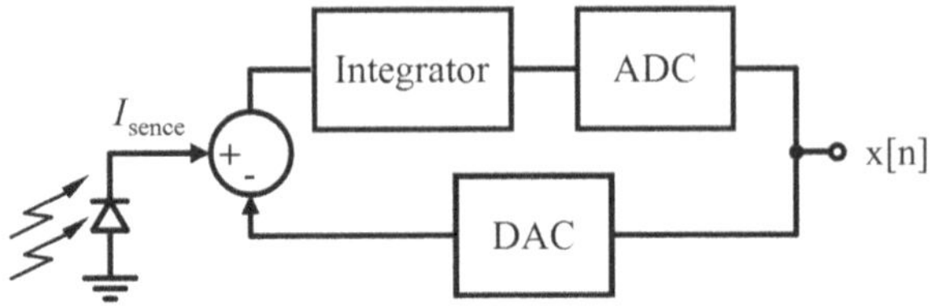

Fig. 4.24 The schema of ΔΣ current sensing

within the loop of a ΔΣ current sensing modulator as the detector [244, 250, 251]. Illustrated Fig. 4.24, the fundamental principle of ΔΣ current sensing involves feeding the photodiode current (input signal) into a high DC gain integrator, which is then connected to an ADC. The sensor output is represented by the digital output from the ADC, which is used to control a DAC. The DAC subsequently adjusts the input signal by subtracting an output-dependent current.

4.5.1.2 Direct Current Integration (DCI)

In the structure of DCI depicted in Fig. 4.25, the photocurrent produced by incident photons is directly integrated over the capacitance of the photodiode over a specified duration and transformed into charge. Then, this charge will be read as a voltage signal V_{Out} [252].

4.5.2 Data Transfer

As modern electronics continue to advance, numerous studies document the integration of miniature optical biosensors using the CMOS process. Miniaturized optical sensors allowed the realization of portable devices for sensitive imaging [253], medical diagnostics [254], gene expression control [247], and environmental sensing [255]. Prior studies have demonstrated that miniaturized CMOS optical sensors rely on wired communication. More recently, along with the advancement of CMOS technology real-time sensing has taken the attention of researchers to introduce a new generation of biosensors as ingestible electronics. In-body ingestible sensors, enabling real-time monitoring of internal targets, offer data that can be leveraged for early treatment assessments, thereby fostering a more personalized approach to medicine. Such sensors rely on wireless interfaces for communication within the body and outside the medium. In this section, we will miniaturize CMOS optical sensors with wire and wireless interfaces.

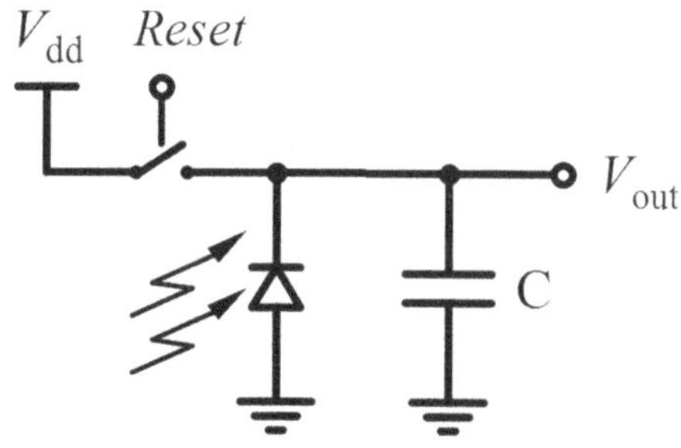

Fig. 4.25 The simplifies scheme showing the principle of DCI

4.5.2.1 CMOS Optical Sensors Located Outside the Body

Recently, there has been substantial research focused on the integration of external components onto a chip to enable fully integrated optical biosensors. This integration streamlines the creation of compact and highly automated testing platforms for point-of-care (PoC) analysis. The emergence of lab-on-a-chip (LoC) technology presents an encouraging avenue for PoC diagnostics. This innovative technology facilitates rapid and accurate analysis of biological samples in a miniaturized form. It integrates and automates the processes of sampling, preparation, analysis, and reporting of diverse chemical compounds. For instance, Eltoukhy et al. [256] introduced a integrated bioluminescence detection LoC for gene expression analysis through reporter gene assays, intracellular adenosine triphosphate (ATP) determination, and deoxyribonucleic acid (DNA) sequencing. The detection system features a fiber-optic faceplate (FOF) that has immobilized luminescent reporters/probes connected directly to an optical CMOS detection system. This setup is fabricated using a 0.18 μm CMOS process. A block diagram illustrating the detection SoC can be found in Fig. 4.26. The system is divided into three key sections: an 8 × 16 pseudo-differential pixel array, a 13-bit 128-channel ADC, and a column-level digital signal processing (DSP) single-instruction multiple-data (SIMD) array. In this study, as shown in Fig. 4.27, a pseudo-differential circuit design utilizing the DCI concept was employed as a readout circuit. This design offers specific capabilities, including the detection of emission rates below 10–6 lux (4 × 105 photons/cm^2) over a 30-second integration period at room temperature, an intrinsic dynamic range of 61 dB, and a static power consumption of 26 mW.

Jang et al. [257] have developed an integrated fluorescent-based biosensor tailored for DNA microarrays. This sophisticated system includes a transducer array, molecular capture probes, a fluorescent emission filter, and readout circuitry incorporating components such as CF-TIA, chopper-stabilized preamp, and a 14-bit ADC. To integrate the biochemical aspect of the assay with the fluorescent detector seamlessly, capturing probes are positioned on the chip and linked to the CMOS detector through a FOF. This sensor is particularly effective for detection in real-time of fluorescent signals emitted from biological targets. It has enabled the authors

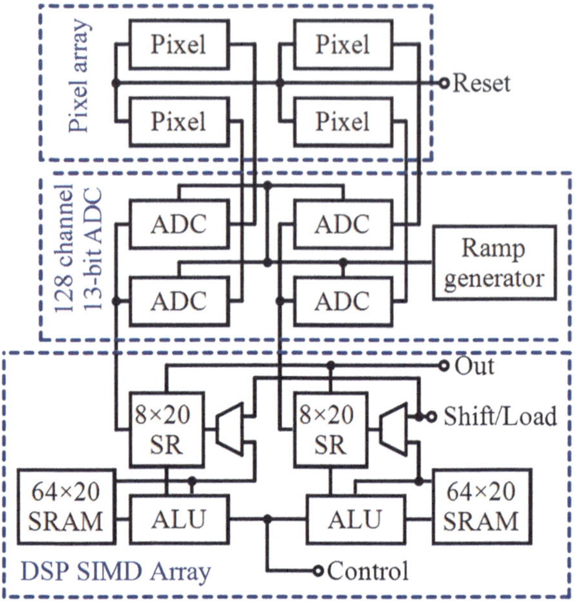

Fig. 4.26 Block diagram of bioluminescence detection arrays

Fig. 4.27 Schema of pseudo-differential pixel

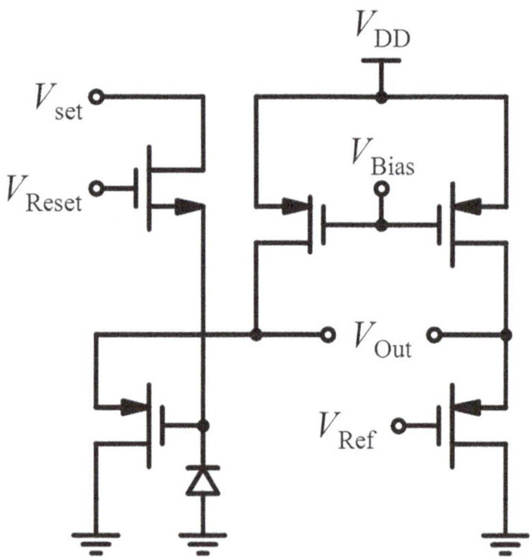

to investigate the kinetics of real-time DNA hybridization across three DNA target concentrations in solution.

In another work, Hong et al. [242] introduced copper-based nanoplasmonic filters for the initial time to actualize a fully integrated fluorescence biosensor in a 65 nm CMOS process. This development has paved the way for conducting vast multiplexed assays on a one chip, with a broad range of applications spanning from in vitro to in vivo settings. Notably, this sensor demonstrates the ability to detect 48 zeptomoles of Qdot-based fluorophores on the surface, while the filter attains over 50 dB of measured rejection.

Another fully integrated fluorescence sensor was presented by Aghlmand et al. [247] for dynamic monitoring of living cells. This design is shown in Fig. 4.28 comprises on-chip bandpass optical filters, photodiodes, CF-TIA, correlated double sampler (CDS), and resistive adder block in 65 nm standard CMOS. This study successfully captures the signals from different optical filters and photodiodes positioned differentially across the central and left/right columns of the chip using six rows of front-end circuitry. In the design, each row utilizes a CF-TIA with a variable feedback capacitor to turn the differential photodiode current into voltage. CDS eliminated low-frequency correlated noise components and offset by sampling the output of the CF-TIA twice in each row [258]. Moreover, a resistive adder is implemented to compound the outputs of multiple rows on the chip, thereby amplifying the signal strength. The sensor further encompasses an on-chip thermal sensor, as well as a clock generator and a digital scan chain block for efficient distribution of all digital control bits within the circuit.

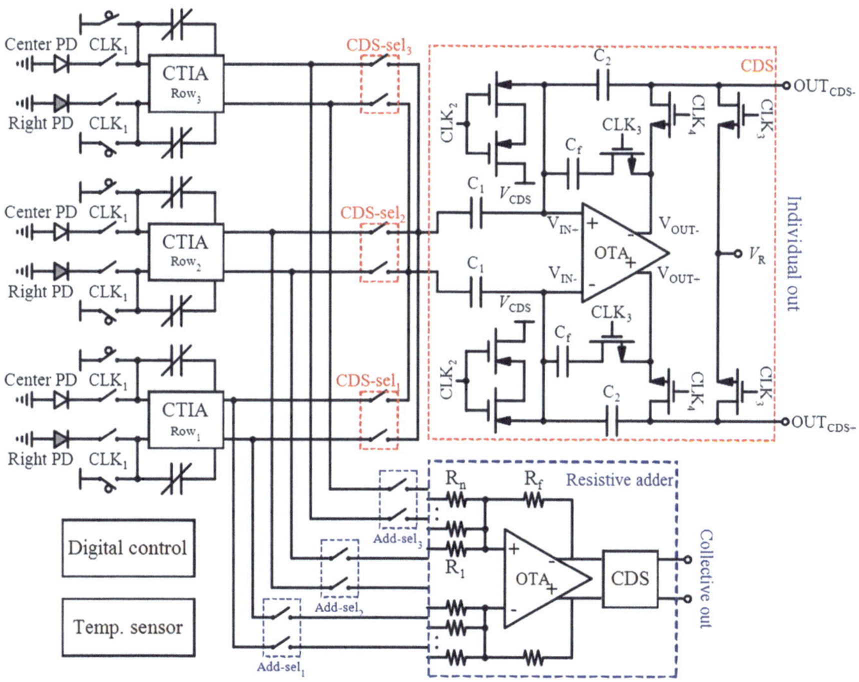

Fig. 4.28 Readout circuit of a fully integrated fluorescence-based sensor for dynamic monitoring of living cells

4.5.2.2 CMOS Optical Sensors Located Inside the Body

The design of implantable optical biosensors has received lots of attention, particularly for real-time monitoring within the body, neural signal monitoring, and brain imaging. For example, in a study by Noormohammadi et al. [250], an advanced optoelectronic biosensor has been proposed for use in wired implantable fiber photometry applications utilizing a 0.18 μm CMOS process. The research involved merging a differential CMOS photodetector with a differential capacitive transimpedance amplifier (DCTIA) to act as an input photo-sensing module, combined with a second order 1-bit CTΔΣM to achieve a wide dynamic range, simplified implementation, and high energy efficiency. Kobayashi et al. [259] introduced another wired implantable sensor for optical communication with brain cells. While wired implantable sensors [250, 259–261] provide high performance, the infection risk arising from the external wiring limits their effectiveness for continuous monitoring.

Rabbani et al. proposed the first wireless implantable fluorescence image sensor [262]. The further explained and expanded this work presented in [253]. Figure 4.29a depicts the block diagram of this design comprising 4 main blocks: (1) power management unit (PMU), (2) imaging front-end, (3) laser driver, and (4) finite state machine (FSM). The PMU includes an active rectifier and multiple low-dropout voltage regulators (LDOs) to power different subcomponents. The imaging front-end comprise of the pixel array (see Fig. 4.29b) and the structure of each pixel along with the sample and hold are demonstrated in Figs. 4.29c and 4.29d, respectively. The imager array is connected to the readout circuitry, buffers, and a differential 8-bit SAR ADC for converting the analog pixel values into digital data. The laser driver delivers a consistent current to the laser diode using the charge stored in C_{Store}. The FSM manages the timing and functions of the chip, coordinating them with the external ultrasound (US) transducer. The operation of this design is as follows [253]. The mote piezo detects US pulses emitted by an external transducer, and an active rectifier transforms the US signal into a DC voltage (V_{Rect}), charging the storage capacitor of C_{Store} to a maximum of 5 V. Upon V_{Rect} reaching 4.2 V, a power-on-reset (POR) signal is activated, leading to the FSM resetting to the charging state. A watchdog signal supervises intervals without ultrasound to direct the FSM state transitions, synchronized by the clock extracted from the US waveform upon detecting the initial rising edge of the watchdog signal, the chip shifts to the imaging state, initiating the laser driver and capturing the image using the pixel array. Following the integration period, which is adjustable within the range of 16–128 ms and can be programmed into the implant, the laser and pixel array are deactivated. Post image capture, the pixels are sampled sequentially by an 8-bit SAR ADC. This image sensor can transmit 11.52 kbits of data in a single measurement cycle by providing power to the 0.26 mW pixel array and the substantial 78 mW power of the laser diode during a 64 ms illumination interval.

In another work, Zhu et al. [245] proposed a 15-pixel fluorescence-based biosensing array with integrated nanoplasmonic filters and transmitter (TX)/receiver (RX) modules for ingestible electronic applications. The structure of the sensor is

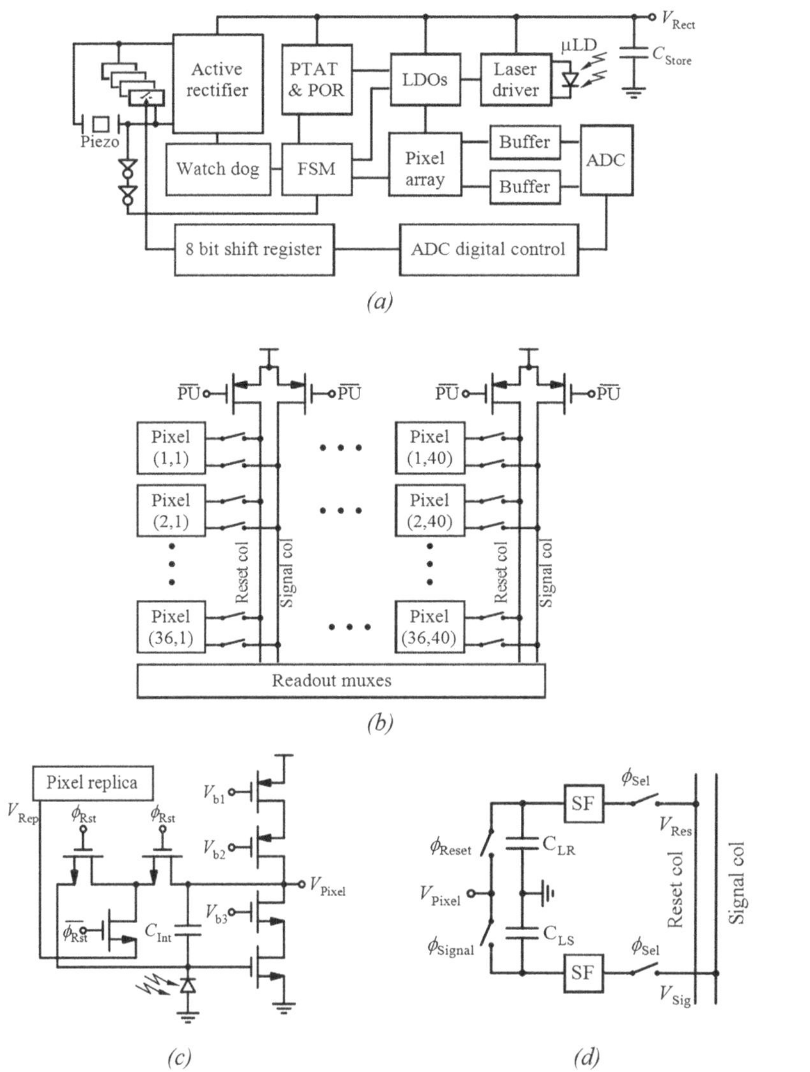

Fig. 4.29 (**a**) Simplifies block diagram of the IC, (**b**) structure of the imager array, (**c**) Schematic of a pixel, (**d**) In-pixel sample and hold

shown in Fig. 4.30a that fabricated in 65 nm CMOS process. The chip's 15-pixel array enables it to conduct multiplex biomolecular assays. The RX decodes amplitude-shift keying (ASK)/ on-off keying (OOK) pulse pause encoding (PPE)-modulated radio frequency (RF) signals, removing the requirement for a high-power clock data recovery (CDR) circuit. After decoding, the serial data is transformed into 20 parallel bits, with 12 of these bits allocated to the timing control module (TCM) to ensure accurate integration timing for the photodiodes. This allows the

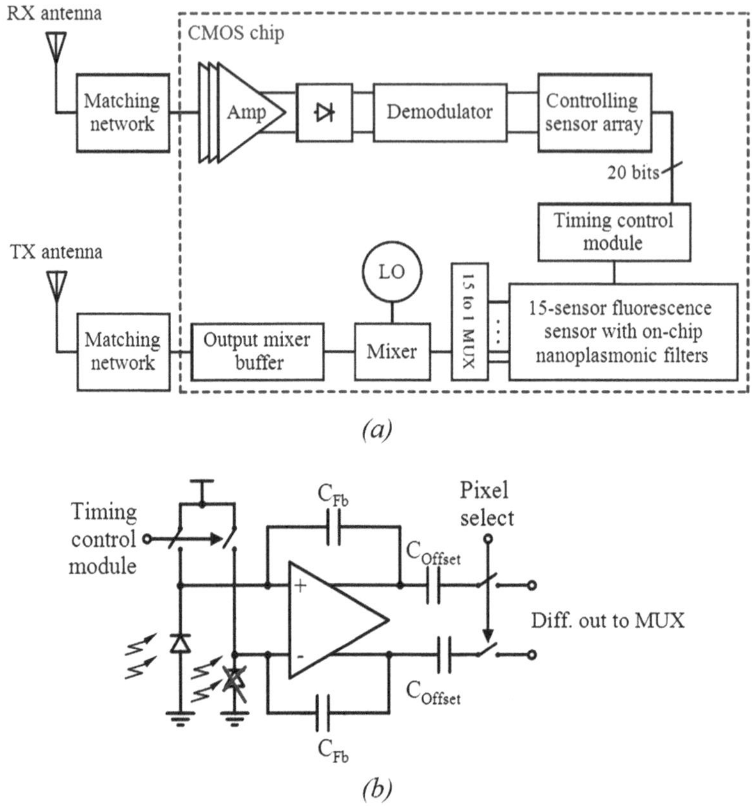

Fig. 4.30 (**a**) Structure of the biomolecular fluorescence-based sensor incorporating an ultra-low power wireless interface (**b**) CF-TIA with differential photodiode with one optically sealed (blue cross)

sensor to effectively adapt to complex biological environments. Four out of the remaining eight bits are assigned for pixel selection by the decoder. The analog output baseband signal originating from the pixel array undergoes modulation at 100 MHz and is then transmitted through a dedicated TX antenna for external reception, serving as an optimal solution for debugging tasks. The structure of each pixel is shown in Fig. 4.30b, which consists of two photodiodes and a CF-TIA to convert the fluorescent signal from photodiodes to a readable voltage signal. The differential structure plays a crucial role in eliminating common mode dark current and eradicating integration time uncertainties. This research marks a pioneering effort in the realm of ingestible electronics, showcasing CMOS ICs with remarkable picomolar sensitivity in protein/DNA assays and wireless transmission capabilities through multiple tissue layers. The project underscores groundbreaking advancements in energy efficiency within this domain.

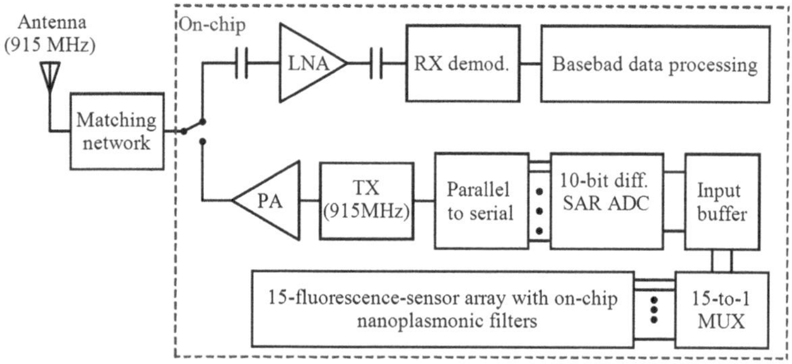

Fig. 4.31 Block diagram of the first ingestible fluorescence sensor chip

An ingestible CMOS fluorescence sensor array presented for the first time by Zhu et al. [248], featuring a bi-directional 915 MHz OOK/frequency shift keying (FSK) wireless interface, and advanced optics packaging for in-vivo bio-molecular sensing. Figure 4.31 illustrate the structure of the ingestible optical sensor chip implemented in a 65 nm LP process. Incorporating a 15-pixel photodiode sensor array, this innovative design features on-chip metal-based nano-optic plasmonic filters (M_4-M_7). These filters showcase an impressive capability to reduce background interference by more than 39 dB.

The output current of the photodiode is integrated with a CTIA and then through a 10-bit SAR ADC is digitized. A FSK/OOK TX consist of a current-starving oscillator and a switching power amplifier (PA) transmit the digitized data to the external base station with output power of −15 dBm. On the other hand, the signal received by RX is utilized to activate a FSM that manages the sensor operations, incorporating all timing generation digital circuitries on the chip. Noteworthy, the sensitivity and power consumption of the RX reported as −59 dBm and 121 μW, respectively. The fluorescence sensor can achieve a detection limit of 40 dots/μm^2 of Qdots and detect target DNA molecules within the range of 100 pM to 1 nM. This design enables real-time monitoring of intricate bio-molecular processes in an in-vivo environment with exceptional sensitivity while maintaining low power consumption. It is notable, this design is powered by a 1.55 V, 12.5 mAh coin-cell battery with a dimension of 0.9 × 2.3 cm^2. Also, Liu et al. [263], in their groundbreaking work unveiled the inaugural ultra-compact bacterial-electronic ingestible capsule. This cutting-edge device features an integrated CMOS threshold-based bioluminescence detector, fueled by a diminutive 5.5 mAh coin-cell battery.

The authors in [264] to eliminate the battery powering, proposed a multicolor fluorescence-based image sensor providing real-time monitoring in cancer therapy relies on power harvesting. This work is introduced as a first implantable fluorescence image sensor capable of both wireless communication and power transfer, operation at 5 cm depth, and 3-color fluorescence imaging while benefit from a the highly small form factor (0.09 cm^3).

4.6 CMOS Magnetic Biosensors

The utilization of magnetic particles in medical diagnostics has garnered considerable attention in recent times. Since their signals remain stable in biological systems and buffer solutions, allowing for reliable detection and extended shelf life [265]. The magnetic biosensors discussed in this section include Hall-effect biosensors, inductive biosensors, and giant magnetoresistance (GMR) biosensors. Overall, this section aims to provide insights into how different types of magnetic sensors are implemented using CMOS technology and their applications in detecting magnetic signals from labeled biological objects.

4.6.1 Hall-Effect Magnetic Biosensors

The combination of high reliability, accuracy, and compatibility with CMOS technology has made silicon-based Hall sensors indispensable for a diverse of applications [266–272]. The market's need for advanced biosensors that can efficiently interface with biological entities in testing and accurately interpret microscopic biochemical processes is consistently on the rise. The Hall magnetic sensors hold significant promise in bio-applications owing to their compact size, affordability, and seamless integration with CMOS technology [266–270, 272–277]. For instance, Besse et al. [273] introduced a high-sensitivity silicon CMOS Hall sensor designed to detect magnetic microbeads of 2.8 μm in diameter, which paving the path for cost-effective microsystems tailored for biochemical applications. Liu et al. [267] designed a CMOS 8 × 8 Hall-effect magnetic sensor that employed a magnetic relaxation technique to characterize and detect magnetic nanoparticles (MNPs) in biomedical applications. Figure 4.32 shows the magnetic relaxation measurements. During phase 1, B_{Ext} is applied for a specified time of t_m and removed for a duration of t_r. Then to omitted the large baseline of B_{Ext}, the magnetic field induced in MNPs (B_{MNPs}) is measured at duration of relaxation time. Noteworthy, during phase 2 the

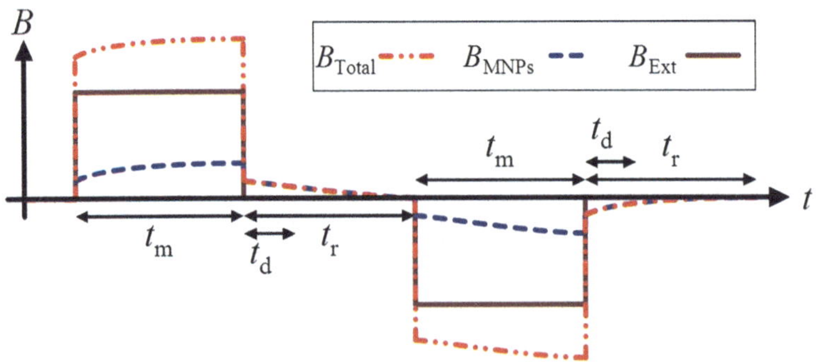

Fig. 4.32 The timing diagram of the detection technique relies on magnetic relaxation

magnetic is applied in the opposite direction in which by achieving difference of phases 1 and 2 through CDS method, the stray magnetic fields can be suppressed. In this research, three MNPs samples were analyzed. The samples included magnetite nanocrystals with 20 nm and 25 nm diameters coated with oleic acid, as well as magnetic beads suspended in double-distilled water at a concentration of 50 mg[solids]/ml. These samples were measured using the CMOS Hall-effect sensor. The samples exhibit distinct relaxation behaviors, indicating variations in their intrinsic magnetic properties. In another design, to detect the concentration of human serum albumin (HAS), a CMOS Hall sensor with 10,240 sensing sites using 2.8 μm Dynal beads as labels is presented by Gambini et al. [268]. This design reduced the readout time by 4 times compared to their previous works [274] by implementing a parallel readout interface instead of a single readout. Another advantage is that the sensitivity of the magnetic beads is improved by more than 50 times compared with a single Hall sensor. In addition, employing nested chopping and auto-zeroing decreases the noise and drifts. Bhalla et al. [275] utilized TSMC's 0.35 μm process to develop a Hall sensor capable of detecting specific proteins within 10 nm magnetic beads.

Kuo et al. [276] implemented a LoC Hall sensor in 0.35 μm CMOS process for human whole blood testing in which a micro-controller unit (MCU) is utilized to control the detection procedure. Figure 4.33 depicts the architecture of the system-on-a-chip (SoC) sensor. It consists of a reference and sensing Hall sensor array

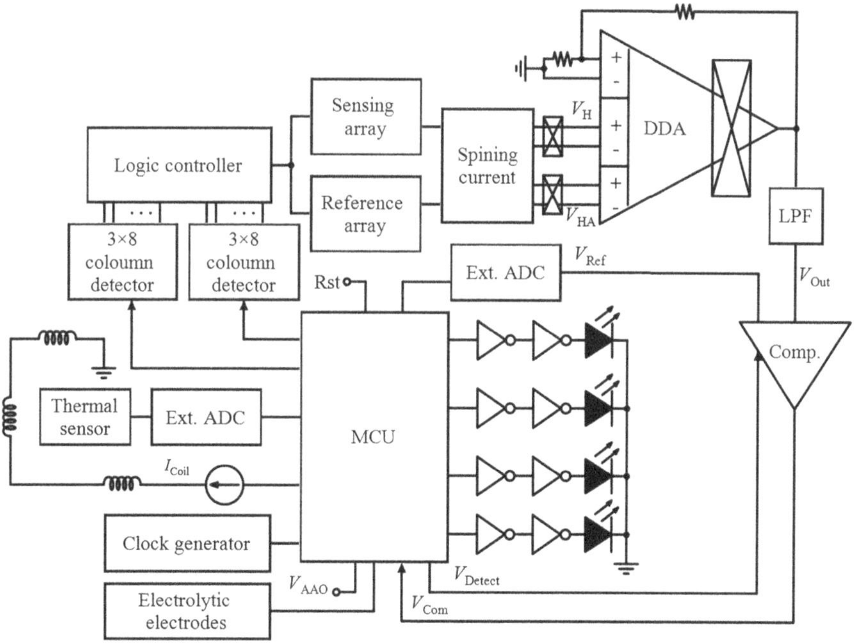

Fig. 4.33 Schematic of the CMOS assay SoC with MCU

(antibodies are immobilized on the sensing part), chopped spinning current circuit, chopper stabilized differential difference amplifier (DDA), low pass filter (LPF), comparator, thermal sensor, clock generator, row and column decoders, logic controller, and MCU. The on-chip polarization coil generates the magnetic field and magnetizes the magnetic beads. The sensor utilized the current spinning technique for offset cancellation. Using DDA, the voltage discrepancy between a Hall sensor primarily for sensing (V_H) and a Hall sensor set as a reference (V_{HA}) is determined. V_H is chopper down-converted to its base frequency while the offset of the Hall sensor and DDA is up-converted to a higher frequency for processing. Then to filter the up-converted offset signal and complete offset cancellation, an LPF is utilized. In the following, to enable a comparison between the V_{Out} and V_{Ref}, MCU sends V_{Detect} to the comparator, and then the comparison voltage (V_{Com}) will be applied to the MCU. The voltage of the V_{Ref} is defined by the relationship between the biomarker concentration curve and the Hall voltage curve. Due to the baseline voltage's sensitivity to temperature, a thermal sensor is utilized to calibrate the thermal-induced offset voltage. In this work, the off-chip components are an external ADC (Ext. ADC), an external DAC (Ext. DAC), a current generator, and four indicating light-emitting diodes (LEDs). In the end, in the case of surpassing of the target biomolecules in the human blood sample from the predetermined statistical threshold, the MCU will transmit a signal, causing the LED to illuminate and alert the user.

Chang et al. [277] presented a Hall sensor for a wearable biomagnetic sensor for SoC in a 0.5 μm CMOS process. In their work to minimize the variation in sensitivity of the Hall probe, the sensor produces a reference magnetic field using an on-chip coil. Furthermore, it uses a calibration technique for compensating of the Hall probe's drift error. In another work, a current-mode CMOS Hall sensor is developed by Heidari et al. [270] to show the feasibility of employing CMOS magnetic sensors for magnetomyography (MMG) applications. The cross-shaping current-mode Hall sensor with the block diagram of the sensor is shown in Fig. 4.34. The bias current I_{Bias} passes from two probes of Hall sensors while differential Hall currents, $I_{M,}$ and I_N are generated at two other probes of Hall sensors. In the following, the output current of the Hall sensors is turned to the voltage by a chopper integrator amplifier and followed by a low-pass filter. This architecture aims to modify the SNR and sensitivity as the reported experimental results show a high sensitivity of approximately 2400 V/A/mT.

4.6.2 Inductive Biosensor

Inductive sensors work according to the principle of electromagnetic induction. They detect changes in the magnetic field by measuring variations in inductance. When a magnetic field interacts with a coil, it induces a voltage or current in the coil, which can be measured to detect the presence and strength of the magnetic field. In the inductive sensors for biomedical applications, MNPs serve as labels

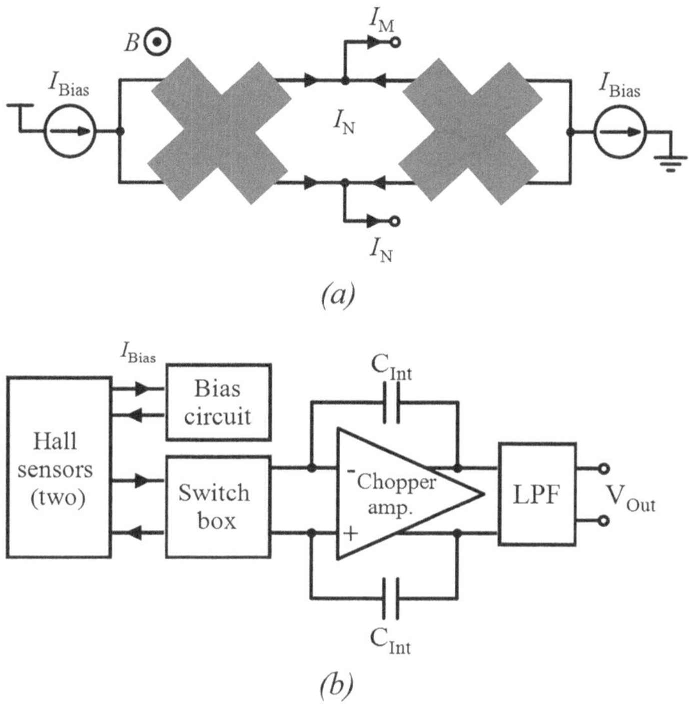

Fig. 4.34 A block diagram for the current-mode Hall sensor for MMG applications

for target detection in which the inductance changes in the effect of targets. For example, Wang et al. [278] presented a CMOS inductive biosensor with an LC-oscillator structure at 1 GHz, which is designed relying on the complementary cross-coupled topology that is shown in Fig. 4.35. The sensor is constructed of 8 arrays for parallel testing in which the frequency of the oscillator is changed in response to the DNA samples. In their work, for 1 nM DNA samples labeled by MNPs with a diameter of 50 nm, the frequency shift is reported as 2.8 ppm. Another 1 GHz inductive biosensor with 64 arrays was developed by Wang et al. [279] in a 65 nm CMOS process that employed a correlated double counting (CdC) configuration to achieve better sensitivity. The sensor is tested with the sample of DynaBeads® MyOneTM Carboxylic Acid diameter of 1 μm and the CdC provides 6 dB noise suppression as the sensor frequency shift without and with CdC are 125 ppm and 63 ppm, respectively. Also, this inductive sensor has been used as a cell sensor that the cardiac progenitor cells labeled by magnetic particles [280]. The authors depicted the real-time monitoring of the periodic and autonomous beating of the progenitors by an on-chip magnetic sensor.

The reviewed inductive sensors [278–280] worked at a specific frequency that limited their detection ability. To provide multiplexed biosensing by utilizing frequency signatures of beads, a sensor capable of operating across a wide frequency

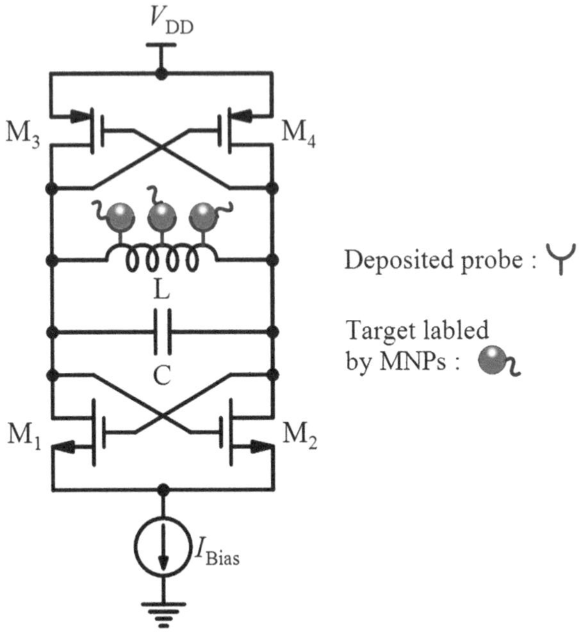

Fig. 4.35 Resonance-shift magnetic sensor sensing schema

range or multi-frequency structure is required. This method capitalizes on the distinct resonance frequencies exhibited by different types of magnetic particles when their induced magnetizations are polarized. Sideris et al. [281] proposed A 2 × 2 array of the magnetic sensor based on transformer operating at 1.44 and 3.65 GHz, which achieves reference-free drift-cancelling. The outcomes of the initial DNA bio-detection experiment have been obtained, confirming the sensor's ability to conduct practical bioassays. In other work, Sideris et al. [282] developed a magnetic spectrometer in 65 nm CMOS that operates in a range of 1.1 to 3.3 GHz. The measured frequency response of different kinds of beads depicted each bead shows a unique response. These results imply that the magnetic spectrometer is a promising method for discerning between different magnetic particles. Sun et al. [283] developed a 2 × 2 magnetic spectrometer array utilized a concurrent dual-frequency (CDF) oscillator. Figure 4.36 shows the structure of the CDF transformer-based oscillator working at a range of frequency 1.2–1.65 / 2.9–4 GHz. The fourth-order transformer tank exhibits two resonance frequencies, denoted as f_{LO} and f_{HI} in which these frequencies are selected as f_{LO} is positioned under the usual resonance frequency of MNPs, and f_{HI} is positioned above it.

The limitation of the drift compensation method with a single-frequency oscillator based on transformer is noteworthy, as it necessitates regular switching of the sensing oscillator between f_{LO} and f_{HI} [281]. By employing continuous frequency division operation, this method effectively addresses the challenge of compensating

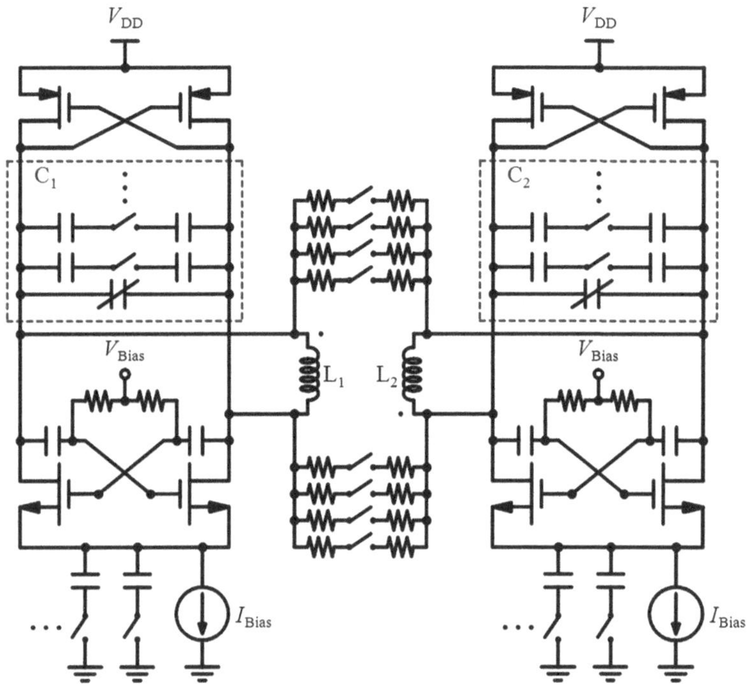

Fig. 4.36 CDF transformer-based oscillator

for the drift of the free-running sensing oscillator with no need for frequent reconfiguration of frequency switching. This development facilitates the execution of wash-free magnetic label assays and single-site multiplexed spectroscopy. The immunoassay carried out in this research integrates biotin-streptavidin and iron oxide magnetic nanoparticle labels, eliminating the requirement for washing steps. This approach demonstrates outstanding sensitivity and proves to be well-suited for PoC diagnostic applications.

One promising approach for detecting and measuring biophysical and biochemical properties of the cell (cell function) is the magnetic flow cytometer (MFC) [284–288]. The implementation of MFC based on an inductive detector versus GMR or μHall detector-based flow cytometers does not require an external magnet for detection [284]. This prevents the possibility of cell lysis from magnetic shear forces, preserving the viability of cells throughout the detection process. This viability allows for optional sorting and culturing, which is essential for certain applications [284]. Murali et al. [286] developed an MFC that relies on an inductive detector in 65 nm CMOS technology incorporated within a microfluidic channel. The cytometer detects variations in magnetic flux density within the spiral coil as the magnetic particles pass over the sensor. This chip identifies cells that are precisely labeled with magnetic markers by assessing changes in coupling between an excitation coil and a pickup coil within a differential spiral transformer operating at frequencies of 0.9 and 2.6 GHz. The performance of the flow cytometer cartridge has been validated for the detection of SKBR-3 breast cancer cells labeled with manganese ferrite magnetic markers using EpCAM-biotin-streptavidin chemistry. Furthermore, it has the capability to classify magnetic labels composed of various materials. The study also presents measurement results for classifying magnetic labels made from different materials.

In another work, Tang et al. [288] presented an MFC with a 2D oscillator 7 × 7 array in a 65 nm CMOS process. The sensor is designed with dual frequencies operating at 1.3 and 3.4 GHz to leverage the frequency-dependent nature of the magnetic susceptibility of the biomarker. Furthermore, a dual-frequency design along with a reference oscillator are employed as drift cancellation mechanisms to mitigate the noise issues typically encountered with individual sensors. The choice of utilizing either or both drift suppression techniques depends on the specific application. The sensor includes 49 arrays of cross-coupled oscillators. Each of the oscillator circuits is realized with a single optimized quality factor inductor and a switchable capacitor to configure the oscillating frequency of each sensor to either 1.3 or 3.4 GHz. The oscillator outputs are buffered to permit two simultaneous sensor readouts at independently selected frequency states. The architecture includes an additional pathway where the outputs of the oscillators (sensor and reference) are directly mixed to suppress correlated noise before readout. If the reference and sensor are set to different frequencies, the higher frequency output (3.4 GHz) is divided by three and then mixed with the other output.

In this design, to achieve high throughput, the flow over a single sensor does not concentrate. Instead, the sample is enabled to flow freely through a microfluidic channel integrated into the chip surface, enabling multisite detection. The functionality of the array is demonstrated with magnetic bead flows and detection of lymphoma cancer cells with Maritriptase, and Anti-maritriptase monoclonal antibody with magnetic bead complex.

4.6.3 GMR Magnetic Biosensors

As it was mentioned in the sensing section, two prevalent detection techniques can be employed for GMR sensors including magnetometry and magneto-relaxometry (MRX). Without a magnetic field (H_A), MNPs' moments are randomly distributed, cause in no net field. In the presence of magnetic field, moments align, generating a stray field opposing the applied field. Magnetometry is utilized to quantify the disparity in the fields with and without MNPs, whereas MRX tracks the alterations in the field as the MNPs revert to their random orientation once the magnetic field is discontinued. The most common techniques to measure the magnetoresistance from the MNPs in magnetometry or MRX include the Wheatstone bridge (WhB) and double modulation schema.

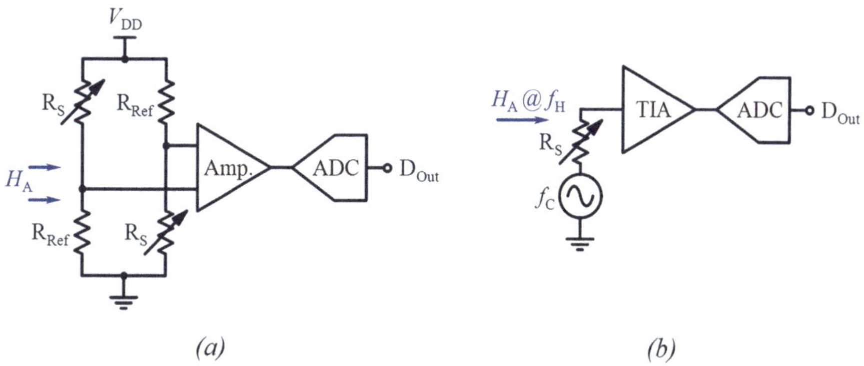

Fig. 4.37 AFE for readout of magnetoresistance (**a**) WhB scheme (**b**) double modulation scheme

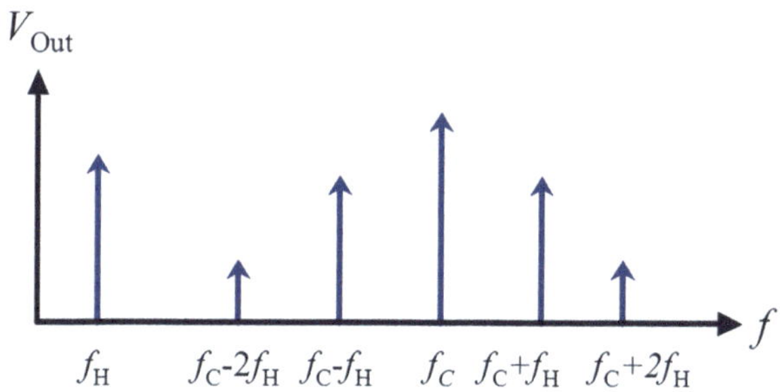

Fig. 4.38 Spectrum showing the double modulation

The WhB is a common architecture for high-precision resistance measurements. Figure 4.37a shows the AFE based on the WhB to a read-out of the magnetic signal. It typically consists of two GMR spin-valve (SV) sensors and two programmable resistors, and a amplifier followed by a ADC. One sensor is biologically active (R_S), while the other serves as a reference (R_{Ref}), magnetically isolated but experiencing the same environment. The bridge's differential output cancels common-mode signals, and a high gain amplifies the small output caused by the MNPs [289].

Figure 4.37b shows the AFE for double modulation that consists of a TIA to amplify the generated current and ADC to cover the signal to digital data. The double modulation scheme uses time-varying excitation voltage (or a current) at frequency f_C and an time-varying magnetic field at frequency f_H to separate resistive and magnetoresistive signal components as depicted in Fig. 4.38 [290]. In other words, the double modulation scheme shifts the signal from the MNPs to a higher frequency, reducing flicker noise in the sensor.

This section will discuss the CMOS GMR biosensor using detection techniques of magnetometry and MRX.

4.6.3.1 GMR Biosensor with Magnetometry Sensing Mechanism

Rapid advancements in DNA microarray technology have significantly expanded their application in both molecular biology research and clinical diagnostics. Han et al. [290] developed 1008 GMR SV biosensors in 0.25 μm BiCMOS technology that are divided into 16 subarrays, each measuring 120 μm × 120 μm, compatible with state-of-the-art DNA spotters. Within the magnetoresistive microarray system, single-stranded DNA of a known sequence is attached to the sensor surface using a sulfur-Au linkage. Complementary probes capture biotinylated analyte DNA, and streptavidin-coated magnetic labels bind to the hybridized DNA. Sensor resistance is altered by stray magnetic fields emitted from the labels, which is detected through a combination of frequency division multiplexing (FDM) and time division multiplexing (TDM). This innovative approach minimizes signal readout duration per pixel. Within the AFE, there is a mixer and PGA present. The on-die mixer enables double modulation that separates the magnetoresistive component and the non-magnetoresistive component of the sensor, leaving only the magnetization configuration term. In another design, Hall et al. [291] proposed a 256 array of GMR SV biosensors in a 0.18 μm CMOS process. In this work, through the combination of FDM and TDM with parallel readout channels, the readout time is diminished by around 15 times compared to the [290]. The AFE comprises two pseudo-differential TIAs, a fully-differential ADC driver, and a ΔΣM. For this sensor, the reported magnetoresistive (MR) ratio is 9.2%. Costa et al. [292] introduced a CMOS front-end with integrated GMR SV sensors using a AMS 0.35 μm technology. The sensor achieves lower noise (16 nV/$\sqrt{\text{Hz}}$) and power consumption (6.5 mW) for biomolecular recognition detection applications.

4.6.3.2 GMR Biosensor with Magnetic Relaxation Sensing Mechanism

In MRX, particles are magnetized and their response is observed after the magnetic field is rapidly removed. This method is robust against magnetic field variations and requires simpler electronics, rendering it suitable for low-power portable applications.

Hall et al. [293] introduced a GMR-based MRX biosensor designed for detecting the relaxation of 30 nm MNPs. Figure 4.39 illustrates the structural layout of the of the proposed MRX detector. The time of magnetization and magnetic field amplitude are determined by a personal computer (PC), which then transmits this information to the field-programmable gate array (FPGA). The FPGA is responsible for controlling the timing of both the electromagnet and the readout circuit. An external PA supplies a constant current I_0 to the electromagnet driver. The driver then generates pulsed current I_{Coil}, which is delivered to the external Helmholtz coil. This setup produces a pulsed magnetic field that interacts with the sensor chip. The sensor response is captured by the AFE, which then transmits the data to the PC for subsequent processing. The AFE comprises a switched integrator, an anti-aliasing filter,

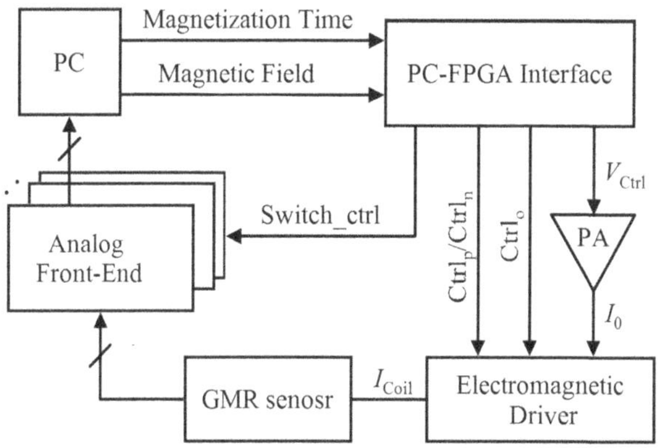

Fig. 4.39 Block diagram of a GMR biosensor for detecting relaxation of MNPs

and an ADC. Additionally, the design includes magnetic correlated double sampling (MCDS) to address sensor-to-sensor variation, temperature variation, circuit offset, and non-linearity. Experimental results with dried MNPs show successful detection of particle relaxation. The biotin-bovine serum albumin (BSA) immunoassay also demonstrates real-time monitoring of binding kinetics.

In GMR biosensors, the high baseline-to-signal ratio and sensor mismatch pose challenges for AFE design. In a study by Zhou et al. [294], a GMR sensor was developed using a 0.18 μm CMOS process. The sensor featured innovative techniques such as duty-cycle resistors (DCRs) to enhance readout speed and high-frequency interference rejection (HFIR) sampling within the ADC. The AFE achieves 46.4 nT/$\sqrt{\text{Hz}}$ noise, <0.235 mT baseline, 0.98 ppm sensitivity, 11 ms readout, and 1.39 mW/channel power consumption.

Another study by Zhou et al. [295] presented a low-noise MRX implementation in a 0.18 μm CMOS process for detecting MNP relaxation. It uses techniques like dynamic element matching (DEM) and magnetoresistive correlated double sampling (MRCDS) to reduce 1/*f* noise and fast-settling miller compensation (FSMC) to lower amplifier power. The design achieves 9.7 nTrms input-referred noise and superior FoM, consuming 4.32 mW from a 1.8 V supply.

4.7 CMOS NMR Biosensors

The capability of nuclear magnetic resonance (NMR) to observe intermolecular and intramolecular interactions, including those involving macromolecules such as nucleic acids, renders the NMR instrument a potent tool in medical applications [296–299]. Components essential for an NMR system include a magnet for producing a consistent magnetic field to polarize nuclear spins, an RF coil encompassing the sample, and an RF transceiver that generates excitation RF magnetic fields and monitors resonance.

Over the last 10 years, substantial research endeavors have been dedicated to scaling down NMR magnets, coils, and electronic components, which will examine in following. This concerted emphasis on scaling down the components essential to NMR technology reflects a growing interest in developing compact and portable NMR systems through CMOS technology with enhanced capabilities and versatility.

4.7.1 Coil

In the NMR system, the coil functions as the intermediary between the droplet samples and electronics, converting the magnetic field generated by the nuclei into the voltage required for the transceiver (TRX). Achieving optimal coil performance in the NMR instrument is a multifaceted task, demanding simultaneous improvements in several key parameters: quality factor, SNR, B_{Ext} (external magnetic field)-homogeneity B_{RF} (RF magnetic field)-homogeneity, minimizations, and concentration sensitivity, self-resonance frequency [300].

The quality factor which is described as the ratio of coil reactance to its parasitic resistance is crucial and significantly influences the SNR. There has been insufficient attention given to developing devices with specific geometries aimed at generating uniform B_{RF} fields over micro-scale samples. On the other hand, NMR coils should be designed according to the target application as a micro-coil or mm-coil. For mass-limited applications such as single-cell NMR, micro-coils are suitable, but their concentration sensitivity is significantly reduced compared to conventional mm-coils [301]. Notably, concentration sensitivity refers to the lowest concentration of a sample needed to achieve a designated SNR objective. In order to enhance NMR coil performance for samples with concentration limitations, one can optimize the detection volume by maximizing the extent of the homogeneous region of the B_{Ext}-field at the specific operating frequency within the magnet [301].

The coils can be implemented with various configurations including the planar, vertical, solenoid, scroll, cone-shaped, helmholtz, standing, etc. [300]. From a dimension point of view, the coil can to be realized on-chip or off-chip, which will be examined in the following.

4.7.1.1 Off-chip Coil

Krüger et al. [302] employed off-chip coils in a portable CMOS-based NMR system with the capability of spectroscopy, relaxometry, and imaging. In this work, three types of off-chip coils are utilized. The solenoidal sample coil generates RF magnetic fields and detects precession signals for further analysis. For spectroscopy length of the sample coil with a 1.4 μL sample is 1.8 mm. For relaxometry larger sample volume of 3.9 μL with a sample coil length of 5 mm is employed and samples with a volume of up to ~200 μL with a sample coil length of 10 mm are used

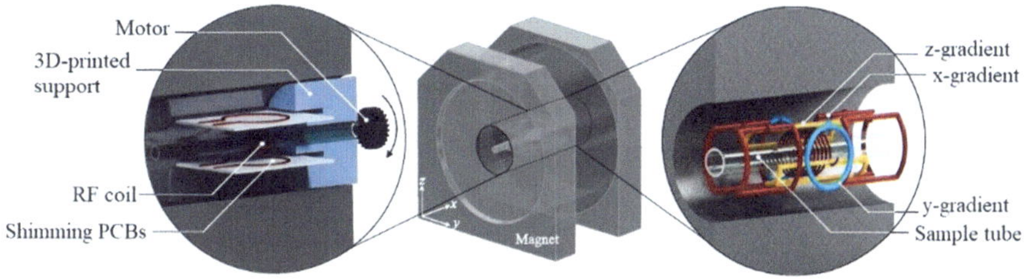

Fig. 4.40 (**a**) shimming coils (left) for NMR spectroscopy and, (**b**) gradient coils (right) for MRI

for MRI. In this study, for NMR spectroscopy, the shimming coils (see Fig. 4.40) are used to compensate for the B_{Ext} inhomogeneity of the permanent magnet to achieve high-resolution [303]. As shown in Fig. 4.40, to introduce gradients to the permanent field for MRI, the sample tube containing the sample coil is enclosed by three sets of gradient coils. These coils are responsible for creating field gradients along the x-axis using a Golay coil pair (red color), along the y-axis with a Maxwell coil pair (blue color), and along the z-axis using a Saddle coil pair (yellow color).

Also, in another MRI system that was miniaturized for in situ monitoring of bacterial growth and biofilm formation introduced by Zhou et al. [299] besides a sample off-chip coil, 5 pairs of shim off-chip coils to correct different orders of the magnetic field and 3 pairs of gradient off-chip coils to introduce field gradients in all three dimensions are employed. The sample coil is a 7-turn solenoid coil with length and diameter of 7 mm, and 9.4 mm, respectively wound with enamel copper wire with a diameter of 1 mm. The measured inductance at 15.7 MHz is 393 nH, with a quality factor of 78. All shim and gradient coils are planar-coil designed and fabricated by PCB. The x and y-direction gradient coil consists of four rectangular planar coils with a width of 21.4 mm and the z-direction gradient coil is a Maxwell coil which consists of two circular coils. Three shim coils are used to generate the gradient along the x-, y-, and z-directions, which are designed similarly to the gradient coils with less turn but wider trace width than gradient coils that provide long-time and large current injection during shim operation. The remaining two pairs of shim coils are used for correcting the quadradic inhomogeneity of the permanent magnetic field.

Pourmodhej et al. [304] introduced at an NMR system with on-chip and off-chip coils an frequency of 21 MHz for NMR spectroscopy. Figure 4.41 illustrates the high frequency structural simulator (HFSS) model and the equivalent circuit for off-chip coil, which includes the parasitic capacitance and resistance among the wires. The primary objective in the coil design is to optimize the strength and uniformity of the RF magnetic field (B_{RF}). Constructed using MW35C copper wire wound around a glass tube, the wire has a diameter of 404 μm, the solenoid's inner diameter is approximately 1 mm, and the pitch among wires is around 500 μm. In this research, the ANSYS HFSS simulator is utilized for modeling and simulating three coils with 30, 50, and 100 turns, respectively. Figure 4.42 showcases the B_{RF} distribution in the x-y-z directions, highlighting the uniformity of the magnetic field

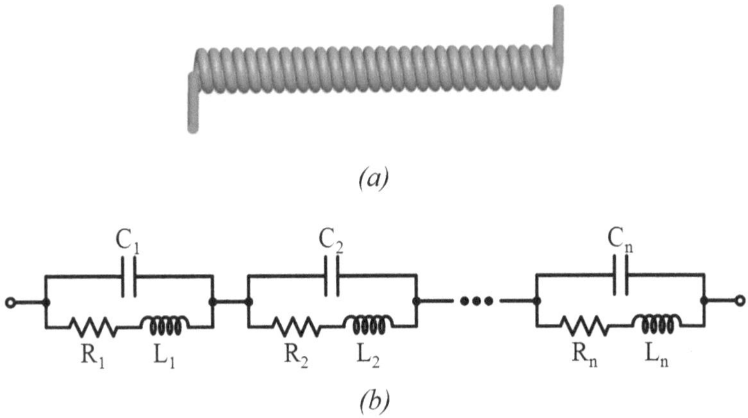

Fig. 4.41 Models of the off-chip coils (**a**) HFSS, (**b**) equivalent circuity

along the z-axis and negligible magnetic field strength along the x and y axes. Furthermore, the characterization of the coils is conducted using a vector network analyzer, and the inductance and quality factor of the coils versus frequency are obtained as depicted in Fig. 4.43. The results indicate that the coil with 100 turns exhibits a peak quality factor (approximately 40) at 21 MHz, making it the optimal choice for the NMR system.

4.7.1.2 On-Chip Coil

CMOS technology, with its multiple metal layers, emerges as the optimal choice for implementing the integrated coil, avoiding the use of bulky equipment and enhancing integration. On the other hand, unlike the off-chip coil, the interconnecting wires in micrometer-scale among the on-chip coil and the electronics minimizes the pickup of parasitic magnetic signals and electromagnetic interference, paving the way for interference-free in vivo experiments within a precisely defined region of interest. By eliminating the necessity for time-consuming spatial encoding, the on-chip coil facilitates continuous recording of magnetic signals in a nanoliter volume with millisecond resolution, revolutionizing experimental capabilities.

For example, Authors in [305], utilized an on-chip planar micro-coil with features, 24-turn, 300 μm outer diameter integrated on a NMR-on-a-chip spectrometer, which is susceptible in vivo measurements of blood oxygenation and flow in nanoliter volumes. Grisi et al. [306] introduced a multilayer 150 μm planar on-chip coil for NMR spectroscopy. The use of a multilayer on-chip coil offers the advantage of achieving high spin sensitivities in extremely small sample volumes, as demonstrated in NMR spectroscopy experiments on single intact ova measuring between 0.1 and 0.5 nL. Lei et al. [307] utilized a planar coil in their study for a multi-type biological/chemical micro-NMR assay, which also acts as a sample heater for

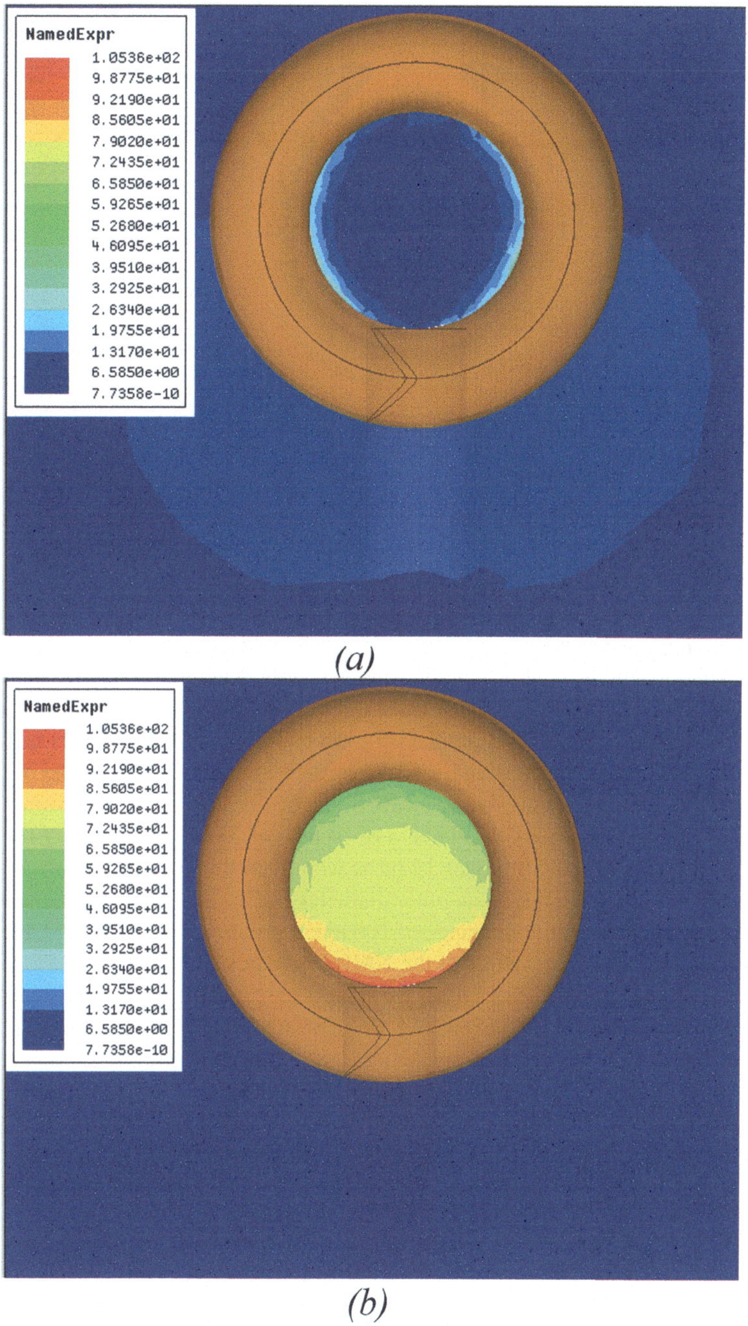

Fig. 4.42 Simulation results of HFSS (**a**) B_{RF} in xy-plane, (**b**) B_{RF} in z direction

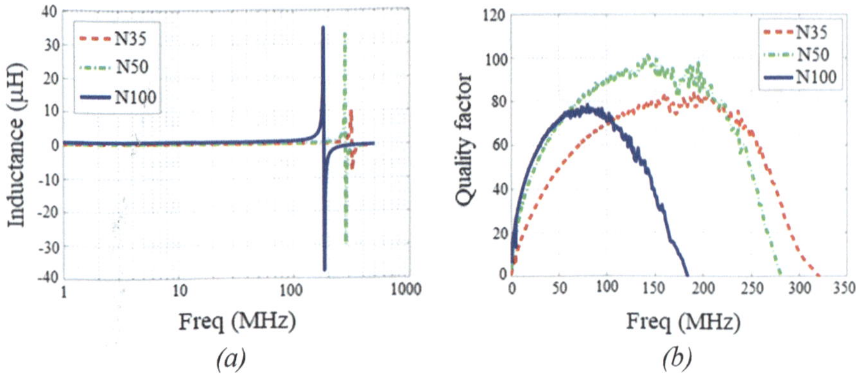

Fig. 4.43 Characterization results of coil (**a**) inductance, and (**b**) quality factor versus frequency

thermal profiling. The on-chip planar coil features 23 turns, a conductor width of 40 µm, and a spacing of 1.85 µm. Other specifications of coils are as follows, a dimension of 2 × 2 mm^2, L of 506 nH, and quality factor of 1.84 at the NMR frequency of 19.6 MHz. The quality factor of the coil in this study was enhanced by implementing a thick top metal layer of 2.5 µm and employing a stacked-metal-layer technique. Remarkably, the samples were loaded onto the on-chip planar coil using a handheld pipette, and the system successfully detected levels of <100 pM of Enterococcus faecalis-derived DNA from a 2.5 µL sample. In another effort, an on-chip planar spiral coil and a solenoidal off-chip coil are used as a sample coil in two different NMR systems. The planar spiral micro-coil contains 25 turns and occupies an area of 2.5 mm × 2.5 mm. At the NMR frequency of 20.9 MHz, the coil in question exhibits an inductance of 430 nH, a resistance of 31 Ω, and a quality factor of 1.9. This solenoidal coil comprises 14 turns wound around a capillary tube with an inner diameter of 0.75 mm and an outer diameter of 1 mm. Upon measurement, the coil was found to have an inductance of 100 nH, a resistance of 0.5 Ω, and a significantly higher quality factor of 28 at the NMR frequency of 23.9 MHz.

In the continuation of the discussion about on-chip coil, to confirm the feasibility of CMOS technology, the design and simulation outcomes of two on-chip coil structures, referred to as serial stacked coil (SSC) and differential stacked coil (DSC) are examined below. These findings stem from the study of Pourmodheji et al. [308] and are conducted at a frequency of 300 MHz utilizing 0.13 µm CMOS technology.

SSD and DSC Structures of Coil

SSC is composed of several planar coils distributed across various metal layers indexed by i where $0 \leq i \leq 8$ as depicted in Fig. 4.44a. This configuration aligns with the 0.13 µm CMOS technology utilized, which incorporates 8 metal layers. In order to attain a high level of inductance, the planar coils, each with multiple

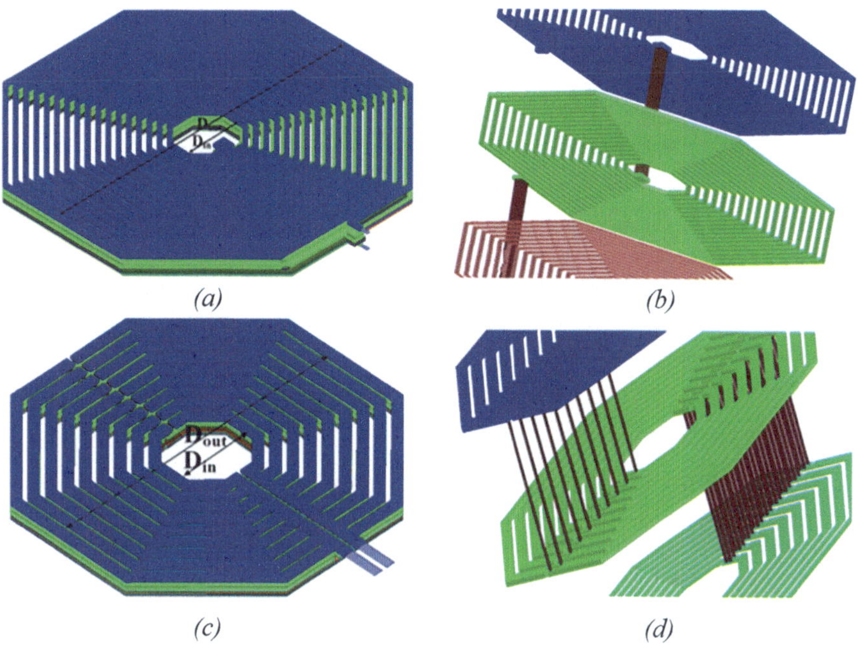

Fig. 4.44 NMR on-chip coil structures: (**a**) SSC, (**b**) SSC with several turns connected through vias (**c**) DSC, (**d**) DSC with several turns connected through vias

turns denoted by the index j ($1 \leq j \leq n$), are interconnected vias, as shown in Fig. 4.44b. According to the HFSS simulation, the best quality factor around 300 MHz is achieved with the value of 9 for n. The equivalent resistance is given by Eq. (4.15) [309].

$$R_{eq-SSC} = \sum_i \sum_j R_{i,j} \tag{4.15}$$

The symmetrical differential structure of DSC is shown in Fig. 4.44c that characterized by a unique design comprising numerous planar coils arranged in a symmetrical pattern. Each coil is configured with i layers and j turns in each layer. This intricate arrangement culminates in the creation of a high inductance within the structure, contributing to its overall functionality and efficiency [310]. In this design, each layer consists of multiple parallel coils to enhance the magnetic field strength (B_{RF}) and reduce resistance. As a result, several vias are employed to connect the coils in parallel between two layers, as depicted in Fig. 4.44d. The Eq. (4.16) is used to calculate the equivalent resistance of a DSC structure.

$$R_{eq-DSC} = \sum_i \left(\sum_j R_{i,j}^{-1} \right)^{-1} \tag{4.16}$$

The quality factor of the equivalent tank circuit of DSC and SSC structures is defined by Eq. (4.17).

$$Q_{L(\omega)} = \frac{\omega L_{eq}}{R_{eq}}\left(1 - \frac{C_{eq}R_{eq}^2}{L} - \omega^2 L_{eq}C_{eq}\right) \tag{4.17}$$

where L_{eq} and C_{eq} represent the equivalent inductance and capacitance, and R_{eq} denotes the equivalent resistance derived from Eqs. (4.15) or (4.16) for SSC and DSC structures, respectively. Since the equivalent resistance for the SSC structure is bigger than the DSC structure, according to Eqs. (4.15, 4.16, and 4.17) and it can be deduced that the quality factor of the DSC structure is greater than that of the SSC structure.

Optimized Geometry Design of SSD and DSC Structures

From a circuit perspective, the key parameters to consider for designing an on-chip coil are the resonant frequency, quality factor, and physical area. Pourmodheji et al. [308] utilized the ANSYS HFSS software to optimize the geometry at a frequency of 300 MHz. The hexagonally shaped DSC structure's optimal inner and outer dimensions are achieved as 80 μm and 365 μm, respectively. The same geometry was applied to the SSC structure. Figure 4.45 illustrates the obtained quality factor of both structures across different frequencies. The simulation results from HFSS indicate that the SSC and DSC structures operate at frequencies of 40 MHz and

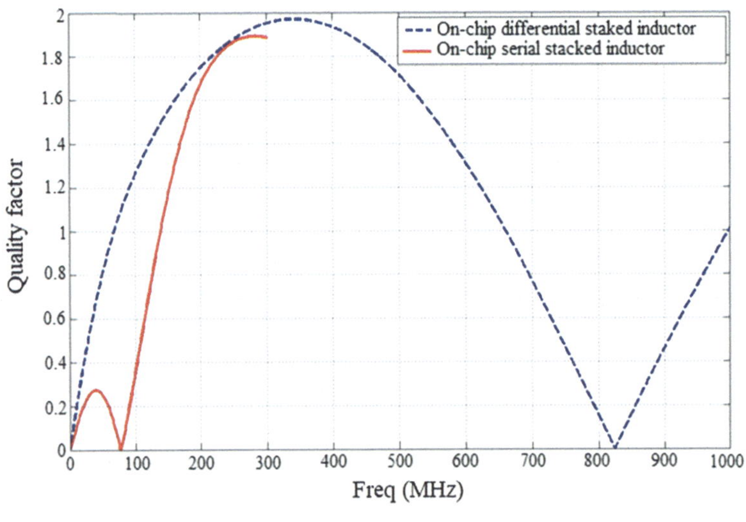

Fig. 4.45 quality factor results versus frequency for DSC and SSC structures

300 MHz, respectively (see Fig. 4.45). Due to the DSC's differential configuration, the inductor exhibits a quality factor of approximately 2, which is 7 times superior to the quality factor of the SSC structure.

Homogenous of the Magnetic Field

An additional benefit of the DSC architecture is the uniformity of the magnetic field B_{RF} produced inside the on-chip coil. It can be seen from Fig. 4.44b, d, the metal vias results in the introduction of horizontal magnetic field components, which in turn impacts the homogeneity of the magnetic field B_{RF}.

In the DSC structure, the currents passing through the vias that connect any two layers' flow in opposite directions. This configuration results in the cancellation of the horizontal magnetic field components. Consequently, it can be posited that the symmetric design of the DSC effectively mitigates magnetic parasitic effects, a feat not achievable with the asymmetric structure of the SSC. The magnetic fields produced by these structures in three distinct directions (B_{RFx}, B_{RFy}, and B_{RFz}) are illustrated in Fig. 4.46a-f.

Upon examination of these figures, it is evident that the intensity of magnetic field in the x and y directions is lower compared to the the z direction within the central region of the coils for both DSC and SSC configurations. At the center point of the SSC and DSC, the ratio of the B_{RFxy} over B_{RFz} is 3.02% and 0.93%, respectively. According to these results, the vertical magnetic field B_{RFz} in both structures is similar, but the DSC demonstrates a lower magnetic field in the xy-plane compared to the SSC configuration.

The Fig. 4.47a, b display the distribution of B_{RFz} within the middle volume of the DSC and SSC structures. Based on the findings, the average B_{RFz} values for the DSC and SSC structures are 1290 A/m and 1115 A/m, respectively. Moreover, the standard deviation for the DSC is around 59.5, significantly lower than the standard deviation for the SSC (108). These results suggest that the magnetic field uniformity in the DSC structure outperforms that of the SSC structure.

4.7.2 *Magnet*

As discussed earlier, the magnetic resonance frequency is directly proportional to the strength of the external permanent magnetic field that is defined by $f_L = \gamma\ B_{Ext}$. According to this equation, a strong magnetic field enables the generation and recording of magnetic resonance at high frequencies. As f_L varies with the temperature-dependent B_{Ext}, implementing a calibration method is essential to bolster the NMR system's robustness [311]. SNR of the NMR is one of the most challenging that affected by the external permanent field given from the following equation [312].

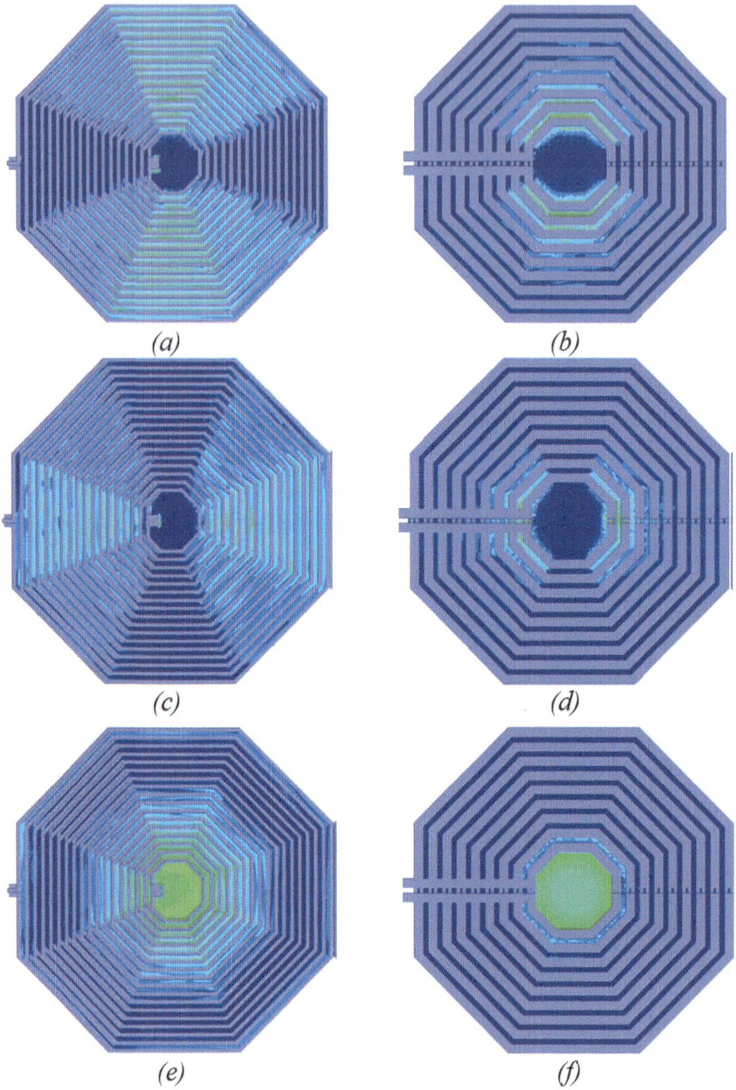

Fig. 4.46 Simulation results of BRF Magnetic field. (**a**) B_{RFx}, (**c**) B_{RFy}, and (**e**) B_{RFz}, generated by SSC, (**b**) B_{RFx}, (**d**) B_{RFy} and (**f**) generated by DSC

$$SNR = \frac{n\gamma^{2.5}\sqrt{tB_{Ext}^{3}}}{\sqrt{2T\left(R_{c}+R_{s}\right)}} \tag{4.18}$$

where n represents the number of spins in the detector, t denotes the total experimental time, γ stands for the gyro-magnetic ratio of the nucleus, R_S and R_C indicate the resistances of the sample and the coil, and T signifies the temperature of the

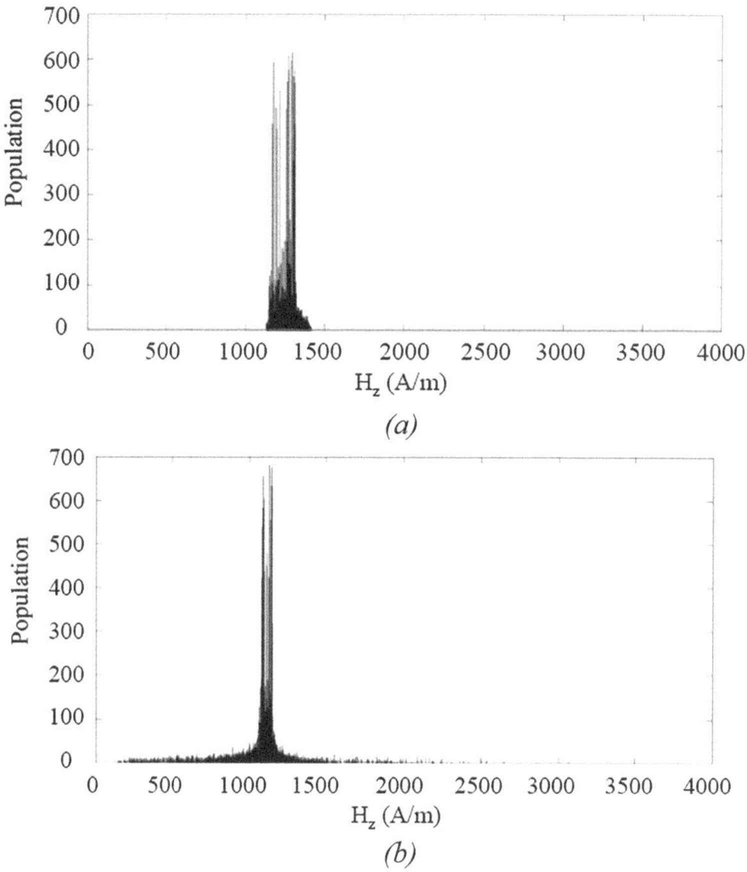

Fig. 4.47 Population of magnetic field strength (**a**) DSC (**b**) SSC

sample, coil, and preamplifier. According to this formula, increased external permanent magnetic field strength enhances sensitivity, while higher temperatures reduce sensitivity. Conversely, a crucial aspect of NMR miniaturization involves the advancement of small permanent magnets characterized by high field homogeneity and stability. Briefly, the most important parameter has to be taken into account in designing magnets for NMR applications comprising the B_{Ext} field strength, the magnetic field homogeneity, and minimizing the size and the weight of the magnet.

A larger magnet produces a more robust NMR signal, thereby reducing the sensitivity demands on the transceiver design. Nevertheless, the downside of a larger magnet is its bulkiness, as the magnet becomes the predominant component in terms of size. As an example, Lei et al. [307] described a handheld NMR system where the dimensions ($14 \times 6 \times 11$ cm^3) and weight (1.4 kg) are primarily influenced by the 0.46 T portable magnet, which weighs 1.25 kg, has a diameter of 8 cm, and a height of 5.5 cm. In this design, to enhance the robustness, a closed-loop B_{Ext}-field stabilization scheme is proposed.

In a separate study, Sun et al. [313] introduced a palm-sized NMR system weighing 0.1 kg. In their pursuit of significant size and cost reductions, they employed a miniature magnet the size of a ping-pong ball (0.56 T). However, the pronounced permanent magnetic field inhomogeneity associated with the ping-pong ball-sized magnet used in the palm system led to a considerable underestimation of the true T_2 value [314]. Dreyer et al. [297] documented a homogeneity of 30 ppm across a sample volume of 35 μL in the NMR system designed for PoC analysis. The magnet used in this system is a custom-designed 0.36 T benchtop NMR magnet, weighing 5.5 kg. Another NMR spectroscopy study conducted by Ha et al. [315] showcased a compact 0.51 T NdFeB permanent magnet. This magnet achieved a remarkable 0.13 ppm field inhomogeneity through six-directional electrical shimming, covering an effective sample volume of 0.8 μL.

In a different approach, by Lei et al. [316] introduced an NMR system that utilized a 2D multi-electrode digital microfluidic device within a compact portable magnet (0.46 T, 1.25 kg). This setup enabled efficient management of multiple samples within a constrained space.

It is important to note that the inherent inhomogeneity of the external permanent magnet in the portable device results in a spatial variation in the precession rate of the nuclei, posing a challenge to accurately measure the original T_2. To address this issue, the spin-echo technique, such as the Carr–Purcell–Meiboom–Gill (CPMG) pulse sequence, can be employed. This method involves flipping the nuclei by 180° at intervals τ to refocus the dephasing effect caused by B_{Ext} inhomogeneity, thus maximizing the spins again [316, 317]. In another study by Krüger et al. [302], a portable NMR system was introduced featuring a NdFeB Halbach permanent magnet with a B_{Ext} strength of 0.51 T. The Halbach magnet demonstrated an inherent B_{Ext} field inhomogeneity of 0.4 ppm across a sample volume of 0.8 μL positioned at the center of the magnet bore. In this configuration, two techniques were employed to enhance the B_{Ext} field inhomogeneity from 0.4 ppm (approximately 8.4 Hz) over a 0.8 μL sample to 0.05 ppm (around 1.1 Hz) across a larger 1.4 μL sample volume. Initially, a magnet equipped with a pair of custom-designed shimming coils, each carrying a dc current, was utilized to create a specific static magnetic field pattern that compensates for the B_{Ext} inhomogeneity [318, 319]. Subsequently, to further enhance homogeneity, the sample tube was rotated at 33 Hz, resulting in motional averaging that effectively reduced the field inhomogeneity among the plane perpendicular to the rotation axis [320].

A promising approach to miniaturizing NMR magnets involves the strategic arrangement of small permanent magnetic blocks combined with a shimming scheme to optimize the magnetic field homogeneity [298, 321]. Dreyer et al. [298] utilized an H-shaped permanent magnet with passive shimming to create a miniaturized NMR magnet operating at a field strength of 0.29 T. This magnet weighed 330 g and had dimensions of 65 × 35 × 35 mm^3. Passive shimming involves the strategic placement of materials to enhance B_{Ext} field homogeneity [322, 323]. In this design, a two-step procedure was implemented to achieve homogeneity in the region of interest (ROI). Initially, COMSOL Multiphysics is employed to model

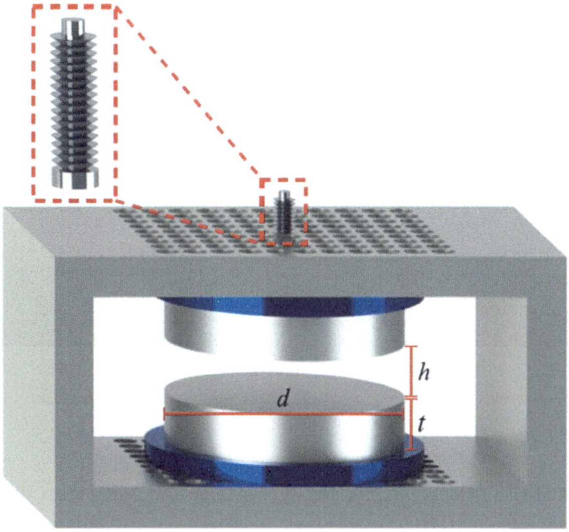

Fig. 4.48 The diagram of the specially designed NMR magnet shows that the blue sections correspond to the NdFeB magnetic blocks, with the remaining components (yoke, pole pieces, and screws) being made from iron

and optimize the core magnet, consisting of the permanent magnet blocks and the yoke. Subsequently, two passive shim techniques, specifically iron pole pieces and adjustable iron screws, are utilized to further enhance the homogeneity of the B_{Ext} field. As illustrated in Fig. 4.48, two iron pole pieces are introduced onto the magnetic blocks, followed by the addition of iron screws to the yoke to further homogenize the magnetic field [324].

Fig. 4.49 shows the magnetic field map after adding iron pole pieces (before iron screws). This method reduces the parabolic profile to achieve a magnetic field homogeneity of 300 ppm, resulting in a decrease in the maximum B_{Ext} field strength within the ROI to 290 mT. Following the incorporation of the iron screws, the field homogeneity improved by 100 ppm within a $5 \times 5\ \mathrm{mm}^2$ area at the central slice. As a result, after both optimization steps, field homogeneity improved to 20 ppm.

4.7.3 Transceiver

In the realm of miniaturized NMR-based sensors, the necessity for a small magnet is evident; however, the reduction in magnet size often leads to a weaker NMR signal output. This challenge underscores the critical role that NMR electronics play in shaping the overall performance of the system. As the size of the magnet decreases, the sensitivity and efficiency of the NMR electronics become increasingly crucial in

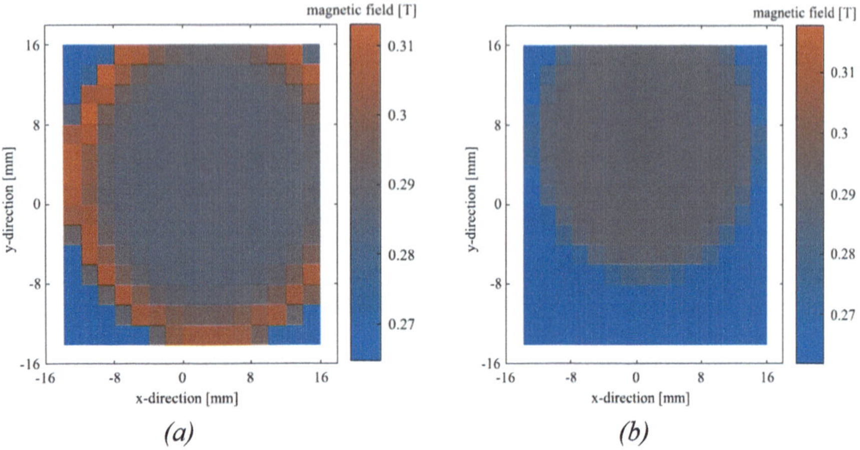

Fig. 4.49 Measured B_{Ext} field in the ROI (**a**) after adding iron pole pieces (**b**) after adding the screws in addition to iron pole pieces

enhancing signal detection and system functionality. To overcome this hurdle, the integration of a highly sensitive RX with CMOS technology is essential. By leveraging this advanced technology combination, it becomes possible to achieve the required sensitivity and signal processing capabilities needed for miniaturized NMR sensors, paving the way for enhanced performance and expanded applications in various fields.

The TRX design is essential to the performance of the NMR system, serving as a critical component of the NMR electronics. This section will delve into the examination of recent advancements in miniaturized NMR-on-a-chip systems tailored for biomedical applications, emphasizing on electronics of TRX. While the primary focus of this section will center on the electronic aspects of the systems, a brief overview of the other essential performance-critical components of the system will also be provided. By reviewing these innovative systems, we aim to showcase their practical applications and performance in various NMR-related fields. Additionally, comparisons between different miniaturized CMOS-based NMR systems will be drawn to provide insights into their respective strengths, limitations, and potential for further development. Through this comprehensive review, we seek to offer a deeper understanding of the evolving landscape of miniaturized NMR technology and its diverse applications across different disciplines.

4.7.3.1 The Conventional Architecture of TRX for NMR System

The basic components of a miniaturized NMR system is shown in Fig. 4.50 that comprising a permanent magnet, an RF coil, and an RF TRX. The permanent magnet generates magnetic field B_{Ext}. The RF NMR coil surrounds a sample and transduces between the electrical signals for the electronics and the magnetic field from the nuclei. The NMR electronic linked to the coil mainly consist of an RF TRX.

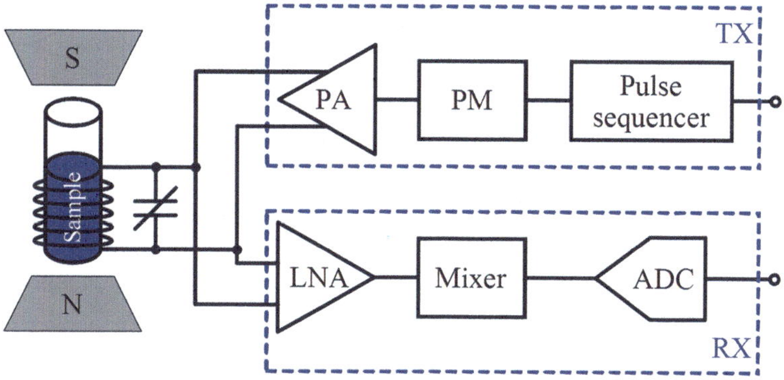

Fig. 4.50 The overall structure of the NMR system

The NMR system works in two mode including excitation mode and receiving mode. For NMR excitation, a pulse sequence at f_L must be applied to the NMR coil to generate the B_{RF} field on the sample and excite the nuclear spins. To achieve this, the conventional NMR system utilizes a TX composed of a pulse-sequence synthesizer and a switching PA. In order to excite coil with sufficiently B_{RF} field, significant currents have to be injected into the NMR coil by the PA. It is notable that for maximum power transfer, the output impedance of PA is to be matched to the coil. The pulse-sequence synthesizer receives external commands and executes various NMR sequences accordingly, and it can be implemented using digital logic gates.

After the excitation, the picks-up coil record the magnetic field produced from the nuclei spin and turn it to a detectible RF voltage signal. Usually the same coil for excitation is utilized for picks up the NMR signal. In the RF RX stage, this coil is connected to a LNA following a down conversion mixer. The LNA enhances the RF voltage signal generated by the precession of proton spins across the sample coil while also providing protection against SNR loss. The LNA amplifies the RF voltage signal induced across the sample coil by the precession of proton spins and mitigates any loss in SNR. To reduce the noise fig. (NF), the LNA should be carefully connected to the coil. On the other hand, usually a variable gain LNA is employed to accommodate the large input dynamic range with no saturation [302]. Mixer down convert the RF signal to the baseband is employed. It is notable, utilizing an active mixer can provide additional gain and relaxing the noise requirement of the subsequent stages.

4.7.3.2 The Related Works of NMR System

Recently, efforts have been made to leverage integrated electronics for NMR applications. An example of a miniaturized electronics for NMR applications, which integrated multiple detection coils and RX on the same IC for the first time was presented by Anders et al. [325]. The co-integration of electronics and reception coils on the same chip enables the adjustment of coil sizes for very small samples,

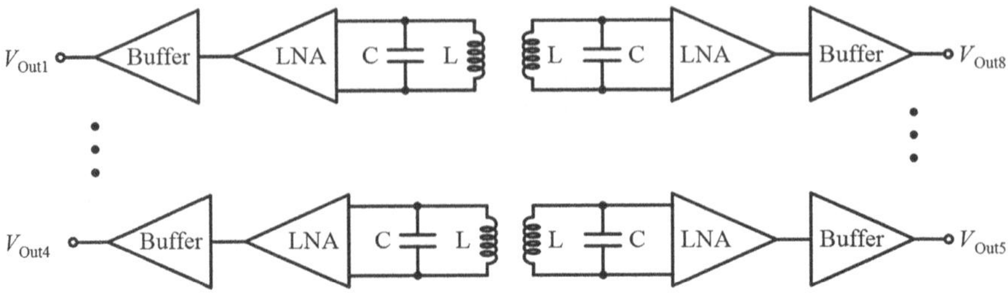

Fig. 4.51 Block-diagram of the integrated RX

facilitating parallel spectroscopy and imaging. At 300 MHz operation, this optimized design comprises eight individual channels. Each channel incorporates a detection coil, tuning capacitor, LNA, and a 50 Ω buffer (refer to Fig. 4.51) The integrated RF- RX demonstrates a measured gain of 28 dB and an input-referred noise of 0.6 nV/$\sqrt{}$Hz at 300 MHz.

As a follow-up to this innovation, the first portable NMR system that combines permanent magnets and spectrometer electronics chips and capable of performing 1D and 2D spectroscopy was developed in [315]. In the same direction, the authors of Sun et al. [313] focused on the design of Palm NMR system and 1-chip NMR system for disease screening using NMR-based biomolecular sensing technology implemented in 0.18 μm CMOS. Figure 4.52 shows the CMOS RF TRX that is common between the palm system and 1-chip NMR system. The integrated TX employed a Class-D PA consisting of differential chains of inverters. In transmission mode, to control the proton excitation rate, the duty cycle of a square-wave RF excitation signal is tuned. The structure of the RX is designed based on the fully differential heterodyne topology that of an LNA, a VGA, and a mixer. In this study, the NF of the RX has been reduced through the minimization of the input-referred noise of the LNA and the optimization of the noise matching with the LNA coil. The measured NF values for the palm and 1-chip system are 0.9 dB and 2.2 dB, respectively.

The 1-chip NMR system integrates the planar coil in the CMOS chip along with the TRX so that the weakening of the SNR ratio raised of the lossy on-chip coil is compensated through the TRX's performance along with a hamburger size magnet. This design directly interfaces the CMOS chip with a sample for LoC operation that enables the detection of human bladder cancer cells and human chorionic gonadotropin (hCG) protein. As mentioned, the palm system uses the same TRX architecture of a 1-chip NMR system with the difference being that a tiny magnet the size of a ping-pong ball and a high-quality solenoidal off-chip coil is employed. Notably, given that the signal is already attenuated by the ping-pong-ball-sized magnet, the palm system incorporates a high-quality solenoidal off-chip coil to prevent any further degradation of the signal. In this design, a sample is placed inside the solenoidal coil and enables to detection of the avidin proteins.

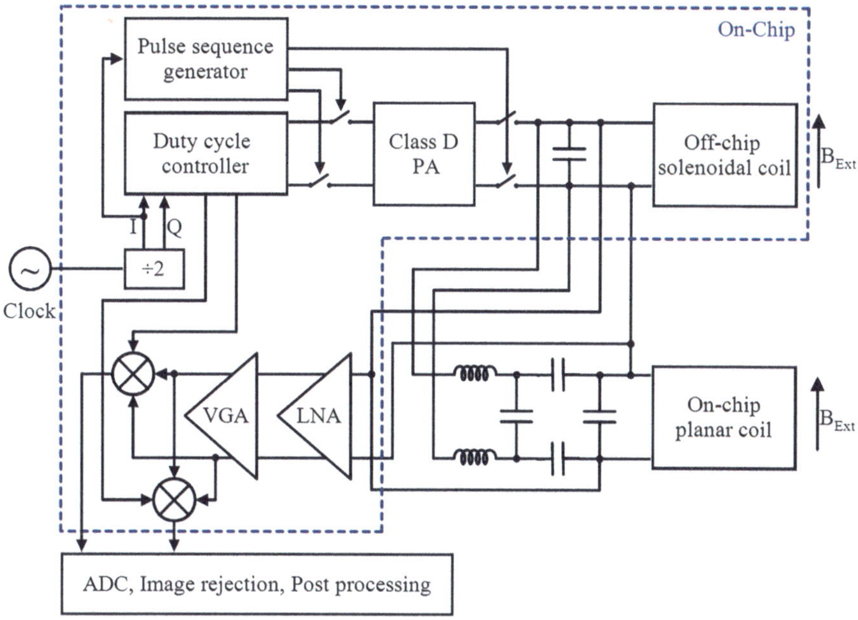

Fig. 4.52 CMOS RF TRX structure of palm and 1-chip NMR system

The brief operation of the detection signal by the NMR system is described as follows. When a sample is positioned inside the coil, it is exposed to the permanent magnetic field B_{Ext}. The hydrogen protons present in the aqueous sample act as nuclear magnets with an NMR frequency denoted by f_L. Specifically, the NMR frequency for protons influenced by B_{Ext} is 23.9 MHz for the palm system and 20.9 MHz for the 1-chip system. The TX generates an RF magnetic field in the coil at frequency f_L to stimulate proton magnets. Upon cessation of RF transmission, the excited proton magnets induce an AC voltage at frequency f_L across the coil, which is then detected by the RX as the NMR signal.

In another effort, Pourmodhej et al. [304] developed a 21 MHz differential NMR spectrometer using a 0.13 μm CMOS. It consists of a dual path RX, two off-chip solenoid mini-coils, and off-chip pulse generators (to excite RF coils). As shown in Fig. 4.53, the introduced RX consists of two differential LNA, phase shifter (PS), variable gain amplifier (VGA), output differential amplifier (ODA) and buffer that briefly discussed as follows. A fully differential cascade push-pull LNA is employed to achieve higher gain and lower noise [325]. The differences between two components, for instance off-chip mini-coils and LNAs are removed through the PS, which is adjusted by external control voltages. The VGA is specifically designed to regulate the output signal level in order to prevent the output stage from saturating. This is crucial as it helps to mitigate potential signal saturation issues that may arise from variations in the NMR signal caused by changes in the target spines in the sample.

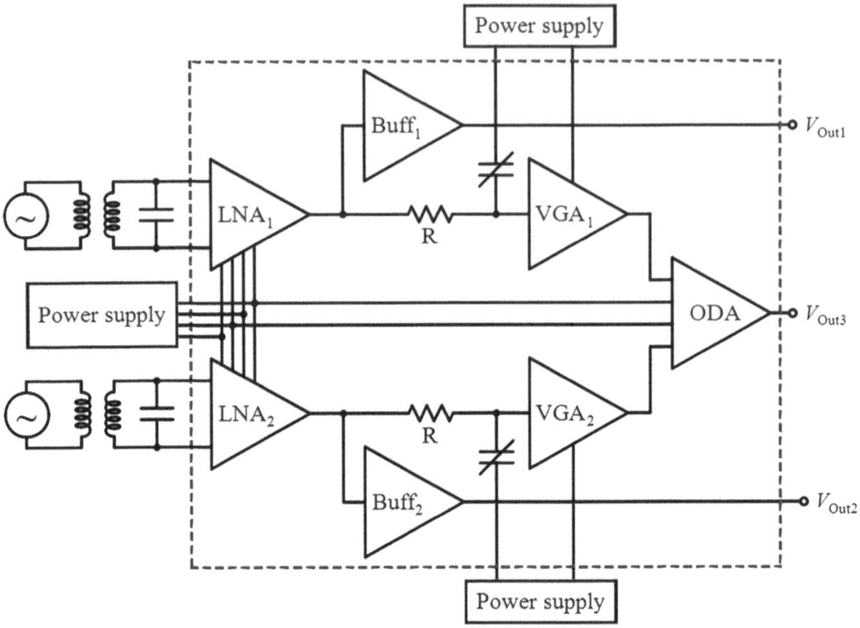

Fig. 4.53 Schematic of a doula path NMR RX

To prevent any additional mistakes in the output signal, PS blocks are employed to adjust the phase discrepancy between two paths. The two different generated signals are differentiating by ODA and buffers enable the testing of an IC without affecting the characteristics of other components within the IC. The measurement result indicates that the front-end RX attains a voltage gain of 80 dB with a low input referred noise of 2.7 $nV/\sqrt{Hz}$.

To address this issue, the dynamic nuclear polarization (DNP) technique [326] can be employed. DNP enhances the intensity of the NMR signal by transferring the significant magnetic moment from electron spins to nuclear spins through microwave irradiation [327].

Recently, Solmaz et al. [328] introduced, for the first time, a DNP microsystem that integrates an on-chip planar micro-coil with CMOS TRX and electron spin resonance (ESR) spectrometers on a single silicon chip smaller than 2 mm^2. This innovative design improves the limit of detection, particularly for samples in the nanoliter and subnanoliter range. In their study, NMR experiments were conducted on liquid samples with a volume of approximately 1 nL. The single-chip DNP microsystem, shown in Fig. 4.54, comprises two main components: the ESR and NMR detectors, fabricated using 0.18 μm CMOS technology. The NMR detector features a broadband (10 MHz to 1 GHz) TRX electronic circuit connected directly to an excitation/detection planar spiral microcoil without a matching network. The ESR detector consists of a differential Colpitts LC oscillator operating at 10.7 GHz. During transmission, the RF signal (16 MHz) is amplified by the TX and delivered

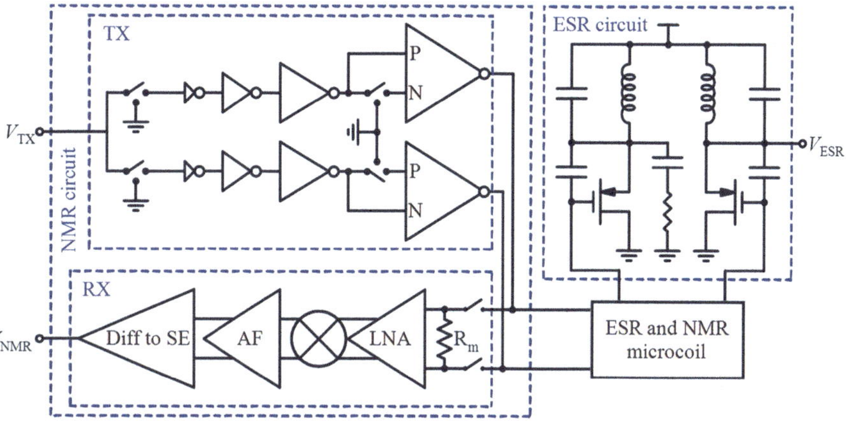

Fig. 4.54 Schematic of the single-chip DNP microsystem

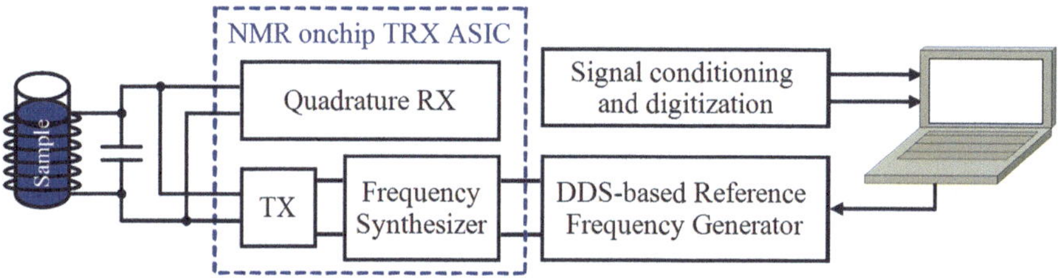

Fig. 4.55 Simplified block diagram of the NMR relaxometry system

to the NMR microcoil. During receive mode, the electromotive force generated in the NMR microcoil as a result of spin precession is first amplified by an RF-RX amplifier, then passed through a mixer operated by the local oscillator signal for down-conversion, and finally boosted by an integrated low-frequency amplifier.

The NMR and ESR detector microcoils are concentric, allowing them to interrogate the same sample volume and perform DNP experiments on a single chip. NMR experiments conducted at 10.7 GHz (ESR)/16 MHz (NMR) on TEMPOL/H_2O solutions demonstrated enhancements as large as 50 at room temperature. The measure of enhancement is determined by comparing the integrals of the NMR signals in the frequency domain between the enhanced and non-enhanced cases.

We will close this section by examining the complete structure of a portable NMR relaxometry system designed by Dreyer et al. [298] in 0.13 μm BiCMOS for the PoC analysis of body liquids. The main building blocks of the NMR relaxometer as shown in Fig. 4.55, include the NMR-on-a-chip TRX application-specific integrated circuit (ASIC), the DDS-based reference frequency generation, the NMR coil, and a custom-designed miniaturized NMR magnet. In this work, since the distance between the NMR sensor coil and the TRX ASIC is short, the conventional

50 Ω impedance matching is removed, which improves power efficiency of the system. The ASIC integrates an on-chip a PLL-based frequency synthesizer, a PA, and a quadrature RX while ADC and the DDS-based reference frequency generator were not integrated to provide greater flexibility.

The system setup includes the ASIC and reference frequency generator, complemented by the back-end electronics. These back-end electronics comprise off-chip anti-aliasing filters (AAFs), buffers for digital control signals, and a commercial data acquisition (DAQ) unit. Specifically, the NMR ASIC's low- intermediate frequency (IF) output signals undergo low-pass filtering by the AAFs with a 350 kHz cutoff frequency, before digitization by an NI PXIe 6366 DAQ unit. Subsequently, post-processing of the captured NMR data occurs on a PC using custom LabVIEW software from National Instruments. The LabVIEW software not only manages NMR experiments but also serves to control both the NMR ASIC and the DDS-based reference frequency generator.

The quadrature RX is composed of an LNA, a quadrature down-conversion mixer, and a VGA output stage featuring automatic DC offset compensation. The LNA employs a cascoded bipolar junction transistor (BJT) differential pair with a resistive load to attain a low input-referred voltage noise of 0.61 $nV/\sqrt{Hz}$ and a significant gain of 31.5 dB. This high gain is essential for mitigating the noise introduced by the following mixer stage. The TX stage utilizes an H-bridge-based PA, controlled by a tapered buffer, to deliver the necessary output current to the tuned NMR coil. The frequency synthesizer features a second-order integer-N PLL with a programmable frequency divider. Input reference frequencies can be adjusted within the range of 5.5 MHz to 12.2 MHz, while the output frequency spans from 5 MHz to 780 MHz, corresponding to B_{Ext} fields from 0.1 T to 18 T for proton NMR. In this setup, the NMR frequency of interest operates at 2.3 MHz. The measurements conducted on human blood samples in this study demonstrate a notable concentration sensitivity of 2.2 $mM/\sqrt{Hz}$. The results confirm the effectiveness of the suggested NMR relaxometry system in reliably detecting biomarkers like proteins and lipids, and in pinpointing alterations caused by fluctuations in blood glucose levels.

4.8 CMOS Temperature Sensors

4.8.1 BJT Temperature Sensors

The temperature-dependent behavior utilized in the design of BJT temperature sensors is achieved by the ratio of a proportional to absolute temperature (PTAT) voltage (ΔV_{BE}) and a temperature-independent voltage ($V_{BE} + \alpha\ \Delta V_{BE}$). Designing a BJT-based temperature sensor faces two main challenges: addressing the V_{BE} spread as the primary error source and developing a cost-effective calibration technique for temperature error due to V_{BE} spread. Various attempts to solve these issues is provided. For example, the discrepancy between transistors and current sources restricts the accuracy of ΔV_{BE}. Meijer et al. [329] addressed this issue using DEM, which dynamically interchanges current sources to reduce mismatch errors. Pertijs et al. [330] proposed a temperature sensor with an on-chip CTΔΣM and digital bus interface in a 0.5 μm CMOS process. In this work, dynamic offset cancellation and DEM are used for high initial accuracy, with second-order curvature correction for wide-range linearity. The V_{BE} spread is trimmed via single-point calibration post-packaging. The sensor achieves ±0.5 °C accuracy (3σ) from −50 °C to 120 °C after calibration. This group proposed another temperature sensor extending the range from −55 °C to 125 °C with an accuracy of ±0.1 °C using 0.7 μm CMOS [331]. This sensor is shown in Fig. 4.56 that consist of a bipolar core to generate the voltages ΔV_{BE} and V_{BE}. These voltages serve as inputs to a ΔΣM, which generates a bitstream, bs. The average value of this bitstream corresponds to the ratio of $\alpha\ \Delta V_{BE}$ and V_{REF}. To reduce temperature errors from circuit non-idealities to ±0.01 °C, the design incorporates CDS, system-level chopping in the ΔΣM and bias circuit chopping, a special bias circuit for insensitivity to current gain and supply voltage variations, and DEM to eliminate mismatch errors. Curvature correction uses a temperature-dependent reference and a nonlinear decimation filter. The remaining significant error, the spread of the base-emitter voltage, is trimmed out using a high-resolution trimming circuit based on a current ΔΣ DAC after a single temperature calibration. Despite effective calibration methods, individual calibration adds significant cost.

In another design, Yousefzadeh et al. [332] presented a BJT-based temperature sensor in 0.16 μm CMOS that achieved ±0.06 °C (3σ) accuracy from −55 °C to 125 °C after a single room-temperature trim. The sensor features PTAT/Resistance biasing to provide less nonlinearity and a supply-independent current, a β-compensating resistor for suppressing the effect of β on V_{BE}, and a two-step SAR-ΔΣ ADC architecture for enhanced accuracy.

The reviewed works utilized an ADC to convert the temperature-sensing signal to digitized information. There have been reports of some temperature sensors that work in the time domain. These type of sensors provides digitized information through frequency-to-digital converter (FDC) [333–337] or duty-cycle-modulated (DCM) [338–342]. For instance, Park et al. [335] introduced a BJT-based temperature-to-frequency converter (TFC) that detects temperature by measuring only the oscillation frequency. This design without any trimming circuit demonstrated a 3σ-inaccuracy of ±1 °C from −40 °C to 140 °C.

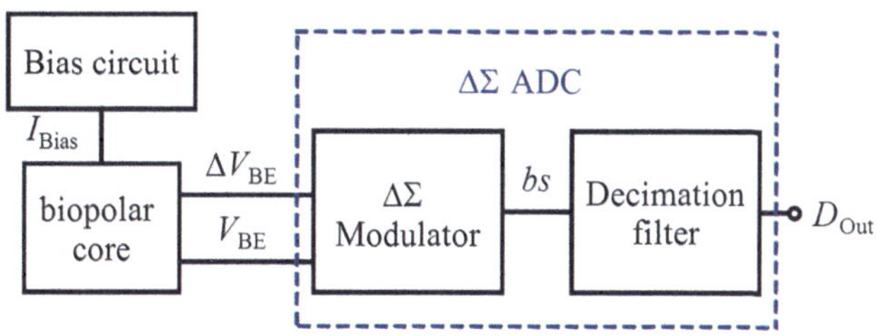

Fig. 4.56 Block diagram of a temperature sensor with ΔΣM

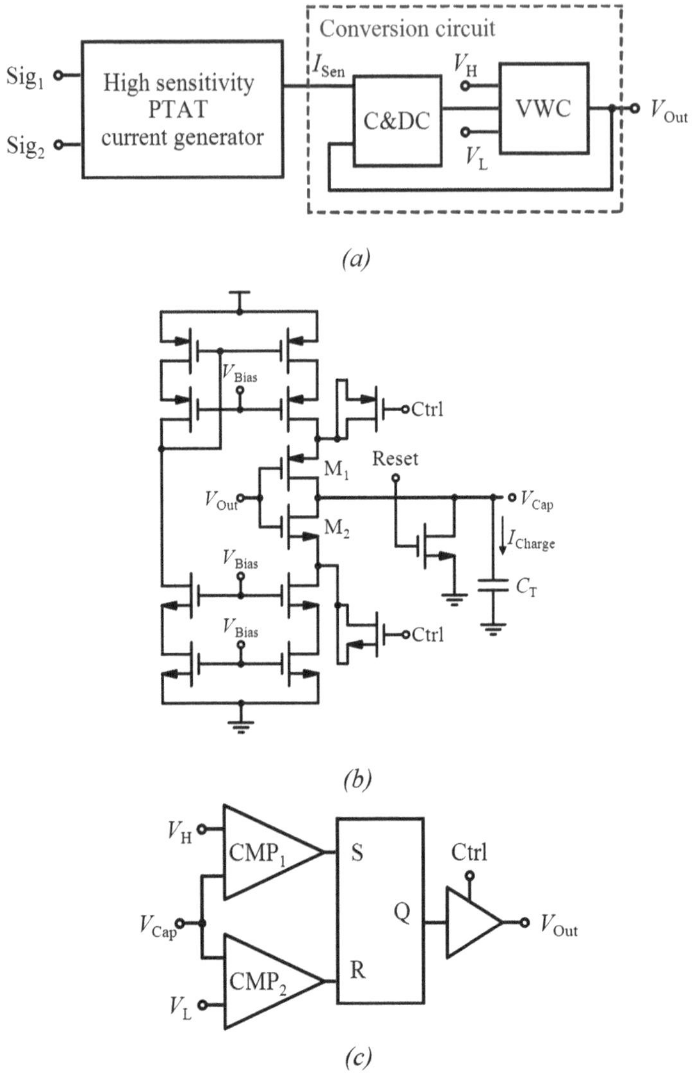

Fig. 4.57 (**a**) The block diagram of the temperature sensor using PTAT and CTAT current subtraction with frequency output (**b**) the schematic of C&DC (**c**) the schematic of VWC

Other work presented a wide dynamic range temperature sensor with frequency output by Lee et al. [336] that its block diagram is shown in Fig. 4.57a. A novel PTAT current generator with high sensitivity is developed that subtracts PTAT and CTAT current raised basically from the BJT transistor. The generated current, I_{sen}, charged and discharged the capacitor of C_T in the charge and discharge circuit (C&DC) as depicted in Fig. 4.57b. The periodic capacitor voltage obtained is subsequently employed to produce the frequency output signal, V_{Out}, through a voltage window comparator (VWC). The schematic of VWC is demonstrated in Fig. 4.57c that act as a voltage-to-frequency converter. When the capacitor voltage V_{Cap} drops below the reference voltage V_L, CMP_1 outputs logic 0 and CMP_2 outputs logic 1. Using the SR latch and the buffer, V_{Out} resets to logic 0, turning on M_1 and off M_2, initiating the charging state. I_{Charge} charges the capacitor until V_{Cap} exceeds V_H, flipping CMP_1 to logic 1 and CMP_2 to logic 0, setting V_{Out} to logic 1, and discharging C_T. This cycle repeats, producing an output frequency proportional to the input current I_{Sen}. The measurement results indicate temperature sensing errors ranging from −0.19 °C to +0.34 °C within a sensing range of −40 °C to 70 °C. The output dynamic range is 2.825.

In temperature sensors with a DCM output signal, the temperature information is modulated to a duty cycle in the time domain, rather than converting complementary to absolute temperature (CTAT) and PTAT voltages to digital values. Figure 4.58 shows a block diagram of a DCM temperature sensor.

The OpAmp (OP_1) and OP_2 generate the PTAT current (I_{PTAT}) and CTAT current (I_{CTAT}), respectively. Then, the combination of these currents is utilized for alternately charging and discharging of a capacitor C. As a result, the cycle of the resulting oscillation has a linear function of the current combination and subsequently a linear function of temperature. By using chopping, DEM, and a single room temperature trim, the sensor also maintains a spread of less than ±0.15 °C (3σ) from −45 to 130 °C. Another DCM sensor is presented by Huang et al. [342] that achieved inaccuracy of ±0.54 °C (3σ) over a temperature range of −40 °C to 125 °C.

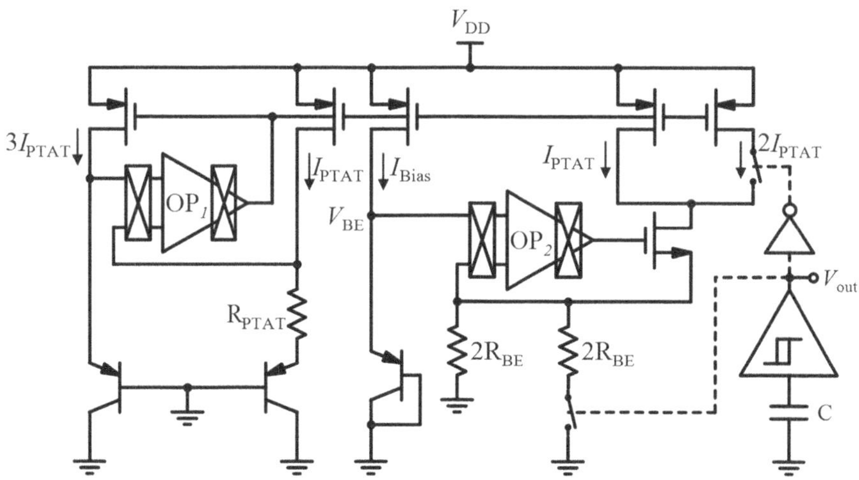

Fig. 4.58 Block diagram of a DCM temperature sensor

4.8.2 MOSFET Temperature Sensors

Recently, MOSFET temperature sensors have become popular for low-power applications due to their use of MOSFETs operating in the subthreshold region. In this mode, MOSFETs exhibit an exponential current-voltage (I-V) relationship, similar to that of BJT devices. Due to the nonlinearity of MOSFET current in the subthreshold region concerning temperature, the approach of utilizing the disparity between two MOSFET currents is employed to achieve a behavior that is PTAT.

The readout circuit has an important role in the accuracy of the sensors. Souri et al. [343] proposed a sub-1 V sensor for radio frequency identification (RFID) applications that utilized a dynamic threshold MOSFET (DTMOS) as a temperature-sensing element. A DTMOS is a MOSFET with connected body and gate terminals,

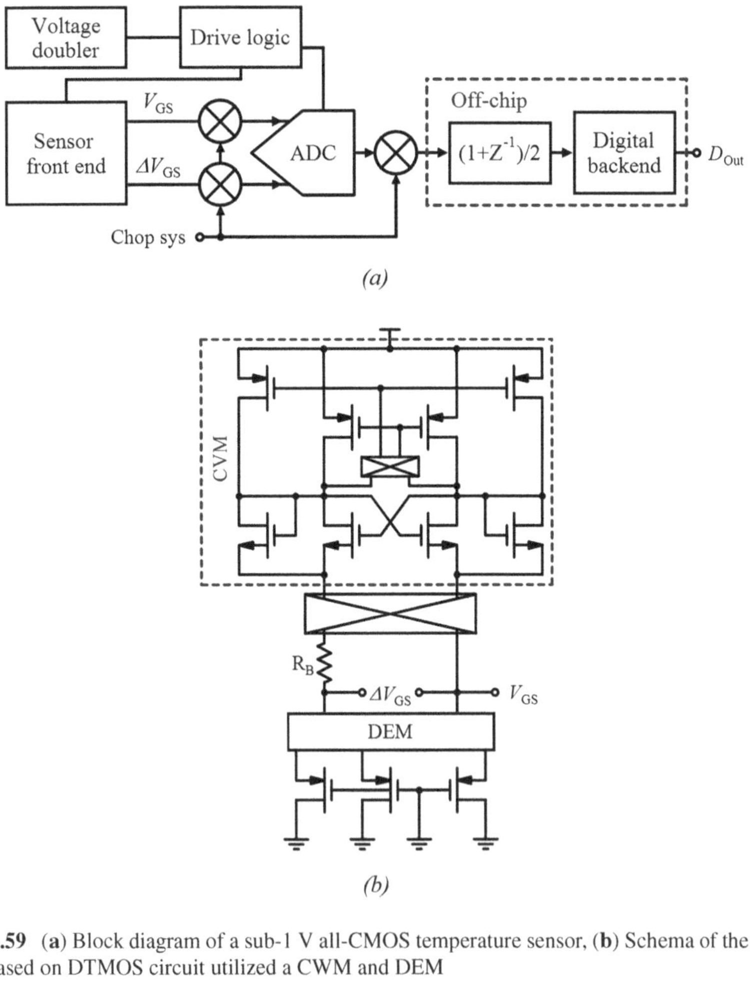

Fig. 4.59 (**a**) Block diagram of a sub-1 V all-CMOS temperature sensor, (**b**) Schema of the front-end based on DTMOS circuit utilized a CWM and DEM

causing dynamic threshold voltage variation [344]. Figure 4.59 shows the block diagram and the front-end circuit of the sensor. The ratio between V_{GS}, (exhibits CTAT behavior) and ΔV_{GS} (exhibits the PTAT behavior) of two DTMOSTs in the front-end is used to measure temperature. The current-voltage mirror (CVM) generates ΔV_{GS} across a resistor, leading to biasing currents with a precise PTAT dependency. To reduce the impact of DTMOS mismatch on the accuracy of ΔV_{GS}, a 1:2 area ratio is implemented by integrating three unit DTMOSTs into a DEM scheme. Then, the zoom ADC digitizes the output of the DTMOST frontend. The sensor achieves high accuracy of a ± 0.4 °C over a temperature range of −40 to 125 °C which consume 700 nA from a 0.85 V supply.

Another temperature sensor is introduced by Bashir et al. [345] employed a MOSFET PTAT circuit operating in the sub-threshold region, along with a second-order ΔΣADC for temperature-to-digital conversion. The sensor is implemented in 65 nm CMOS standard process and draws a power consumption of 27.8 μW, while achieving an accuracy of ±0.25 °C across a temperature range of −55 °C to 125 °C. In another design, a differential voltage readout scheme utilizing MOSFET transistors is implemented by Li et al. [346] to address the process variation issues in MOSFET circuits. Additionally, DEM is employed to minimize circuit mismatch. The sensor is manufactured using a 55 nm process. Measurement results indicate an error range of −0.69/0.85 °C among 16 samples tested across temperatures ranging from 0 °C to 100 °C.

In a different adaptation, a novel temperature sensor design is suggested, incorporating a transducer and readout circuit as a unified unit rather than distinct components by Kim et al. [347]. The core structure of the temperature sensor is depicted in Fig. 4.60 that consist of a temperature to voltage comparator, a SAR logic, and a capacitive-DAC (CDAC). The readout component of this sensor employs a clocked comparator engineered with a PTAT input offset voltage to compare the current temperature with the expected value. The outcome of the comparator, in the form of an on-bit result, is then quantized by a successive approximation register (SAR) to create a multibit output code. Essentially, in operational mode, the sensor explores the ambient temperature by modulating the test temperature (or the corresponding differential input voltage, V_{REF}-V_{DAC}) using SAR. Given that the SAR's digital output is proportional to the PTAT offset and exhibits a linear relationship with temperature, the sensor functions effectively without the necessity of intricate digital processing.

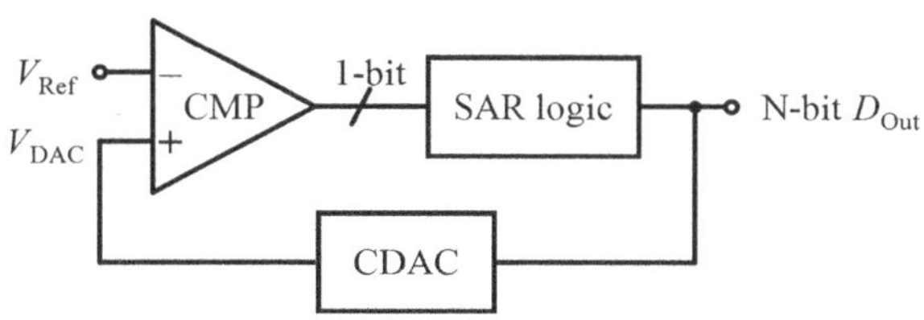

Fig. 4.60 Core block diagram of a SAR temperature sensor

This fusion intends to optimize temperature reliability and stability by simplifying the temperature conversion process, obviating the need for analog signal generation, and facilitating the direct translation of temperature measurements into digital data. This innovation allows for an expansion of the temperature range beyond the limitations of previous circuits. The temperature sensor, manufactured using a 0.18 μm CMOS process, exhibits a broad temperature detection span ranging from −50 °C to +130 °C, while maintaining a low energy consumption rate of 38.69 pJ/conv. Following a two-point calibration, the sensor demonstrates a 3-sigma temperature precision with an inaccuracy of −2.54 °C to +2.16 °C.

For wireless system applications frequency-to-digital conversion is preferred compared to the ADCs due to the low power operation [348]. In a study by Jeong et al. [348], a 71nW temperature sensor designed for wireless sensor nodes was presented, fabricated using a 0.18 μm CMOS process. The proposed temperature sensor comprises three main components as illustrated in Fig. 4.61; (1) a temperature sensing core, (2) a current to frequency converter, and (3) a frequency to digital converter,. The sensing core converts temperature to current, the oscillator converts current to frequency, and the counter translates frequency to digital output. The sensor achieved an inaccuracy of +1.5 °C/−1.4 °C after 2-point calibration across 0 °C to 100 °C. In another effort by Yang et al. [349], a subthreshold ring oscillator is used as an exponential temperature-to-frequency converter. In this sensor, instead of a counter as a frequency-to-digital converter, a sampling schema utilized to achieve better performance across temperature. The temperature sensor implemented in a 0.18 μm CMOS process and shows inaccuracy of −0.22/0.19 °C across −20 °C to 100 °C. Another temperature sensor for wireless sensor networks with frequency output is proposed by Azcona et al. [350]. The sensor is devised to detect the temperature of the PTAT current, which is subsequently converted to frequency through the implementation of a source-coupled multi-vibrator circuit. Following a single-point calibration, the temperature sensor attains a maximum temperature inaccuracy of under 1 °C. It operates at an average power consumption of 600 nW at +85 °C with a 0.9 V supply voltage.

In another study, a temperature sensor developed by Someya et al. [351] utilized a current ratio involving two sub-threshold NMOS transistors. The drain voltages of these transistors are carefully controlled to remain sub-thermal drain voltage (STV) and above thermal drain voltage (AVT). This approach enhances the linearity and

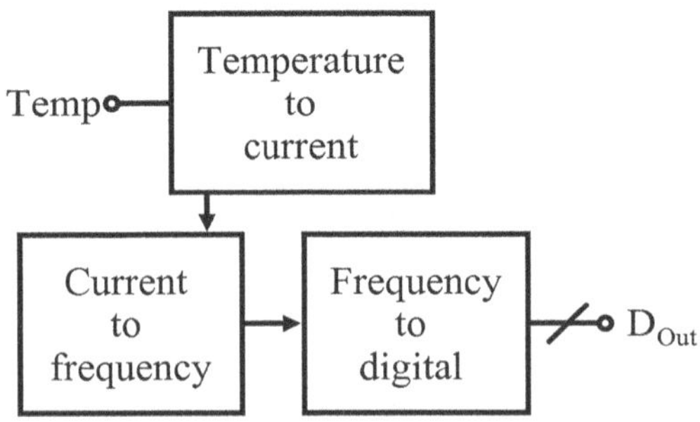

Fig. 4.61 Block diagram of a temperature sensor for wireless sensor nodes

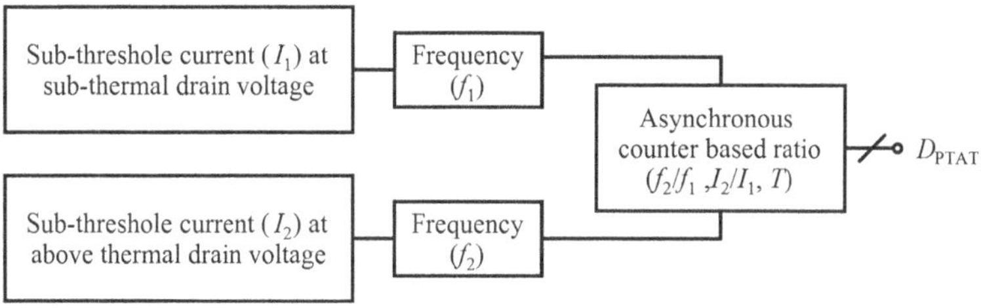

Fig. 4.62 Flowchart of a temperature sensor based on sub-threshold NMOS transistors

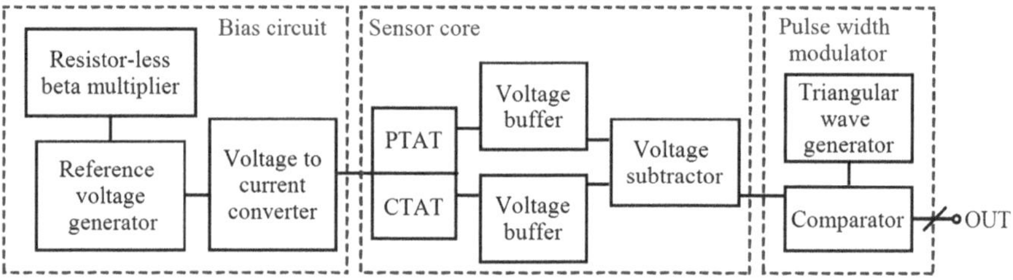

Fig. 4.63 A DCM temperature sensor utilized PWM

sensitivity of the temperature sensor design. The conversion process of the sensor is shown in Fig. 4.62, The generated currents form STV and ATV turn to frequency by current-to-frequency converter designed based on relaxation oscillators. Then, the frequency ratio (f_2/f_1) is calculated to obtain the PTAT digital output. As a result, the current ratio I_2/I_1 exhibits a PTAT characteristic in the −20 °C to 80 °C range. The sensor is fabricated in a 0.18 μm CMOS process and consumes only 11 nW and show −0.9/+1.2 °C peak-to-peak inaccuracy. In this study, to improve the linearity of I_2/I_1 a new current generator is developed. In addition, a frequency-locked loop (FLL)-based current-to-frequency converter is introduced that enhances power consumption and supply voltage tolerance of the temperature sensor. The results obtained from the prototype, fabricated using a 65 nm CMOS process, demonstrate that the proposed temperature sensor consumes only 6.4 nW and has an inaccuracy range of −1 °C to +0.7 °C.

In the realm of temperature sensors, those featuring DCM outputs offer digital-friendly interfaces and simple control logic, proving superior to frequency-based counterparts due to the linearity of ratio values over absolute frequency values [340, 352]. Chouhan et al. [353] introduced a 7.2 μW DCM temperature sensor implemented in a 0.18 μm CMOS process. The system's block diagram, as shown in Fig. 4.63, illustrates a temperature sensing setup that produces a pulse output with a duty cycle directly proportional to temperature. Within its design, a bias circuit generator is composed of three sub-blocks: a resistorless beta multiplier, a reference voltage generator, and a voltage-to-current converter. The sensor core integrates

MOSFET-based temperature sensors and a voltage buffer to counteract loading effects. The buffered voltages undergo subtraction through an operational amplifier-based voltage subtractor. The resultant signal is transformed into pulses using a PWM system with a triangular wave generator and comparator. For further insights, detailed discussions are provided in subsequent sections. Post single-point calibration, the temperature sensor achieves an inaccuracy of within ±1.5 °C across the temperature range from −30 °C to +70 °C. Another DCM temperature sensor employs a PTAT current generator as the front end and incorporates a temperature-dependent oscillator, where the output characteristic is the duty cycle rather than frequency [352].

4.8.3 ETF Temperature Sensors

In the context of electrothermal filter (ETF) temperature sensors, the phase shift ($\varnothing_{ETF}$) of the ETF when driven at a frequency f_{drive} is proportional to $(S\sqrt{f_{\text{drive}}})T^{0.9}$. It can be deducted from the mentioned equation, ETF temperature sensors can operate in two mode including constant phase shift (CTP) or constant frequency (CTF). At CTP, the frequency (as an output signal) is proportional to $1/T^{1.8}$, which implies a non-linear function of temperature. While, at CTF the phase shift is proportional to $T^{0.9}$, which indicate a linear functionality of phase shift and temperate. In this section, the ETF temperature sensors operated at CTF and CTP are reviewed.

4.8.3.1 ETF Temperature Sensor Driving at CTP

A temperature-to-frequency converter was implemented using an ETF within a FLL by Makinwa et al. [354]. By maintaining a CTP in the ETF, the frequency output becomes temperature-dependent. The FLL configuration, depicted in Fig. 4.64, includes an ETF, preamplifier, synchronous demodulator (transconductance, chopper, and external integrating capacitor), and a voltage-controlled oscillator (VCO). The first chopper modulated the offset of amplifiers in the input of the demodulator to f_{VCO} and then integrator filtered out of offset. An extra off-chip chopper at lower frequency of (f_{VCO}/128) chopped again the thermal filter, preamp and gm_1 to reduce

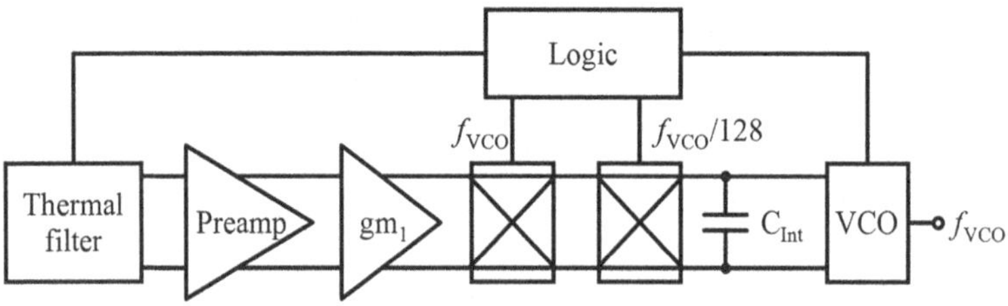

Fig. 4.64 ETF temperate sensor based on the FLL

phase error erased from chopper's charge injection mismatch. The VCO generates a square wave to drive the ETF, with the phase-shifted output undergoing amplification and synchronous demodulation. The demodulator's output is further amplified to adjust the VCO. The VCO achieves frequency stabilization when the chopper's DC output reaches zero, indicating a 90-degree phase shift in the ETF. This temperature sensor has been developed using a 0.7 μm CMOS process, delivering an accuracy of 0.5 °C across the temperature span of −40 °C to 105 °C, with a power consumption of 2.5 mW from a 5 V supply. Zhang et al. [355] presented an enhanced FLL architecture featuring an on-chip integrator capacitor, showcasing a temperature-sensing inaccuracy of under 0.7 °C over the range of −40 °C to 100 °C.

4.8.3.2 ETF Temperature Sensor Driving at Constant Frequency

In the field of temperature sensors, the phase-domain delta-sigma modulator (PDΔΣM) is notable for its capability to convert the temperature-dependent phase shift into a digital signal within an ETF system. Vroonhoven et al. [356] introduced an ETF temperature sensor utilizing a PDΔΣM operated at 85 kHz, as depicted in Fig. 4.65. The amplified ETF output signal undergoes multiplication with a phase-shifted φ_0 or φ_1 copy to form the summing node. The chopper-based multiplier at the gm-stage output generates a DC output current that varies in proportion to the cosine of the phase discrepancy between the inputs, reaching zero at a 90-degree phase difference. Post-demodulation, the integrating capacitor C_{Int} captures this current. The modulator's average bitstream output offers a representation of the ETF's phase shift, facilitating temperature measurement. Implemented using a 0.7 μm CMOS process, this sensor attains an accuracy of ±0.5 °C (3σ) over the temperature span of −55 °C to 125 °C.

Kashmiri et al. [357] adopt a similar topology with an optimized ETF layout to minimize lithographic inaccuracies' impact on thermal phase spread. Moreover, a new front-end design is proposed to leverage the anticipated decrease in electrical

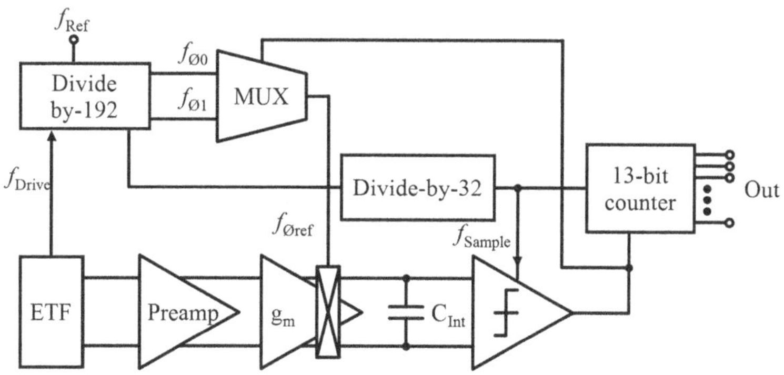

Fig. 4.65 ETF temperature sensor employed the PDΔΣM

phase spread. Tests on 16 samples from a single batch demonstrate an untrimmed inaccuracy of under ±0.7 °C (3σ) over the temperature range spanning −55 °C to 125 °C. In another endeavor, Vroonhoven et al. [358] utilize the same PDΔΣM as in [356] but introduce a new schematic layout for the ETF to boost accuracy. By enhancing interface electronics and leveraging more precise lithography, they achieve higher precision, with an untrimmed inaccuracy of ±0.2 °C (3σ) across the −55 °C to 125 °C range. The PDΔΣM 's power consumption is 500 μW from a 1.8 V supply, marking a substantial fivefold reduction compared to [356].

4.8.4 Resistor Temperature Sensors

4.8.4.1 Wheatstone Bridge Temperature Sensors

Pan et al. [359] introduced a Wheatstone bridge (WhB) temperature sensor with current readout, where the temperature-dependent sensing current from the WhB is digitized by a single-bit CTΔΣM. This sensor achieves an inaccuracy of ±100 mK (3σ) across the temperature range of −40 °C to 85 °C while consuming 180 μW from a 1.8 V supply. Figure 4.66 illustrates the basic structure of the CTΔΣM-based readout for the WhB sensor [360]. The configuration comprises a WhB composed of resistors with positive R_p(T) and negative R_n(T) temperature coefficients. The DAC integrated within the CTΔΣM drives the average value of I_{err} to zero by toggling the DAC's resistors between V_{DD} and GND, effectively balancing the bridge setup.

In a subsequent design by Pan et al. [360], a multi-bit zoom CTΔΣM is employed for the readout circuit. Additionally, a multi-bit resistor DAC is utilized to reduce the magnitude of I_{err}, leading to a diminished swing at the input of the modulator's loop filter. Consequently, the integration capacitor size and power dissipation of the ADC can be significantly decreased. This enhancement results in an inaccuracy of

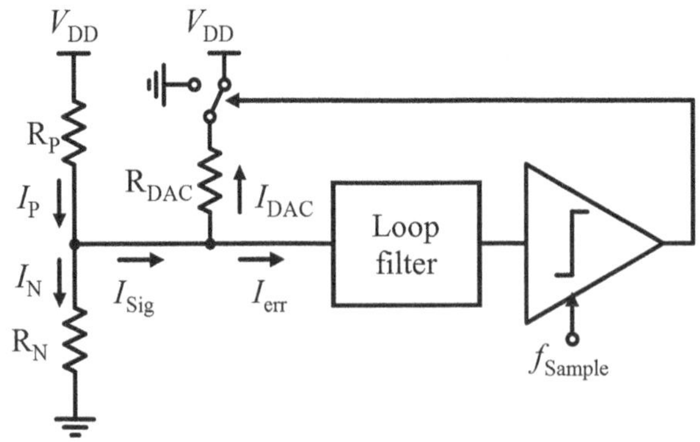

Fig. 4.66 WhB temperature sensor with CTΔΣM readout

±0.12 °C (3σ) over the range of −55 °C to 125 °C, with a power consumption of 52 μA from a 1.8 V supply. In another work by Pan et al. [361], a finite impulse response (FIR) DAC is used to reduce the swing of I_{err}, leading to improved energy efficiency and area reduction. The system achieves an inaccuracy of ±0.14 °C (3σ) over the temperature range of −55 °C to 125 °C, offering a resolution of 0.16 mK and consuming 79 μW of power. Furthermore, in an additional effort by Pan et al. [362], the sensor's accuracy is enhanced to ±0.1 °C (3σ) across −55 °C to 125 °C by employing a sensitivity-preserving return-to-common-mode (RCM) DAC switching scheme and an energy-efficient operational OTA with a tail-resistor linearization scheme. The sensor dissipates only 55 μW from a 1.8 V supply. To achieve a significant reduction in power consumption, Pan et al. [363] leveraged the duty cycle concept to develop a μW-power temperature sensor tailored for biomedical applications, which only draws 6.6 μW from a 1.6 V supply.

Some other design of WhB based sensor read out the temperature through its output frequency [364, 365]. For instance, Jiang et al. [364] developed a temperature sensor that convert the resistance into a time-based signal through a FLL. It achieves an inaccuracy of 0.55 °C over the −40 °C to 85 °C range while consumes 15.6 μW.

4.8.4.2 Wien Bridge Temperature Sensors

In a scenario that an WB driven by a fixed frequency, the amplitude of the WB output will be remaining relatively constant, while the output phase will vary over temperature. To readout the temperature-dependent phase response a precision phase read-out circuit is necessary. Shahmohammadi et al. [366] utilized PDΔΣM to digitize of the phase shift. The sensor was developed using 0.18 μm CMOS technology, with a power consumption of 36 μW. Following batch calibration and a 3-point trim process, the sensor achieves an inaccuracy of ±0.15 °C (3σ) across the industrial temperature range of −40 °C to 85 °C. In a different study by Pan et al. [367], a second-order modulator was employed instead of a first-order modulator to attain sub-mK resolution in a brief conversion time. As shown in Fig. 4.67, the proposed temperature sensor utilizes complementary square waves for driving the sensor, enhancing simplicity and reducing energy consumption. It employs a continuous-time (CT)-PDΔΣM to digitize the output current phase with high resolution, using a single-bit quantizer for simplicity and linearity. By down-converting the phase to a DC current through multiplication with a phase reference at the same frequency, the multiplier determines the output's polarity. The integrated output is then quantized after passing through a loop filter. Through a negative feedback loop, the quantizer adjusts reference phases to maintain a zero average input for the loop filter, thereby providing a digital representation of the sensor's output phase. The sensor, fabricated using 0.18 μm CMOS technology, consumes 87 μA from a 1.8 V supply. It delivers an inaccuracy of ±0.03 °C (3σ) across the temperature range of −40 °C to 85 °C following a first-order fit.

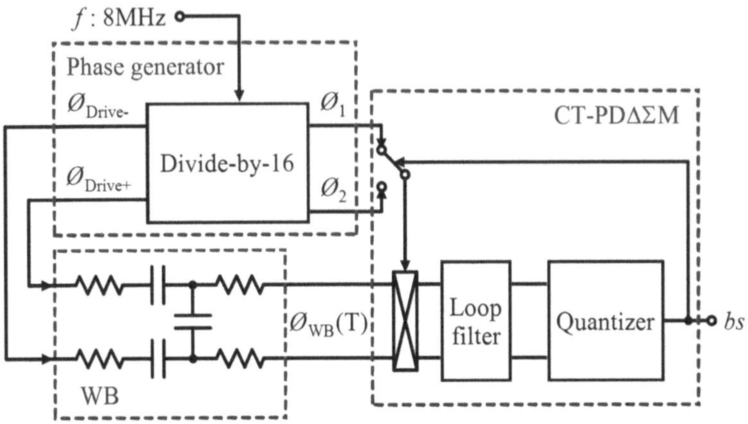

Fig. 4.67 WB temperature sensor with CT-PDΔΣM readout

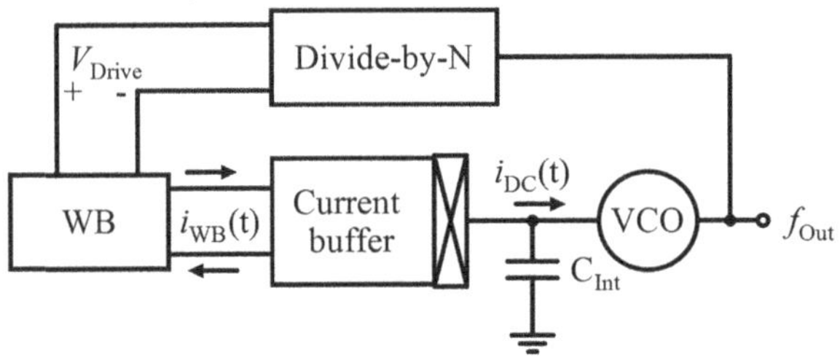

Fig. 4.68 WB temperature sensor whit FLL readout

In another work by Pan et al. in [368], a WB sensor based PDΔΣM featured a first integrator constructed using a two-stage miller compensated OpAmp with current-reuse amplifiers. This design allowed for a reduction in the integration capacitor (C_{Int}) around 8 time compared to [367]. Consequently, the sensor occupies 6 times less area while achieving comparable relative accuracy over a 76% wider operating range compared to the previous design. The sensor achieves a 0.1 °C (3σ) inaccuracy from −40 °C to 180 °C. Another work proposed by Pan et al. [369] is a hybrid ETF/WB temperature sensor with second-order PΔΣM readout circuit been realized in a 0.18 μm CMOS technology that the inaccuracy of the WB sensor is 0.03 °C over −35 °C and 105 °C.

An alternate time-based method for reading the WB is via a FLL approach, as depicted in Fig. 4.68 [370]. The VCO output is divided by N to obtain in-phase and quadrature-phase signals. These in-phase signals are used to drive the WB, producing a filtered and phase-shifted output current. Subsequently, this current is demodulated by the quadrature-phase signals. The resulting DC output current ($i_{\mathrm{DC}}(\mathrm{t})$) is approximately proportional to the cosine of the phase shift of the WB, φ_{WB}. This current is integrated on capacitor C_{Int}, causing the voltage adjustment that tunes the VCO's output frequency. When the system reaches a stable state, the phase shift of the WB becomes negligible, indicating that the output frequency is locked to $N.\omega_0$ (where ω_0 is the WB's center frequency). The sensor exhibits an accuracy of less than 0.12 °C over a temperature range from −40 °C to 85 °C. Furthermore, the sensor attains a resolution of 2.8 mK while consuming 31 μW.

4.8.4.3 Poly-Phase Filter Temperature Sensor

In the case that poly-phase filter (PPF) temperature sensor driven by a f_{Drive}, the output of the PPF displays a phase shift that is temperature-dependent and can be easily digitized using a PDΔΣM. Angevare et al. [371], employed 2-bit first-order PDΔΣM. This design has inaccuracy ±1.3 °C (3σ) over the temperature range of −55 °C to 125 °C and dissipated 28 μW from a 0.9 V supply. In another work introduced by Martin et al. [372] the phase shift of PPF is read out by a FLL. The phase shift of the PPF is established by a zero-crossing (ZC) detector, enabling the implementation of the remaining FLL components in a space-efficient manner. The sensor has an accuracy of ±0.12 °C (3σ) over the temperature range of −40 °C to 85 °C and a resolution of 2.5 mK. It operates on 68 μW from a 0.85 V power supply. Another PPF sensor based on FLL is introduced by Lee et al. [373] shown in Fig. 4.69. The FLL uses an XOR gate instead of a phase-frequency detector and a switched-capacitor loop filter (SCLF) instead of a charge pump, that significantly improving the sensor's accuracy. Moreover, this design integrates a multi-phase counter at the output of the FLL to enable effective conversion of frequency to digital signals. The sensor, developed using a 65 nm CMOS process, occupies an area of 6400 μm^2 and operates at a power consumption of 40 μW with a supply voltage of 0.9 V. Following a single-point trimming procedure, it achieves a temperature accuracy of ±0.64 °C (3σ) over a wide temperature range spanning from −50 to 125 °C.

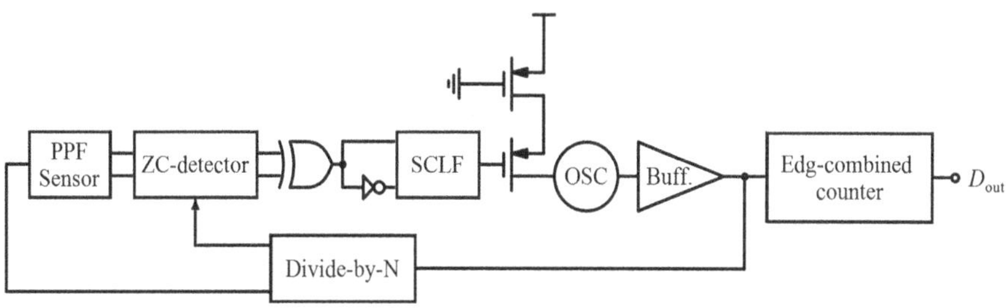

Fig. 4.69 PPF temperature sensor based on FLL

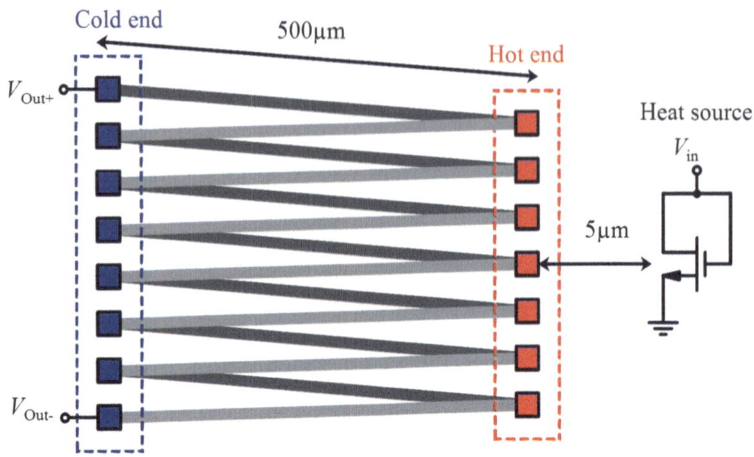

Fig. 4.70 Schema showing the setup of a thermopile with the dissipating transistor functioning as a heat source

4.8.5 Seebeck Effect Temperature Sensors

Temperature sensors utilizing the Seebeck effect have been developed with various configurations and materials [374–382]. Jaeggi et al. [378] introduced a microsystem with two CMOS thermal converters on a single oxide/nitride membrane, each consisting of a polysilicon heating resistor and a bidoped polysilicon thermopile. Koll et al. [379] presented a sensor for temperature variations caused by analyte sorption using gas-sensitive polymer-coated membranes. Another design by the same group [380] improved mechanical stability and temperature distribution, featuring N-well island structures and on-membrane diodes. Voiculescu et al. [381] optimized thermopile sensitivity by arranging thermocouples alongside the heater on the same membrane. In another design, a differential temperature sensor utilizing the Seebeck effect was developed by Aldrete-Vidrio et al. [382]. The sensor featured two thermopiles with identical structures but made of different materials. In the first thermopile, 8 thermocouples (16 stripes) were connected in series, constructed from $poly_1$ (N-doped) and $poly_2$ (N-doped). The second thermopile included thermocouples made of poly1 and P+ diffusion. Both thermopiles had a hot junction-to-cold junction distance of 500 µm. An NMOS transistor, configured in a diode connection setup, served as a heat source and was positioned 5 µm from the hot junction on the same silicon die as the thermopiles that is shown Fig. 4.70. Activation of the diode-connected transistor resulted in an increase in temperature around the device, which was captured by the differential temperature sensors. The output voltage of the sensor was observed using an Agilent 34,401 A Digital Multi-meter. Experimental findings indicated sensitivities of 0.10155 V/W for the $poly_1$-$poly_2$ thermopile and 0.26722 V/W for the $poly_1$-P+ diffusion thermopile.

4.9 Summary

This chapter has dissected the interface circuits integral to a wide range of CMOS biosensors. By delving into the operational principles and circuit designs behind voltammetric, impedimetric, capacitive, FET-based, optical, magnetic, NMR, and temperature sensors, as well as neural stimulation and recording systems, we have underscored the technological advancements that enable precise and efficient biosensing.

The comprehensive understanding gained from this exploration not only showcases the versatility and adaptability of CMOS technology in addressing complex biological challenges but also emphasizes its critical contribution to the future of medical diagnostics, therapeutic interventions, and bioanalytical research. As we move forward, the continued innovation in CMOS biosensor interface circuits will undoubtedly drive the development of more sophisticated, sensitive, and integrated systems, paving the way for breakthroughs in health care and biological sciences.

References

1. Jafari HM, Genov R (2013) Chopper-stabilized bidirectional current acquisition circuits for electrochemical amperometric biosensors. IEEE Trans Circuits Syst I: Regul Pap 60(5):1149–1157
2. Kim BN, Herbst AD, Kim SJ, Minch BA, Lindau M (2013) Parallel recording of neurotransmitters release from chromaffin cells using a 10× 10 CMOS IC potentiostat array with on-chip working electrodes. Biosens Bioelectron 41:736–744
3. Chien J-C, Baker SW, Soh HT, Arbabian A (2020) Design and analysis of a sample-and-hold cmos electrochemical sensor for aptamer-based therapeutic drug monitoring. IEEE J Solid State Circuits 55(11):2914–2929
4. Nazari MH, Mazhab-Jafari H, Leng L, Guenther A, Genov R (2012) CMOS neurotransmitter microarray: 96-channel integrated potentiostat with on-die microsensors. IEEE Trans Biomed Circuits Syst 7(3):338–348
5. Viswam V et al (2018) Impedance spectroscopy and electrophysiological imaging of cells with a high-density CMOS microelectrode Array system. IEEE Trans Biomed Circuits Syst 12:1356–1368
6. Manickam A, Johnson CA, Kavusi S, Hassibi A (2012) Interface design for CMOS-integrated electrochemical impedance spectroscopy (EIS) biosensors. Sensors 12(11):14467–14488
7. Manickam A, Chevalier A, McDermott M, Ellington AD, Hassibi A (2010) A CMOS electrochemical impedance spectroscopy (EIS) biosensor array. IEEE Trans Biomed Circuits Syst 4(6):379–390
8. Ghodsevali E, Gosselin B, Boukadoum M, Miled A (2015) High accuracy and sensitivity differential potentiostat with amplifier-based error cancellation feedback loop. In: Biomedical Circuits and Systems Conference (BioCAS), 2015 IEEE. IEEE, pp 1–4
9. Manickam A et al (2019) A CMOS electrochemical biochip with 32×32 three-electrode voltammetry pixels. IEEE J Solid State Circuits 54(11):2980–2990
10. Ghoreishizadeh SS, Baj-Rossi C, Cavallini A, Carrara S, De Micheli G (2014) An integrated control and readout circuit for implantable multi-target electrochemical biosensing. IEEE Trans Biomed Circuits Syst 8(6):891–898

11. Li L, Liu X, Qureshi WA, Mason AJ (2011) CMOS amperometric instrumentation and packaging for biosensor array applications. IEEE Trans Biomed Circuits Syst 5(5):439–448
12. Buscaglia LA, Oliveira ON, Carmo JP (2021) Roadmap for electrical impedance spectroscopy for sensing: a tutorial. IEEE Sensors J 21(20):22246–22257
13. Sutula S, Cuxart JP, Gonzalo-Ruiz J, Muñoz-Pascual FX, Terés L, Serra-Graells F (2014) A 25-μw all-mos potentiostatic delta-sigma adc for smart electrochemical sensors. IEEE Trans Circuits Syst I: Regul Pap 61(3):671–679
14. Busoni L, Carla M, Lanzi L (2002) A comparison between potentiostatic circuits with grounded work or auxiliary electrode. Rev Sci Instrum 73(4):1921–1923
15. Wang W-S, Kuo W-T, Huang H-Y, Luo C-H (2010) Wide dynamic range CMOS potentiostat for amperometric chemical sensor. Sensors 10(3):1782–1797
16. Al Mamun KA, McFarlane N (2015) A CMOS potentiostatic glucose monitoring system for VACNF amperometric biosensors. In: Circuits and Systems (ISCAS), 2015 IEEE International Symposium on. IEEE, pp 477–480
17. Martin SM, Gebara FH, Strong TD, Brown RB (2004) A low-voltage, chemical sensor interface for systems-on-chip: the fully-differential potentiostat. In: Circuits and systems, 2004. ISCAS'04. Proceedings of the 2004 international symposium on, vol 4. IEEE, p IV-892-5
18. Nazari MH, Genov R (2009) A fully differential CMOS potentiostat. In: Circuits and systems, 2009. ISCAS 2009. IEEE international symposium on. IEEE, pp 2177–2180
19. Martin SM, Gebara FH, Strong TD, Brown RB (2009) A fully differential potentiostat. IEEE Sensors J 9(2):135–142
20. Martin SM, Gebara FH, Strong TD, Brown RB (2004) A low-voltage, chemical sensor interface for systems-on-chip: the fully-differential potentiostat. In: 2004 IEEE international symposium on circuits and systems (IEEE Cat. No. 04CH37512), vol 4. IEEE, p IV-892
21. Ghodsevali E, Gosselin B, Boukadoum M, Miled A (2015) High accuracy and sensitivity differential potentiostat with amplifier-based error cancellation feedback loop. In: 2015 IEEE Biomedical Circuits and Systems Conference (BioCAS). IEEE, pp 1–4
22. Augustyniak, M. et al. (2006) 2.1 A 24 × 16 CMOS-based Chronocoulometric DNA microarray.
23. Martin SM, Gebara FH, Strong TD, Brown RB (2009) A fully differential potentiostat. Sens J, IEEE 9(2):135–142
24. Martin SM, Gebara FH, Larivee BJ, Brown RB (2005) A CMOS-integrated microinstrument for trace detection of heavy metals. IEEE J Solid-State Circuits 40(12):2777–2786
25. Liu X (2014) CMOS instrumentation for electrochemical biosensor array microsystems. Michigan State University, Doctor of Philosophy Electrical Engineering
26. Hassibi A, Lee TH (2006) A programmable 0.18-μm CMOS electrochemical sensor microarray for biomolecular detection. IEEE Sensors J 6(6):1380–1388
27. Boutet P-A, Manen S (2011) Low power CMOS potentiostat for three electrodes amperometric chemical sensor. In: 2011 Faible Tension Faible Consommation (FTFC). IEEE, pp 15–18
28. Kim J, Dunbar W (2014) Nanopore-application CMOS potentiostat design with input parasitic compensation. Electron Lett 50(8):578–579
29. Carrara S, Torre MD, Cavallini A, De Venuto D, De Micheli G (2010) Multiplexing pH and temperature in a molecular biosensor. In: 2010 Biomedical Circuits and Systems Conference (BioCAS). IEEE, pp 146–149
30. Chung W-Y, Silverio AA, Tsai VF (2014) An amperometric sensor readout circuit for multiple electrochemical sensor cells. In: 2014 International Symposium on Integrated Circuits (ISIC). IEEE, pp 528–531
31. De Venuto D, Torre MD, Boero C, Carrara S, De Micheli G (2010) A novel multi-working electrode potentiostat for electrochemical detection of metabolites. In: SENSORS, 2010 IEEE. IEEE, pp 1572–1577
32. Li H, Parsnejad S, Ashoori E, Thompson C, Purcell EK, Mason AJ (2017) Ultracompact microwatt CMOS current readout with picoampere noise and kilohertz bandwidth for biosensor arrays. IEEE Trans Biomed Circuits Syst 12(1):35–46

33. Narula HS, Harris JG (2006) A time-based VLSI potentiostat for ion current measurements. IEEE Sensors J 6(2):239–247
34. Massicotte G, Sawan M (2013) An efficient time-based CMOS potentiostat for neurotransmitters sensing. In: 2013 IEEE international symposium on medical measurements and applications (MeMeA). IEEE, pp 274–277
35. Ayers S, Gillis KD, Lindau M, Minch BA (2007) Design of a CMOS potentiostat circuit for electrochemical detector arrays. IEEE Trans Circuits Syst I: Regul Pap 54(4):736–744
36. White KA, Mulberry G, Kim BN (2019) Parallel 1024-ch cyclic voltammetry on monolithic CMOS electrochemical detector array. IEEE Sensors J 20(8):4395–4402
37. Huang M, Dorta-Quiñones CI, Minch BA, Lindau M (2021) On-chip cyclic voltammetry measurements using a compact 1024-electrode CMOS IC. Anal Chem 93(22):8027–8034
38. Huang C-W, Lu MS-C (2011) Electrochemical detection of the neurotransmitter dopamine by nanoimprinted interdigitated electrodes and a CMOS circuit with enhanced collection efficiency. IEEE Sensors J 11(9):1826–1831
39. White KA et al (2018) Single-cell recording of vesicle release from human neuroblastoma cells using 1024-ch monolithic CMOS bioelectronics. IEEE Trans Biomed Circuits Syst 12(6):1345–1355
40. Rosenstein JK, Wanunu M, Merchant CA, Drndic M, Shepard KL (2012) Integrated nanopore sensing platform with sub-microsecond temporal resolution. Nat Methods 9(5):487–492
41. Rosenstein JK, Ramakrishnan S, Roseman J, Shepard KL (2013) Single ion channel recordings with CMOS-anchored lipid membranes. Nano Lett 13(6):2682–2686
42. Dorta-Quiñones CI et al (2018) A bidirectional-current CMOS potentiostat for fast-scan cyclic voltammetry detector arrays. IEEE Trans Biomed Circuits Syst 12(4):894–903
43. Tedjo W, Chen T (2019) An integrated biosensor system with a high-density microelectrode array for real-time electrochemical imaging. IEEE Trans Biomed Circuits Syst 14(1):20–35
44. Levine PM, Gong P, Levicky R, Shepard KL (2008) Active CMOS sensor array for electrochemical biomolecular detection. IEEE J Solid State Circuits 43(8):1859–1871
45. Schienle M et al (2004) A fully electronic DNA sensor with 128 positions and in-pixel A/D conversion. IEEE J Solid State Circuits 39(12):2438–2445
46. Laifi A, Abaji A, Adib M, Thewes R (2015) A 96 dB SNDR current-mode continuous-time $\Delta\Sigma$ modulator for electrochemical sensor arrays. In: Mixed design of integrated circuits & systems (MIXDES), 2015 22nd international conference. IEEE, pp 239–242
47. Levine PM, Gong P, Levicky R, Shepard KL (2009) Real-time, multiplexed electrochemical DNA detection using an active complementary metal-oxide-semiconductor biosensor array with integrated sensor electronics. Biosens Bioelectron 24(7):1995–2001
48. Kruppa P et al (2010) A digital CMOS-based 24×16 sensor array platform for fully automatic electrochemical DNA detection. Biosens Bioelectron 26(4):1414–1419
49. Liu X, Li L, Mason AJ (2014) High-throughput impedance spectroscopy biosensor array chip. Phil Trans R Soc A 372(2012):20130107. (1–14)
50. Dragas J et al (2017) In vitro multi-functional microelectrode Array featuring 59 760 electrodes, 2048 electrophysiology channels, stimulation, impedance measurement, and neurotransmitter detection channels. IEEE J Solid State Circuits 52(6):1576–1590. [Online]. Available: https://ieeexplore.ieee.org/abstract/document/7913669
51. Jafari H, Soleymani L, Genov R (2012) 16-channel CMOS impedance spectroscopy DNA analyzer with dual-slope multiplying ADCs. IEEE Trans Biomed Circuits Syst 6(5):468–478
52. Bajestan MM, Helmy AA, Hedayati H, Entesari K (2014) A 0.62–10GHz CMOS dielectric spectroscopy system for chemical/biological material characterization. In: 2014 IEEE MTT-S International Microwave Symposium (IMS). IEEE, pp 1–4
53. Bajestan MM, Helmy AA, Hedayati H, Entesari K (2014) A 0.62–10 GHz complex dielectric spectroscopy system in CMOS. IEEE Trans Microw Theory Tech 62(12):3522–3537
54. Vlachogiannakis G, Pertijs MA, Spirito M, de Vreede LC (2018) A 40-nm CMOS complex permittivity sensing pixel for material characterization at microwave frequencies. IEEE Trans Microw Theory Tech 66(3):1619–1634

55. Kassanos P, Triantis IF, Demosthenous A (2013) A CMOS magnitude/phase measurement chip for impedance spectroscopy. IEEE Sensors J 13(6):2229–2236
56. Hedayatipour A, Aslanzadeh S, McFarlane N (2019) CMOS based whole cell impedance sensing: challenges and future outlook. Biosens Bioelectron 143:111600
57. Hamilton TJ, Nelson NM, Sander D, Abshire P (2009) A cell impedance sensor based on a silicon cochlea. In: 2009 IEEE biomedical circuits and systems conference. IEEE, pp 117–120
58. Lu MS-C, Chen Y-C, Huang P-C (2010) 5 × 5 CMOS capacitive sensor array for detection of the neurotransmitter dopamine. Biosens Bioelectron 26(3):1093–1097
59. Chang A-Y, Lu MS-C (2013) A CMOS magnetic microbead-based capacitive biosensor array with on-chip electromagnetic manipulation. Biosens Bioelectron 45:6–12
60. Stagni C et al (2006) CMOS DNA sensor array with integrated A/D conversion based on label-free capacitance measurement. IEEE J Solid State Circuits 41(12):2956–2964. [Online]. Available: https://ieeexplore.ieee.org/abstract/document/4014638
61. Mohammad K, Buchanan DA, Thomson DJ (2016) Integrated 0.35 pm CMOS capacitance sensor with atto-farad sensitivity for single cell analysis. In: Biomedical Circuits and Systems Conference (BioCAS), 2016 IEEE. IEEE, pp 22–25
62. Couniot N, Bol D, Poncelet O, Francis LA, Flandre D (2014) A capacitance-to-frequency converter with on-chip passivated microelectrodes for bacteria detection in saline buffers up to 575 MHz. IEEE Trans Circuits Syst II: Express Briefs 62(2):159–163
63. Mohammad K, Thomson DJ (2017) Differential ring oscillator based capacitance sensor for microfluidic applications. IEEE Trans Biomed Circuits Syst 11(2):392–399
64. Senevirathna B, Lu S, Abshire P (2017) Characterization of a high dynamic range lab-on-CMOS capacitance sensor array. In: 2017 IEEE International Symposium on Circuits and Systems (ISCAS). IEEE, pp 1–4
65. Gaggatur JS, Banerjee G (2017) High gain capacitance sensor interface for the monitoring of cell volume growth. In: 2017 30th international conference on VLSI design and 2017 16th international conference on embedded systems (VLSID). IEEE, pp 201–206
66. Senevirathna B, Castro A, Dandin M, Smela E, Abshire P (2016) Lab-on-CMOS capacitance sensor array for real-time cell viability measurements with I2C readout. In: 2016 IEEE international symposium on circuits and systems (ISCAS). IEEE, pp 2863–2866
67. Naviasky E, Datta-Chaudhuri T, Abshire P (2014) High resolution capacitance sensor array for real-time monitoring of cell viability. In: 2014 IEEE International Symposium on Circuits and Systems (ISCAS). IEEE, pp 634–637
68. Senevirathna BP, Lu S, Dandin MP, Basile J, Smela E, Abshire PA (2018) Real-time measurements of cell proliferation using a lab-on-CMOS capacitance sensor array. IEEE Trans Biomed Circuits Syst 12(3):510–520. [Online]. Available: https://ieeexplore.ieee.org/abstract/document/8359302
69. Helmy AA et al (2012) A self-sustained CMOS microwave chemical sensor using a frequency synthesizer. IEEE J Solid State Circuits 47(10):2467–2483
70. Nehring J, Bartels M, Weigel R, Kissinger D (2015) A permittivity sensitive PLL based on a silicon-integrated capacitive sensor for microwave biosensing applications. In: 2015 IEEE topical conference on biomedical wireless technologies, networks, and sensing systems (BioWireleSS). IEEE, pp 1–3
71. Guha S, Schmalz K, Wenger C, Herzel F (2015) Self-calibrating highly sensitive dynamic capacitance sensor: towards rapid sensing and counting of particles in laminar flow systems. Analyst 140(9):3262–3272
72. Elhadidy O, Elkholy M, Helmy AA, Palermo S, Entesari K (2013) A CMOS fractional- N PLL-based microwave chemical sensor with 1.5% permittivity accuracy. IEEE Trans Microw Theory Tech 61(9):3402–3416
73. Mitsunaka T et al (2016) CMOS biosensor IC focusing on dielectric relaxations of biological water with 120 and 60 GHz oscillator arrays. IEEE J Solid State Circuits 51(11):2534–2544
74. Chien J-C, Anwar M, Yeh E-C, Lee LP, Niknejad AM (2014) A 6.5/17.5-GHz dual-channel interferometer-based capacitive sensor in 65-nm CMOS for high-speed flow cytometry. In: 2014 IEEE MTT-S International Microwave Symposium (IMS). IEEE, pp 1–4

75. Chien J-C, Yeh E-C, Lee LP, Anwar M, Niknejad AM (2015) A near-field modulation chopping stabilized injection-locked oscillator sensor for protein conformation detection at microwave frequency. In: 2015 Symposium on VLSI Circuits (VLSI Circuits). IEEE, pp C332–C333
76. Chien J-C, Niknejad AM (2016) Oscillator-based reactance sensors with injection locking for high-throughput flow cytometry using microwave dielectric spectroscopy. J Solid-State Circuits 51(2):457–472
77. Elhadidy O, Shakib S, Krenek K, Palermo S, Entesari K (2015) A wide-band fully-integrated CMOS ring-oscillator PLL-based complex dielectric spectroscopy system. IEEE Trans Circuits Syst I: Regul Pap 62(8):1940–1949
78. Ciccarella P, Carminati M, Sampietro M, Ferrari G (2016) Multichannel 65 zF rms resolution CMOS monolithic capacitive sensor for counting single micrometer-sized airborne particles on chip. IEEE J Solid State Circuits 51(11):2545–2553
79. Ciccarella P, Carminati M, Sampietro M, Ferrari G (2016) CMOS monolithic airborne-particulate-matter detector based on 32 capacitive sensors with a resolution of 65zF rms. In: 2016 IEEE International Solid-State Circuits Conference (ISSCC). IEEE, pp 486–488
80. Prakash SB, Abshire P (2007) On-chip capacitance sensing for cell monitoring applications. IEEE Sensors J 7(3):440–447
81. Prakash SB, Abshire P (2008) Tracking cancer cell proliferation on a CMOS capacitance sensor chip. Biosens Bioelectron 23(10):1449–1457. [Online]. Available: https://www.sciencedirect.com/science/article/abs/pii/S0956566307005064
82. Couniot N, Francis LA, Flandre D (2016) A 16 ×16 CMOS capacitive biosensor Array towards detection of single bacterial cell. IEEE Trans Biomed Circuits Syst 10(2):364–374. [Online]. Available: https://ieeexplore.ieee.org/abstract/document/7106573
83. De Venuto D, Carrara S, Riccò B (2009) Design of an integrated low-noise read-out system for DNA capacitive sensors. Microelectron J 40(9):1358–1365
84. Petrellis N, Spathis C, Georgakopoulou K, Birbas A (2013) Capacitive sensor estimation based on self-configurable reference capacitance. Recent Patents on Signal Processing 3(1):12–21
85. Romani A et al (2004) Capacitive sensor array for localization of bioparticles in CMOS lab-on-a-chip. In: 2004 IEEE international solid-state circuits conference, 2004. Digest of technical papers. ISSCC. IEEE, pp 224–225
86. Georgakopoulou K, Spathis C, Petrellis N, Birbas A (2016) A capacitive-to-digital converter with automatic range adaptation for readout instrumentation. IEEE Trans Instrum Meas 65(2):336–345
87. Ha H, Sylvester D, Blaauw D, Sim J-Y (2014) 12.6 A 160nW 63.9 fJ/conversion-step capacitance-to-digital converter for ultra-low-power wireless sensor nodes. In: Solid-state circuits conference digest of technical papers (ISSCC), 2014 IEEE International. IEEE, pp 220–221
88. Tanaka K, Kuramochi Y, Kurashina T, Okada K, Matsuzawa A (2007) A 0.026 mm2 capacitance-to-digital converter for biotelemetry applications using a charge redistribution technique. In: IEEE Asian solid-state circuits conference, vol ASSCC'07. IEEE, 2007, pp 244–247
89. Alhoshany A, Salama KN (2018) A precision, energy-efficient, oversampling, noise-shaping differential SAR capacitance-to-digital converter. IEEE Trans Instrum Meas 99
90. Alhoshany A, Sivashankar S, Mashraei Y, Omran H, Salama KN (2017) A Biosensor-CMOS Platform and Integrated Readout Circuit in 0.18-μm CMOS Technology for Cancer Biomarker Detection. Sensors 17(9):1942 (1–12)
91. Guiducci C et al (2004) DNA detection by integrable electronics. Biosens Bioelectron 19(8):781–787
92. Ghafar-Zadeh E, Sawan M (2010) CMOS capacitive sensors for lab-on-chip applications. Springer, New York

93. Widdershoven F et al (2010) CMOS biosensor platform. In: 2010 IEEE International Electron Devices Meeting (IEDM). IEEE, pp 36.1. 1–36.1. 4. [Online]. Available: https://ieeexplore.ieee.org/abstract/document/5703484
94. Evans I, York T (2004) Microelectronic capacitance transducer for particle detection. IEEE Sensors J 4(3):364–372
95. Tanskanen A, Bahreyni B, Syrzycki M (2016) Charge-based femto-farad capacitance measurement technique for MEMS applications. In: 2016 IEEE Canadian Conference on Electrical and Computer Engineering (CCECE). IEEE, pp 1–4
96. York T, Evans I, Pokusevski Z, Dyakowski T (2001) Particle detection using an integrated capacitance sensor. Sensors Actuators A Phys 92(1–3):74–79
97. Ghafar-Zadeh E, Sawan M (2005) A high precision and linearity differential capacitive sensor circuit dedicated to bioparticles detection. In: The 3rd International IEEE-NEWCAS Conference, 2005. IEEE, pp 299–302
98. Ghafar-Zadeh E, Sawan M, Therriault D (2008) A 0.18-μm CMOS capacitive sensor lab-on-chip. Sensors Actuators A Phys 141(2):454–462
99. Ghafar-Zadeh E, Sawan M (2008) A Core-CBCM sigma delta capacitive sensor array dedicated to lab-on-chip applications. Sensors Actuators A Phys 144(2):304–313
100. Prakash SB, Abshire P (2007) A fully differential rail-to-rail capacitance measurement circuit for integrated cell sensing. In: 2007 IEEE Sensors. IEEE, pp 1444–1447
101. Prakash SB, Abshire P (2009) A fully differential rail-to-rail CMOS capacitance sensor with floating-gate trimming for mismatch compensation. IEEE Trans Circuits Syst I: Regul Pap 56(5):975–986
102. Nabovati G, Ghafar-Zadeh E, Mirzaei M, Ayala-Charca G, Awwad F, Sawan M (2015) A new fully differential CMOS capacitance to digital converter for lab-on-Chip applications. IEEE Trans Biomed Circuits Syst 9(3):353–361
103. Forouhi S, Dehghani R, Ghafar-Zadeh E (2018) Toward high throughput core-CBCM CMOS capacitive sensors for life science applications: a novel current-mode for high dynamic range circuitry. Sensors 18(10):3370 (1–29)
104. Tabrizi HO, Farhanieh O, Owen Q, Magierowski S, Ghafar-Zadeh E (2021) Wide input dynamic range fully integrated capacitive sensor for life science applications. IEEE Trans Biomed Circuits Syst 15(2):339–350
105. Forouhi S, Farhanieh O, Dehghani R, Ghafar-Zadeh E (2017) A current based capacitance-to-frequency converter for lab-on-chip applications. IEEE
106. Tabrizi HO, Forouhi S, Ghafar-Zadeh E (2022) A high dynamic range dual 8× 16 capacitive sensor Array for life science applications. IEEE Trans Biomed Circuits Syst
107. Druart S, Flandre D, Francis LA (2014) A self-oscillating system to measure the conductivity and the permittivity of liquids within a single triangular signal. J Sensors 2014
108. Lee K-H et al (2010) One-chip electronic detection of DNA hybridization using precision impedance-based CMOS array sensor. Biosens Bioelectron 26(4):1373–1379
109. Noorsal E, Sooksood K, Xu H, Hornig R, Becker J, Ortmanns M (2011) A neural stimulator frontend with high-voltage compliance and programmable pulse shape for epiretinal implants. IEEE J Solid State Circuits 47(1):244–256
110. Butz N, Taschwer A, Nessler S, Manoli Y, Kuhl M (2018) A 22 V compliant 56 μW twin-track active charge balancing enabling 100% charge compensation even in monophasic and 36% amplitude correction in biphasic neural stimulators. IEEE J Solid State Circuits 53(8):2298–2310
111. Lee H-M, Park H, Ghovanloo M (2013) A power-efficient wireless system with adaptive supply control for deep brain stimulation. IEEE J Solid State Circuits 48(9):2203–2216
112. Ortmanns M, Rocke A, Gehrke M, Tiedtke H-J (2007) A 232-channel epiretinal stimulator ASIC. IEEE J Solid State Circuits 42(12):2946–2959
113. Li J, Liu X, Mao W, Chen T, Yu H (2021) Advances in neural recording and stimulation integrated circuits. Front Neurosci 15:663204

114. Ballini M et al (2014) A 1024-channel CMOS microelectrode array with 26,400 electrodes for recording and stimulation of electrogenic cells in vitro. IEEE J Solid State Circuits 49(11):2705–2719. [Online]. Available: https://ieeexplore.ieee.org/abstract/document/6923484.
115. Hsu W-Y, Schmid A (2017) Compact, energy-efficient high-frequency switched capacitor neural stimulator with active charge balancing. IEEE Trans Biomed Circuits Syst 11(4):878–888
116. Van Dongen MN, Hoebeek FE, Koekkoek S, De Zeeuw CI, Serdijn WA (2015) High frequency switched-mode stimulation can evoke post synaptic responses in cerebellar principal neurons. Front Neuroengineering:2
117. Lee H-M, Kwon KY, Li W, Ghovanloo M (2014) A power-efficient switched-capacitor stimulating system for electrical/optical deep brain stimulation. IEEE J Solid State Circuits 50(1):360–374
118. Yao L, Li P, Je M (2015) A pulse-width-adaptive active charge balancing circuit with pulse-insertion based residual charge compensation and quantization for electrical stimulation applications. In: 2015 IEEE Asian solid-state circuits conference (A-SSCC). IEEE, pp 1–4
119. Chen Z, Liu X, Wang Z (2020) A charge balancing technique for neurostimulators. Analog Integr Circ Sig Process 105:483–496
120. Gosselin B (2011) Recent advances in neural recording microsystems. Sensors 11:4572–4597
121. Zou X, Xu X, Yao L, Lian Y (2009) A 1-V 450-nW fully integrated programmable biomedical sensor interface chip. IEEE J Solid State Circuits 44(4):1067–1077
122. Liu X et al (2017) A microfluidic cytometer for complete blood count with a 3.2-megapixel, 1.1-μm-pitch super-resolution image sensor in 65-nm BSI CMOS. IEEE Trans Biomed Circuits Syst 11(4):794–803
123. Yu H, Yan M, Huang X (2018) CMOS integrated lab-on-a-chip system for personalized biomedical diagnosis. Wiley
124. Park S-Y, Cho J, Na K, Yoon E (2017) Modular 128-channel Δ-$\Delta\sum$ analog front-end architecture using spectrum equalization scheme for 1024-channel 3-D neural recording microsystems. IEEE J Solid State Circuits 53(2):501–514
125. Harrison RR, Charles C (2003) A low-power low-noise CMOS amplifier for neural recording applications. IEEE J Solid State Circuits 38(6):958–965
126. Harrison RR et al (2006) A low-power integrated circuit for a wireless 100-electrode neural recording system. IEEE J Solid State Circuits 42(1):123–133
127. Kipke DR et al (2008) Advanced neurotechnologies for chronic neural interfaces: new horizons and clinical opportunities. J Neurosci 28(46):11830–11838
128. Olsson RH, Buhl DL, Sirota AM, Buzsáki G, Wise KD (2005) Band-tunable and multiplexed integrated circuits for simultaneous recording and stimulation with microelectrode arrays. IEEE Trans Biomed Eng 52(7):1303–1311
129. Lee SB, Lee H-M, Kiani M, Jow U-M, Ghovanloo M (2010) An inductively powered scalable 32-channel wireless neural recording system-on-a-chip for neuroscience applications. IEEE Trans Biomed Circuits Syst 4(6):360–371
130. Mollazadeh M, Murari K, Cauwenberghs G, Thakor N (2009) Micropower CMOS integrated low-noise amplification, filtering, and digitization of multimodal neuropotentials. IEEE Trans Biomed Circuits Syst 3(1):1–10
131. Farshchi S, Pesterev A, Nuyujukian P, Guenterberg E, Mody I, Judy JW (2010) Embedded neural recording with TinyOS-based wireless-enabled processor modules. IEEE Trans Neural Syst Rehabil Eng 18(2):134–141
132. Xiao Z, Tang C-M, Dougherty CM, Bashirullah R (2010) A 20μW neural recording tag with supply-current-modulated AFE in 0.13 μm CMOS. In: 2010 IEEE International Solid-State Circuits Conference-(ISSCC). IEEE, pp 122–123
133. Wattanapanitch W, Fee M, Sarpeshkar R (2007) An energy-efficient micropower neural recording amplifier. IEEE Trans Biomed Circuits Syst 1(2):136–147

134. Shen L, Lu N, Sun N (2018) A 1-V 0.25-μW inverter stacking amplifier with 1.07 noise efficiency factor. IEEE J Solid State Circuits 53(3):896–905
135. Gosselin B, Sawan M, Chapman CA (2007) A low-power integrated bioamplifier with active low-frequency suppression. IEEE Trans Biomed Circuits Syst 1(3):184–192
136. Verma N, Shoeb A, Bohorquez J, Dawson J, Guttag J, Chandrakasan AP (2010) A micropower EEG acquisition SoC with integrated feature extraction processor for a chronic seizure detection system. IEEE J Solid State Circuits 45(4):804–816
137. Avestruz A-T et al (2008) A 5 μW/channel spectral analysis IC for chronic bidirectional brain–machine interfaces. IEEE J Solid State Circuits 43(12):3006–3024
138. Mollazadeh M, Murari K, Cauwenberghs G, Thakor N (2009) Wireless micropower instrumentation for multimodal acquisition of electrical and chemical neural activity. IEEE Trans Biomed Circuits Syst 3(6):388–397
139. Perlin GE, Sodagar AM, Wise KD (2008) A neural amplifier with high programmable gain and tunable bandwidth. In: 2008 30th annual international conference of the ieee engineering in medicine and biology society. IEEE, pp 3154–3157
140. Mohseni P, Najafi K (2004) A fully integrated neural recording amplifier with DC input stabilization. IEEE Trans Biomed Eng 51(5):832–837
141. Horiuchi T, Swindell T, Sander D, Abshire P (2004) A low-power CMOS neural amplifier with amplitude measurements for spike sorting. In: 2004 IEEE international symposium on circuits and systems (ISCAS), vol 4. IEEE, pp IV–29
142. Yin M, Ghovanloo M (2007) A low-noise preamplifier with adjustable gain and bandwidth for biopotential recording applications. In: 2007 IEEE international symposium on circuits and systems. IEEE, pp 321–324
143. Chae MS, Yang Z, Yuce MR, Hoang L, Liu W (2009) A 128-channel 6 mW wireless neural recording IC with spike feature extraction and UWB transmitter. IEEE Trans Neural Syst Rehabil Eng 17(4):312–321
144. Zou X, Liew W-S, Yao L, Lian Y (2010) A 1V 22μW 32-channel implantable EEG recording IC. In: 2010 IEEE International Solid-State Circuits Conference-(ISSCC). IEEE, pp 126–127
145. Gosselin B, Ghovanloo M (2011) A high-performance analog front-end for an intraoral tongue-operated assistive technology. In: 2011 IEEE International Symposium of Circuits and Systems (ISCAS). IEEE, pp 2613–2616
146. Rieger R et al (2006) Very low-noise ENG amplifier system using CMOS technology. IEEE Trans Neural Syst Rehabil Eng 14(4):427–437
147. Holleman J, Otis B (2007) A sub-microwatt low-noise amplifier for neural recording. In: 2007 29th annual international conference of the IEEE engineering in medicine and biology society. IEEE, pp 3930–3933
148. Jochum T, Denison T, Wolf P (2009) Integrated circuit amplifiers for multi-electrode intracortical recording. J Neural Eng 6(1):012001
149. Jeon H, Bang J-S, Jung Y, Choi I, Je M (2019) A high DR, DC-coupled, time-based neural-recording IC with degeneration R-DAC for bidirectional neural interface. IEEE J Solid State Circuits 54(10):2658–2670
150. Heer F, Hafizovic S, Franks W, Blau A, Ziegler C, Hierlemann A (2006) CMOS microelectrode array for bidirectional interaction with neuronal networks. IEEE J Solid State Circuits 41(7):1620–1629
151. Johnson B, Peace ST, Cleland TA, Molnar A (2013) A 50μm pitch, 1120-channel, 20kHz frame rate microelectrode array for slice recording. In: 2013 IEEE Biomedical Circuits and Systems Conference (BioCAS). IEEE, pp 109–112
152. Frey U et al (2010) Switch-matrix-based high-density microelectrode array in CMOS technology. IEEE J Solid State Circuits 45(2):467–482. [Online]. Available: https://ieeexplore.ieee.org/abstract/document/5405139
153. Lopez CM et al (2013) An implantable 455-active-electrode 52-channel CMOS neural probe. IEEE J Solid State Circuits 49(1):248–261

154. Xu J, Wu T, Liu W, Yang Z (2014) A frequency shaping neural recorder with 3 pF input capacitance and 11 plus 4.5 bits dynamic range. IEEE Trans Biomed Circuits Syst 8(4):510–527
155. Jiang W, Hokhikyan V, Chandrakumar H, Karkare V, Marković D (2016) A±50-mV linear-input-range VCO-based neural-recording front-end with digital nonlinearity correction. IEEE J Solid State Circuits 52(1):173–184
156. Nikas A, Jambunathan S, Klein L, Voelker M, Ortmanns M (2019) A continuous-time delta-sigma modulator using a modified instrumentation amplifier and current reuse DAC for neural recording. IEEE J Solid State Circuits 54(10):2879–2891
157. Park K-T, Cho D-G, Park J-W, Hong S, Hwang J (2015) Detection of airborne viruses using electro-aerodynamic deposition and a field-effect transistor. Sci Rep 5(1). https://doi.org/10.1038/srep17462
158. Kim JY et al (2013) Surface engineering for enhancement of sensitivity in an underlap-FET biosensor by control of wettability," (in eng). Biosens Bioelectron 41:867–870. https://doi.org/10.1016/j.bios.2012.08.036
159. Shariati M (2018) The field effect transistor DNA biosensor based on ITO nanowires in label-free hepatitis B virus detecting compatible with CMOS technology. Biosens Bioelectron 105:58–64. https://doi.org/10.1016/j.bios.2018.01.022
160. Dastagir T et al (2007) Electrical detection of hepatitis C virus RNA on single wall carbon nanotube-field effect transistors. Analyst 132(8):738–740
161. Rothberg JM et al (2011) An integrated semiconductor device enabling non-optical genome sequencing. Nature 475(7356):348–352
162. Nikkhoo N, Gulak PG, Maxwell K (2013) Rapid detection of E. Coli bacteria using potassium-sensitive FETs in CMOS. IEEE Trans Biomed Circuits Syst 7(5):621–630
163. Jiang Y et al (2018) A high-sensitivity potentiometric 65-nm CMOS ISFET sensor for Rapid E. Coli screening. IEEE Trans Biomed Circuits Syst 12(2):402–415. [Online]. Available: https://ieeexplore.ieee.org/abstract/document/8310573
164. Malpartida-Cardenas K et al (2019) Quantitative and rapid plasmodium falciparum malaria diagnosis and artemisinin-resistance detection using a CMOS lab-on-Chip platform. Biosens Bioelectron 145:111678
165. Lee KH, Lee JO, Choi S, Yoon JB, Cho GH (2012) A CMOS label-free DNA sensor using electrostatic induction of molecular charges. Biosens Bioelectron 31(1):343–348. https://doi.org/10.1016/j.bios.2011.10.042
166. Bausells J, Carrabina J, Errachid A, Merlos A (1999) Ion-sensitive field-effect transistors fabricated in a commercial CMOS technology. Sensors Actuators B Chem 57(1–3):56–62
167. Bergveld P (1981) The operation of an ISFET as an electronic device. Sensors Actuators 1:17–29
168. Miscourides N, Georgiou P (2016) Linear current-mode ISFET arrays. In: 2016 IEEE International Symposium on Circuits and Systems (ISCAS). IEEE, pp 2827–2830
169. Milgrew MJ, Cumming DR (2008) Matching the transconductance characteristics of CMOS ISFET arrays by removing trapped charge. IEEE Trans Electron Dev 55(4):1074–1079
170. Georgiou P, Toumazou C (2009) ISFET threshold voltage programming in CMOS using hot-electron injection. Electron Lett 45(22):1112–1113
171. Wong H-S, White MH (1989) A CMOS-integrated'ISFET-operational amplifier'chemical sensor employing differential sensing. IEEE Trans Electron Dev 36(3):479–487
172. Aw C-Y, Cheung PW (1988) A pH-ISFET sensor with on-chip temperature sensing. In: Engineering in medicine and biology society, 1988. Proceedings of the Annual International Conference of the IEEE. IEEE, pp 772–773
173. Sohbati M, Toumazou C (2014) A temperature insensitive continuous time ΔpH to digital converter. In: *2014 IEEE International Symposium on Circuits and Systems (ISCAS)*. IEEE, pp 37–40
174. Jakobson C, Nemirovsky Y (1999) 1/f noise in ion sensitive field effect transistors from sub-threshold to saturation. IEEE Trans Electron Dev 46(1):259–261

175. Morgenshtein A, Sudakov-Boreysha L, Dinnar U, Jakobson CG, Nemirovsky Y (2004) Wheatstone-bridge readout interface for ISFET/REFET applications. Sensors Actuators B Chem 98(1):18–27
176. Georgiou P, Toumazou C (2009) An adaptive CMOS-based PG-ISFET for pH sensing. In: 2009 IEEE international symposium on circuits and systems. IEEE, pp 557–560
177. Jamasb S (2004) An analytical technique for counteracting drift in ion-selective field effect transistors (ISFETs). IEEE Sensors J 4(6):795–801
178. Bergveld P (2003) Thirty years of ISFETOLOGY: What happened in the past 30 years and what may happen in the next 30 years. Sensors Actuators B Chem 88(1):1–20
179. Moser N, Lande TS, Toumazou C, Georgiou P (2016) ISFETs in CMOS and emergent trends in instrumentation: a review. IEEE Sensors J 16(17):6496–6514
180. Ravezzi L, Conci P (1998) ISFET sensor coupled with CMOS read-out circuit microsystem. Electron Lett 34(23):2234–2235
181. Duan M, Zhong X, Xu J, Lee Y-K, Bermak A (2020) A high offset distribution tolerance high resolution ISFET array with auto-compensation for long-term bacterial metabolism monitoring. IEEE Trans Biomed Circuits Syst 14(3):463–476
182. Liu Y, Constandinou TG, Georgiou P (2019) Ultrafast large-scale chemical sensing with CMOS ISFETs: a level-crossing time-domain approach. IEEE Trans Biomed Circuits Syst 13(6):1201–1213
183. Milgrew M, Hammond P, Cumming D (2004) The development of scalable sensor arrays using standard CMOS technology. Sensors Actuators B Chem 103(1–2):37–42
184. Hammond PA, Ali D, Cumming DR (2004) Design of a single-chip pH sensor using a conventional 0.6 μm CMOS process. IEEE Sensors J 4(6):706–712
185. Milgrew M, Riehle M, Cumming D (2005) A large transistor-based sensor array chip for direct extracellular imaging. Sensors Actuators B Chem 111:347–353
186. Hammond PA, Ali D, Cumming DR (2005) A system-on-chip digital pH meter for use in a wireless diagnostic capsule. IEEE Trans Biomed Eng 52(4):687–694
187. Rothberg JM, Hinz W, Johnson KL, Bustillo J (2011) Methods and apparatus for measuring analytes using large scale FET arrays. Google Patents
188. Uzzal MM, Zarkesh-Ha P, Edwards JS, Coelho E, Rawat P (2014) A highly sensitive ISFET using pH-to-current conversion for real-time DNA sequencing. In: 2014 27th IEEE international system-on-chip conference (SOCC). IEEE, pp 410–414
189. Shepherd L, Toumazou C (2005) Weak inversion ISFETs for ultra-low power biochemical sensing and real-time analysis. Sensors Actuators B Chem 107(1):468–473
190. Georgiou P, Toumazou C (2009) Chemical log-domain filter. Electron Lett 45(8):391–392
191. Premanode B, Silawan N, Chan WP, Toumazou C (2007) A composite ISFET readout circuit employing current feedback. Sensors Actuators B Chem 127(2):486–490
192. Miscourides N, Georgiou P (2016) A linear programmable-gate ISFET array operating in velocity saturation. In: 2016 IEEE Biomedical Circuits and Systems Conference (BioCAS). IEEE, pp 292–295
193. Miscourides N, Georgiou P (2018) ISFET arrays in CMOS: a head-to-head comparison between voltage and current mode. IEEE Sensors J 19(4):1224–1238
194. Miscourides N, Yu L-S, Rodriguez-Manzano J, Georgiou P (2018) A 12.8 k current-mode velocity-saturation ISFET array for on-chip real-time DNA detection. IEEE Trans Biomed Circuits Syst 12(5):1202–1214
195. Toumazou C, Lidgey FJ, Haigh D (1990) Analogue IC design: the current-mode approach. Presbyterian Publishing Corp
196. Pookaiyaudom P, Toumazou C, Lidgey F (2008) The chemical current-conveyor: a new microchip biosensor. In: 2008 IEEE international symposium on circuits and systems. IEEE, pp 3166–3169
197. Zeng J, Kuang L, Miscourides N, Georgiou P (2020) A 128×128 current-mode ultra-high frame rate ISFET array with in-pixel calibration for real-time ion imaging. IEEE Trans Biomed Circuits Syst 14(2):359–372

198. Juffali W, Georgiou P, Toumazou C (2010) ISFET based urea: creatinine translinear sensor. Electron Lett 46(11):746–748
199. Kalofonou M, Georgiou P, Ou C-P, Toumazou C (2012) An ISFET based translinear sensor for DNA methylation detection. Sensors Actuators B Chem 161(1):156–162
200. Premanode B, Chan W, Toumazou C (2006) Ultra-low power precision ISFET readout using global current feedback. Electron Lett 42(22):1264–1265
201. Chan W, Premanode B, Toumazou C (2009) 64 pH-ISFET averaging array employing global negative current feedback. Electron Lett 45(11):536–537
202. Georgiou P, Toumazou C (2009) ISFET characteristics in CMOS and their application to weak inversion operation. Sensors Actuators B Chem 143(1):211–217
203. Shepherd LM, Toumazou C (2005) A biochemical translinear principle with weak inversion ISFETs. IEEE Trans Circuits Syst I: Regul Pap 52(12):2614–2619
204. Georgiou P, Toumazou C (2007) A silicon pancreatic beta cell for diabetes. IEEE Trans Biomed Circuits Syst 1(1):39–49
205. Wong W, Shepherd L, Georgiou P, Toumazou C (2009) Towards ISFET based DNA logic for rapid nucleic acid detection. In: Sensors, 2009 IEEE. IEEE, pp 1451–1454
206. AlAhdal A, Toumazou C (2012) ISFET-based chemical Schmitt trigger. Electron Lett 48(10):549–551
207. Al-Ahdal A, Toumazou C (2011) ISFET-based chemical switch. IEEE Sensors J 12(5):1140–1146
208. Al-Ahdal A, Toumazou C (2012) High gain ISFET based νMOS chemical inverter. Sensors Actuators B Chem 171:110–117
209. Nabovati G, Ghafar-Zadeh E, Sawan M (2015) A 64 pixel ISFET-based biosensor for extracellular pH gradient monitoring. In: 2015 IEEE international symposium on circuits and systems (ISCAS). IEEE, pp 1762–1765
210. Liu Y, Al-Ahdal A, Georgiou P, Toumazou C (2012) Minimal readout scheme for ISFET sensing arrays based on pulse width modulation. Electron Lett 48(10):548–549
211. Moser N, Lande TS, Georgiou P (2015) A novel pH-to-time ISFET pixel architecture with offset compensation. In: *2015 IEEE International Symposium on Circuits and Systems (ISCAS)*. IEEE, pp 481–484
212. Moser N, Lande TS, Georgiou P (2016) A robust ISFET array with in-pixel quantisation and automatic offset calibration. In: 2016 IEEE Biomedical Circuits and Systems Conference (BioCAS). IEEE, pp 50–53
213. Moser N, Rodriguez-Manzano J, Lande TS, Georgiou P (2018) A scalable ISFET sensing and memory array with sensor auto-calibration for on-chip real-time DNA detection. IEEE Trans Biomed Circuits Syst 12(2):390–401
214. Cacho-Soblechero M, Malpartida-Cardenas K, Moser N, Georgiou P (2019) Programmable ion-sensing using oscillator-based isfet architectures. IEEE Sensors J 19(19):8563–8575
215. Chan WP, Premanode B, Toumazou C (2010) An integrated ISFETs instrumentation system in standard CMOS technology. IEEE J Solid State Circuits 45(9):1923–1934
216. Wang K, Liu Y, Toumazou C, Georgiou P (2012) A TDC based ISFET readout for large-scale chemical sensing systems. In: 2012 IEEE biomedical circuits and systems conference (BioCAS). IEEE, pp 176–179
217. Livi P et al (2014) Sensor system including silicon nanowire ion sensitive FET arrays and CMOS readout. Sensors Actuators B Chem 204:568–577
218. Chang C-F, Lu MS-C (2020) CMOS ion sensitive field effect transistors for highly sensitive detection of DNA hybridization. IEEE Sensors J 20(16):8930–8937
219. Georgiou P, Toumazou C (2008) An adaptive ISFET chemical imager chip. In: *2008 IEEE international symposium on circuits and systems*. IEEE, pp 2078–2081
220. Lee C, Chen Y-W, Lu MS-C (2020) CMOS biosensors for the detection of DNA hybridization in high ionic-strength solutions. IEEE Sensors J 21(4):4135–4142
221. Jiang Y, Coquet P, Yu H (2017) Fast food safety screening with CMOS high-sensitivity large-arrayed ISFET sensor. In: 2017 IEEE Biomedical Circuits and Systems Conference (BioCAS). IEEE, pp 1–4

222. Do AT, Minkyu J, Yeo KS (2013) Improved inverter-based read-out scheme for low-power ISFET sensing array. Electron Lett 49(24):1517–1518
223. Futagawa M, Otake R, Dasai F, Ishida M, Sawada K (2015) Realization of 1 million pixel charge transfer type ion image sensor with 12 μm pixel pitch. In: 2015 transducers-2015 18th international conference on solid-state sensors, actuators and microsystems (TRANSDUCERS). IEEE, pp 236–239
224. Hizawa T, Sawada K, Takao H, Ishida M (2006) Fabrication of a two-dimensional pH image sensor using a charge transfer technique. Sensors Actuators B Chem 117(2):509–515
225. Huang X, Yu H, Liu X, Jiang Y, Yan M, Wu D (2015) A dual-mode large-arrayed CMOS ISFET sensor for accurate and high-throughput pH sensing in biomedical diagnosis. IEEE Trans Biomed Eng 62(9):2224–2233
226. Goh ZDC, Georgiou P, Constandinou TG, Prodromakis T, Toumazou C (2011) Live demonstration: a CMOS-based lab-on-chip array for combined magnetic manipulation and opto-chemical sensing. In: 2011 IEEE international symposium of circuits and systems (ISCAS). IEEE, pp 1997–2001
227. Nemeth B, Piechocinski MS, Cumming DR (2012) High-resolution real-time ion-camera system using a CMOS-based chemical sensor array for proton imaging. Sensors Actuators B Chem 171:747–752
228. Hu Y, Georgiou P (2014) 3-T ISFET front-end utilising parasitic device capacitance. Electron Lett 50(21):1507–1509
229. Maruyama Y, Terao S, Sawada K (2009) Label free CMOS DNA image sensor based on the charge transfer technique. Biosens Bioelectron 24(10):3108–3112
230. Sawada K, Shimada T, Ohshina T, Takao H, Ishida M (2004) Highly sensitive ion sensors using charge transfer technique. Sensors Actuators B Chem 98(1):69–72
231. Lee Y-N et al (2019) High-density 2-μm-pitch pH image sensor with high-speed operation up to 1933 fps. IEEE Trans Biomed Circuits Syst 13(2):352–363
232. Matsuo T, Nakajima H (1984) Characteristics of reference electrodes using a polymer gate ISFET. Sensors Actuators 5(4):293–305
233. Nabovati G, Ghafarzadeh E, Awwad F, Sawan M (2013) A sigma delta ISFET readout circuit for Lab-on-Chip applications. In: New circuits and systems conference (NEWCAS), 2013 IEEE 11th International. IEEE, pp 1–4
234. Liu Y, Toumazou C (2010) An ISFET based sensing array with sensor offset compensation and pH sensitivity enhancement. In: Proceedings of 2010 IEEE international symposium on circuits and systems. IEEE, pp 2283–2286
235. Palan B, Santos F, Karam J, Courtois B, Husak M (1999) New ISFET sensor interface circuit for biomedical applications. Sensors Actuators B Chem 57(1–3):63–68
236. Kalofonou M, Toumazou C (2013) A low power sub-μW chemical Gilbert cell for ISFET differential reaction monitoring. IEEE Trans Biomed Circuits Syst 8(4):565–574
237. Chodavarapu V, Titus A, Cartwright A (2005) Differential read-out architecture for CMOS ISFET microsystems. Electron Lett 41(12):698–699
238. Seong-Jin K, Euisik Y (2012) Label-free CMOS bio sensor with on-chip noise reduction scheme for real-time quantitative monitoring of biomolecules. IEEE Trans Biomed Circuits Syst 6(3):189–196
239. Chudy M, Wróblewski W, Brzózka Z (1999) Towards REFET. Sensors Actuators B Chem 57(1–3):47–50
240. Chovelon J et al (1992) Sensitization of dielectric surfaces by chemical grafting: application to pH ISFETs and REFETs. Sensors Actuators B Chem 8(3):221–225
241. Nakajima H, Esashi M, Matsuo T (1982) The cation concentration response of polymer gate ISFET. J Electrochem Soc 129(1):141
242. Hong L, Li H, Yang H, Sengupta K (2017) Fully integrated fluorescence biosensors on-chip employing multi-functional nanoplasmonic optical structures in CMOS. IEEE J Solid State Circuits 52(9):2388–2406. [Online]. Available: https://ieeexplore.ieee.org/abstract/document/7983353

243. Hong L, Li H, Yang H, Sengupta K (2018) Integrated angle-insensitive nanoplasmonic filters for ultraminiaturized fluorescence microarray in a 65 nm digital CMOS process. ACS Photonics 5(11):4312–4322
244. Khiarak MN, Martel S, De Koninck Y, Gosselin B (2019) High-DR CMOS fluorescence biosensor with extended counting ADC and noise cancellation. IEEE Trans Circuits Syst I: Regul Pap 66(6):2077–2087
245. Zhu C, Hong L, Yang H, Sengupta K (2022) A packaged multiplexed fluorescent biomolecular sensor array and ultralow-power wireless interface in CMOS for ingestible electronic applications. IEEE Sensors J 22(24):24060–24074
246. Aghimand F, Hu C, Sharma S, Pochana KK, Murray RM, Emami A (2023) 21.1 A 65nm CMOS living-cell dynamic fluorescence sensor with 1.05 fA sensitivity at 600/700nm wavelengths. In: 2023 IEEE International Solid-State Circuits Conference (ISSCC). IEEE, pp 312–314
247. Aghlmand F, Hu CY, Sharma S, Pochana K, Murray RM, Emami A (2023) A 65-nm CMOS fluorescence sensor for dynamic monitoring of living cells. IEEE J Solid State Circuits
248. C. Zhu, Y. Wen, T. Liu, H. Yang, and K. Sengupta, "An ingestible pill with CMOS fluorescence sensor array, bi-directional wireless interface and packaged optics for in-vivo biomolecular sensing,". IEEE Trans Biomed Circuits Syst, 2023.
249. Awan MA, Wang B, Quadir NA, Bermak A (2021) Review and analysis of CMOS current readout circuits for biosensing applications. In: 2021 IEEE international symposium on circuits and systems (ISCAS). IEEE, pp 1–5
250. Khiarak MN, Martel S, De Koninck Y, Gosselin B (2017) A high-sensitivity CMOS biophotometry sensor with embedded continuous-time ΣΔ modulation. In: 2017 IEEE international symposium on circuits and systems (ISCAS). IEEE, pp 1–4
251. Manickam A et al (2017) A fully integrated CMOS fluorescence biochip for DNA and RNA testing. IEEE J Solid State Circuits 52:2857–2870
252. Salama K (2005) CMOS luminescence detection lab-on-chip: modeling, design, and characterization. Stanford University
253. Rabbani R et al (2023) Towards a wireless image sensor for real-time fluorescence microscopy in cancer therapy. bioRxiv
254. Alam MW, Vedaei SS, Wahid KA (2020) A fluorescence-based wireless capsule endoscopy system for detecting colorectal cancer. Cancers 12(4):890
255. Lee Y-C et al (2021) CMOS-MEMS technologies for the applications of environment sensors and environment sensing hubs. J Micromech Microeng 31(7):074004
256. Eltoukhy H, Salama K, Gamal AE (2006) A 0.18 um CMOS bioluminescence detection lab-on-chip. IEEE J Solid State Circuits 41(3):651–662
257. Jang B, Cao P, Chevalier A, Ellington A, Hassibi A. A CMOS fluorescent-based biosensor microarray
258. Seo M-W et al (2015) A 10 ps time-resolution CMOS image sensor with two-tap true-CDS lock-in pixels for fluorescence lifetime imaging. IEEE J Solid State Circuits 51(1):141–154
259. Kobayashi T et al (2016) Optical communication with brain cells by means of an implanted duplex micro-device with optogenetics and Ca2+ fluoroimaging. Sci Rep 6(1):21247
260. Choi J et al (2020) Fully integrated time-gated 3D fluorescence imager for deep neural imaging. IEEE Trans Biomed Circuits Syst 14(4):636–645
261. Pollmann EH *et al.*, Subdural CMOS optical probe (SCOPe) for bidirectional neural interfacing. BioRxiv, p. 2023.02. 07.527500, 2023.
262. Rabbani R et al (2022) A 36 $\times$ 40 wireless fluorescence image sensor for real-time microscopy in cancer therapy. In: 2022 IEEE custom integrated circuits conference (CICC). IEEE, pp 1–2
263. Liu Q et al (2022) A threshold-based bioluminescence detector with a CMOS-integrated photodiode array in 65 nm for a multi-diagnostic ingestible capsule. IEEE J Solid State Circuits 58(3):838–851

264. Rabbani R et al (2024) 17.3 a fully wireless, miniaturized, multicolor fluorescence image sensor implant for real-time monitoring in cancer therapy. In: 2024 IEEE international solid-state circuits conference (ISSCC), vol 67. IEEE, pp 318–320
265. Skucha K, Gambini S, Liu P, Megens M, Kim J, Boser BE (2013) Design considerations for CMOS-integrated Hall-effect magnetic bead detectors for biosensor applications. J Microelectromech Syst 22:1327–1338
266. Aytur T, Beatty PR, Boser B, Anwar M, Ishikawa T (2002) An immunoassay platform based on CMOS Hall sensors. In: Solid-state sensor, Actuator and Microsystems Workshop, pp 2–6
267. Liu P, Skucha K, Megens M, Boser B (2011) A CMOS Hall-effect sensor for the characterization and detection of magnetic nanoparticles for biomedical applications. IEEE Trans Magn 47(10):3449–3451
268. Gambini S, Skucha K, Liu PP, Kim J, Krigel R (2012) A 10 kPixel CMOS hall sensor array with baseline suppression and parallel readout for immunoassays. IEEE J Solid State Circuits 48(1):302–317
269. Skucha K, Gambini S, Liu P, Megens M, Kim J, Boser B (2013) Design considerations for CMOS-integrated Hall-effect magnetic bead detectors for biosensor applications. J Microelectromech Syst 22(6):1327–1338
270. Heidari H, Zuo S, Krasoulis A, Nazarpour K (2018) CMOS magnetic sensors for wearable magnetomyography. In: 2018 40th annual international conference of the IEEE engineering in medicine and biology society (EMBC). IEEE, pp 2116–2119
271. Girgin A, Bilmez M, Amin HY, Karalar TC (2019) A silicon Hall sensor SoC for current sensors. Microelectron J 90:12–18
272. Fan H et al (2021) Detection techniques of biological and chemical Hall sensors. RSC Adv 11(13):7257–7270
273. Besse P-A, Boero G, Demierre M, Pott V, Popovic R (2002) Detection of a single magnetic microbead using a miniaturized silicon Hall sensor. Appl Phys Lett 80(22):4199–4201
274. Liu PP et al (2012) Magnetic relaxation detector for microbead labels. IEEE J Solid State Circuits 47(4):1056–1064
275. Bhalla N et al (2013) Microfluidic platform for enzyme-linked and magnetic particle-based immunoassay. Micromachines 4(2):257–271
276. Kuo P-H et al (2015) A smart CMOS assay SoC for rapid blood screening test of risk prediction. IEEE Trans Biomed Circuits Syst 9(6):790–800
277. Chang T, Juang K-C (2016) CMOS hall sensor with reduced sensitivity drift by synchronous excitation calibration for wearable biomagnetic sensor in system-on-chip. In: 2016 IEEE Sensors. IEEE, pp 1–3
278. Wang H, Chen Y, Hassibi A, Scherer A, Hajimiri A. A frequency-shift CMOS magnetic biosensor array with single-bead sensitivity and no external magnet
279. Wang H, Kosai S, Sideris C, Hajimiri A. An ultrasensitive CMOS magnetic biosensor array with correlated double counting noise suppression
280. Wang H, Mahdavi A, Tirrell DA, Hajimiri A (2012) A magnetic cell-based sensor. Lab Chip 12:4465–4471
281. Sideris C, Khial PP, Hajimiri A (2018) Design and implementation of reference-free drift-cancelling CMOS magnetic sensors for biosensing applications. IEEE J Solid State Circuits 53(11):3065–3075
282. Sideris C, Hajimiri A. An integrated magnetic spectrometer for multiplexed biosensing
283. Sun J-H, Ling B, Abdullah-Al Kaiser M, Sideris C (2022) A drift-compensated magnetic spectrometer for point-of-care wash-free immunoassays using a concurrent dual-frequency oscillator. In: ESSCIRC 2022-IEEE 48th european solid state circuits conference (ESSCIRC). IEEE, pp 173–176
284. Murali P, Izyumin I, Cohen D, Chien J-C, Niknejad AM, Boser B. A CMOS micro-flow cytometer for magnetic label detection and classification
285. Murali P, Niknejad AM, Boser BE (2016) CMOS microflow cytometer for magnetic label detection and classification. IEEE J Solid State Circuits 52:543–555

286. Reisbeck M, Helou MJ, Richter L, Kappes B, Friedrich O, Hayden O (2016) Magnetic fingerprints of rolling cells for quantitative flow cytometry in whole blood. Sci Rep 6(1):32838
287. Soares R et al (2019) Go with the flow: advances and trends in magnetic flow cytometry. Anal Bioanal Chem 411:1839–1862
288. Tang H et al (2024) High sensitivity and high throughput magnetic flow CMOS cytometers with 2D oscillator Array and inter-sensor spectrogram cross-correlation. IEEE Trans Biomed Circuits Syst
289. Hall DA (2011) GMR spin-valve biochips and interface electronics for ultrasensitive in-vitro diagnostics. Stanford University
290. Han S-J, Yu H, Murmann B, Pourmand N, Wang SX. A high-density magnetoresistive biosensor array with drift-compensation mechanism
291. Hall DA, Gaster RS, Makinwa KAA, Wang SX, Murmann B (2013) A 256 pixel magnetoresistive biosensor microarray in 0.18 μm CMOS. IEEE J Solid State Circuits 48:1290–1301
292. Costa T, Cardoso FA, Germano J, Freitas PP, Piedade MS (2017) A CMOS front-end with integrated magnetoresistive sensors for biomolecular recognition detection applications. IEEE Trans Biomed Circuits Syst 11:988–1000
293. Zhou X, Huang C-C, Hall DA (2017) Giant magnetoresistive biosensor array for detecting magnetorelaxation. IEEE Trans Biomed Circuits Syst 11:755–764
294. Zhou X, Sveiven M, Hall DA (2019) A CMOS magnetoresistive sensor front-end with mismatch-tolerance and sub-ppm sensitivity for magnetic immunoassays. IEEE Trans Biomed Circuits Syst 13:1254–1263
295. Zhou X et al (2021) A 9.7-nTrms, 704-ms magnetic biosensor front-end for detecting magneto-relaxation. IEEE J Solid State Circuits 56:2171–2181
296. Pourmodheji H, Ghafar-Zadeh E, Magierowski S (2015) Active nuclear magnetic resonance probe: a new multidiciplinary approach toward highly sensitive biomolecoular spectroscopy. In: 2015 IEEE International Symposium on Circuits and Systems (ISCAS). IEEE, pp 473–476
297. Dreyer F, Yang Q, Krüger D, Anders J (2022) A chip-based NMR relaxometry system for point-of-care analysis. In: 2022 IEEE biomedical circuits and systems conference (BioCAS). IEEE, pp 183–187
298. Dreyer F, Yang Q, Alnajjar B, Krüger D, Blümich B, Anders J (2023) A portable chip-based NMR relaxometry system with arbitrary phase control for point-of-care blood analysis. IEEE Trans Biomed Circuits Syst
299. Zhou Q, Fan S, Lei K-M, Ham D, Martins RP, Mak P-I (2024) Miniature magnetic resonance imaging system for in situ monitoring of bacterial growth and biofilm formation. IEEE Trans Biomed Circuits Syst
300. Barne A, Malhari S, Lakhani T, Mehendale N 2022) A review on types of NMR micro-coil designs.. Available at SSRN 4116746.
301. Anders J, Dreyer F, Krüger D (2022) On-chip nuclear magnetic resonance. In: Handbook of biochips: integrated circuits and systems for biology and medicine. Springer, pp 667–698
302. Krüger D et al (2023) A portable CMOS-based spin resonance system for high-resolution spectroscopy and imaging. IEEE J Solid State Circuits
303. M. Weiger and T. Speck, "shimming for high-resolution NMR spectroscopy," *eMagRes*, 2007.
304. Pourmodheji H, Ghafar-Zadeh E, Magierowski S (2017) A CMOS differential receiver dedicated to nuclear magnetic resonance applications. Analog Integr Circ Sig Process 91:97–109
305. Handwerker J et al (2020) A CMOS NMR needle for probing brain physiology with high spatial and temporal resolution. Nat Methods 17(1):64–67
306. Grisi M et al (2017) NMR spectroscopy of single sub-nL ova with inductive ultra-compact single-chip probes. Sci Rep 7(1):44670
307. Lei K-M, Heidari H, Mak P-I, Law M-K, Maloberti F, Martins RP (2016) A handheld high-sensitivity micro-NMR CMOS platform with B-field stabilization for multi-type biological/chemical assays. IEEE J Solid State Circuits 52(1):284–297

308. Pourmodheji H, Ghafar-Zadeh E, Magierowski S (2016) A multidisciplinary approach to high throughput nuclear magnetic resonance spectroscopy. Sensors 16(6):850
309. Watzlaw J, Müntjes J, Mokwa W, Schnakenberg U (2011) Multilayer micro coils for thin film analysis with mobile NMR arrays. Procedia Eng 25:395–398
310. Zolfaghari A, Chan A, Razavi B (2001) Stacked inductors and transformers in CMOS technology. IEEE J Solid State Circuits 36(4):620–628
311. Metz K, Lam M, Webb A (2000) Reference deconvolution: a simple and effective method for resolution enhancement in nuclear magnetic resonance spectroscopy. Concepts Magn Reson 12(1):21–42
312. Hoult DI, Richards R (1969) The signal-to-noise ratio of the nuclear magnetic resonance experiment. J Magn Reson 24(1):71–85
313. Sun N, Yoon T-J, Lee H, Andress W, Weissleder R, Ham D (2010) Palm NMR and 1-chip NMR. IEEE J Solid State Circuits 46(1):342–352
314. Slichter CP (2013) Principles of magnetic resonance. Springer Science & Business Media
315. Ha D, Paulsen J, Sun N, Song Y-Q, Ham D (2014) Scalable NMR spectroscopy with semiconductor chips. Proc Natl Acad Sci 111(33):11955–11960
316. Lei K-M, Mak P-I, Law M-K, Martins RP (2016) A uNMR CMOS transceiver using a butterfly-coil input for integration with a digital microfluidic device inside a portable magnet. IEEE J Solid State Circuits 51(10):2274–2286
317. Carr HY, Purcell EM (1954) Effects of diffusion on free precession in nuclear magnetic resonance experiments. Phys Rev 94(3):630
318. Weiger M, Moskau D, Kerssebaum R, Hull WE (2005) Gradient shimming: principles and practical aspects. Bruker Spin Report:1–27
319. Blasche M, Fischer D, Healthineers S (2017) Magnet homogeneity and shimming. In: Siemens healthineers: siemens healthcare GmbH. White Paper, Erlangen
320. Günther H (2013) NMR spectroscopy: basic principles, concepts and applications in chemistry. Wiley
321. Leupold HA, Potenziani E, Tilak A (1993) Adjustable multi-tesla permanent magnet field sources. IEEE Trans Magn 29(6):2902–2904
322. Danieli E, Mauler J, Perlo J, Blümich B, Casanova F (2009) Mobile sensor for high resolution NMR spectroscopy and imaging. J Magn Reson 198(1):80–87
323. Alnajjar BM, Buchau A, Baumgärtner L, Anders J (2021) NMR magnets for portable applications using 3D printed materials. J Magn Reson 326:106934
324. Hibino Y, Sugahara K, Muro Y, Tanaka H, Sato T, Kondo Y (2018) Simple and low-cost tabletop NMR system for chemical-shift-resolution spectra measurements. J Magn Reson 294:128–132
325. Anders J, Chiaramonte G, SanGiorgio P, Boero G (2009) A single-chip array of NMR receivers. J Magn Reson 201(2):239–249
326. Saunders MG (2011) Enhancing the sensitivity of NMR by dynamic nuclear polarisation. University of Birmingham
327. Ardenkjaer-Larsen JH (2016) On the present and future of dissolution-DNP. J Magn Reson 264:3–12
328. Sahin Solmaz N, Grisi M, Matheoud AV, Gualco G, Boero G (2020) Single-chip dynamic nuclear polarization microsystem. Anal Chem 92(14):9782–9789
329. Meijer GC, Wang G, Fruett F (2001) Temperature sensors and voltage references implemented in CMOS technology. IEEE Sensors J 1(3):225–234
330. Pertijs MA, Niederkorn A, Ma X, McKillop B, Bakker A, Huijsing JH (2005) A CMOS smart temperature sensor with a 3σ inaccuracy of ±0.5 °C from 50 °C to 120 °C. IEEE J Solid State Circuits 40(2)
331. Pertijs MA, Makinwa KA, Huijsing JH (2005) A CMOS smart temperature sensor with a 3σ inaccuracy of ±0.1 °C from −55 °C to 125 °C. IEEE J Solid State Circuits 40(12)
332. Yousefzadeh B, Shalmany SH, Makinwa KA (2017) A BJT-based temperature-to-digital converter with ±60 mK (3σ) inaccuracy from −55 °C to +125 °C in 0.16-μm CMOS. IEEE J Solid State Circuits 52(4):1044–1052

333. Hedayatipour A, Shanta AS, McFarlane N (2017) A sub-μW CMOS temperature to frequency sensor for implantable devices. In: 2017 IEEE 60th international midwest symposium on circuits and systems (MWSCAS). IEEE, pp 253–256
334. Hong HP (2017) A 0.5 V BJT-based CMOS thermal sensor in 10-nm FinFET technology. In: 2017 IEEE asian solid-state circuits conference (A-SSCC). IEEE, pp 41–44
335. Park J-H, Hwang J-H, Shin C, Kim S-J (2022) A BJT-based temperature-to-frequency converter with ±1 °C (3σ) inaccuracy from −40 °C to 140 °C for on-Chip thermal monitoring. IEEE J Solid State Circuits 57(10):2909–2918
336. Lee T-J, Tu K-H (2023) High-sensitivity PTAT current generator using PTAT and CTAT current subtraction method for temperature sensor with frequency-output. IEEE Trans Circuits Syst II: Express Briefs
337. Xu Z, Zhang X, Chen S, Cheong J, Yao L (2023) A temperature-to-frequency converter-based on-Chip temperature sensor with an inaccuracy of +0.65 °C/ – 0.49 °C. Sensors 23(11):5169
338. Heidary A, Wang G, Makinwa K, Meijer G (2014) 12.8 A BJT-based CMOS temperature sensor with a 3.6 pJ· K 2-resolution FoM. In: 2014 IEEE international solid-state circuits conference digest of technical papers (ISSCC). IEEE, pp 224–225
339. Wang G, Heidari A, Makinwa KA, Meijer GC (2016) An accurate BJT-based CMOS temperature sensor with duty-cycle-modulated output. IEEE Trans Ind Electron 64(2):1572–1580
340. Tang Z, Fang Y, Yu X, Shi Z, Tan N (2018) Capacitor-reused CMOS temperature sensor with duty-cycle-modulated output and 0.38 °C (3σ) inaccuracy. Electron Lett 54(9):568–570
341. Guo A-Q, Sun Q, Qi M, Qiao D (2020) A CMOS temperature sensor based on duty-cycle modulation with calibration. Analog Integr Circ Sig Process 102(1):79–89
342. Huang Z, Tang Z, Yu X-P, Shi Z, Lin L, Tan NN (2021) A BJT-based CMOS temperature sensor with duty-cycle-modulated output and ±0.5 °C (3σ) inaccuracy from− 40 °C to 125 °C. IEEE Trans Circuits Syst II: Express Briefs 68(8):2780–2784
343. Souri K, Chae Y, Thus F, Makinwa K (2014) 12.7 A 0.85 V 600nW all-CMOS temperature sensor with an inaccuracy of±0.4° C (3σ) from− 40 to 125° C. In: 2014 IEEE international solid-state circuits conference digest of technical papers (ISSCC). IEEE, pp 222–223
344. Assaderaghi F, Sinitsky D, Parke SA, Bokor J, Ko PK, Hu C (1997) Dynamic threshold-voltage MOSFET (DTMOS) for ultra-low voltage VLSI. IEEE Trans Electron Dev 44(3):414–422
345. Bashir M, Sreehari Rao P, "A low power, miniature temperature sensor with one-point calibrated accuracy of ±0.25 °C from −55 °C to 125 °C in 65 nm CMOS process.
346. Li H, Yang Z, Kong D, Yin A, Peng J, Zhang P (2024) A 840-μm2 low-power all-MOS temperature sensor front-end with real-time voltage calibration. IEICE Electron Express:21.20240055
347. Kim J, Kim J, Park C, Yang M, Jung W (2023) A wide range, energy-efficient temperature sensor based on direct temperature–voltage comparison. IEEE Solid-State Circuits Lett 6:113–116
348. Jeong S, Foo Z, Lee Y, Sim J-Y, Blaauw D, Sylvester D (2014) A fully-integrated 71 nW CMOS temperature sensor for low power wireless sensor nodes. IEEE J Solid State Circuits 49(8):1682–1693
349. Yang K et al (2017) 9.2 A 0.6 nJ -0.22/+0.19 °C inaccuracy temperature sensor using exponential subthreshold oscillation dependence. In: 2017 IEEE International Solid-State Circuits Conference (ISSCC). IEEE, pp 160–161
350. Azcona C, Calvo B, Medrano N, Celma S (2015) 1.2 V–0.18 μm CMOS temperature sensors with quasi-digital output for portable systems. IEEE Trans Instrum Meas 64(9):2565–2573
351. Someya T, Islam AM, Sakurai T, Takamiya M (2019) An 11-nW CMOS temperature-to-digital converter utilizing sub-threshold current at sub-thermal drain voltage. IEEE J Solid State Circuits 54(3):613–622
352. Zhu D, Siek L, Zheng Y (2016) High-accuracy time-mode duty-cycle-modulation-based temperature sensor for energy-efficient system applications. Circuits, Syst Signal Process 35(7):2317–2330
353. Chouhan SS, Halonen K (2015) Design and implementation of micro-power temperature to duty cycle converter using differential temperature sensing. Microelectron J 46(6):482–489

354. Makinwa KA, Snoeij MF (2006) A CMOS temperature-to-frequency converter with an inaccuracy of less less than ±0.5 °C (3σ) from −40 °C to 105 °C. IEEE J Solid State Circuits 41(12):2992–2997
355. Zhang C, Makinwa KA (2008) Interface electronics for a CMOS electrothermal frequency-locked-loop. IEEE J Solid State Circuits 43(7):1603–1608
356. van Vroonhoven CP, Makinwa KA (2008) A CMOS Temperature-to-Digital Converter with an Inaccuracy of±0.5°C (3σ) from-55 to 125°C. In: 2008 IEEE international solid-state circuits conference-digest of technical papers. IEEE, pp 576–637
357. Kashmiri SM, Xia S, Makinwa KA (2009) A temperature-to-digital converter based on an optimized electrothermal filter. IEEE J Solid State Circuits 44(7):2026–2035
358. van Vroonhoven CP, d'Aquino D, Makinwa KA (2010) A thermal-diffusivity-based temperature sensor with an untrimmed inaccuracy of ±0.2°C (3s) from −55°C to 125°C. In: 2010 IEEE international solid-state circuits conference-(ISSCC). IEEE, pp 314–315
359. Pan S, Jiang H, Makinwa KA (2017) A CMOS temperature sensor with a 49fJK 2 resolution FoM. In: 2017 Symposium on VLSI circuits. IEEE, pp C82–C83
360. Pan S, Makinwa KA (2018) A 0.25 mm 2-resistor-based temperature sensor with an inaccuracy of 0.12° C (3 σ) from− 55° C to 125° C. IEEE J Solid State Circuits 53(12):3347–3355
361. Pan S and Makinwa KA 10.4 A wheatstone bridge temperature sensor with a resolution FoM of 20fJ. K 2. In: 2019 IEEE International Solid-State Circuits Conference-(ISSCC), 2019: IEEE, pp. 186–188.
362. Pan S, Makinwa KA (2020) A 10 fJ K 2 Wheatstone bridge temperature sensor with a tail-resistor-linearized OTA. IEEE J Solid State Circuits 56(2):501–510
363. Pan S, Makinwa KA (2020) A 6.6-μW wheatstone-bridge temperature sensor for biomedical applications. IEEE Solid-State Circuits Letters 3:334–337
364. Jiang H, Huang C-C, Chan MR, Hall DA (2020) A 2-in-1 temperature and humidity sensor with a single FLL wheatstone-bridge front-end. IEEE J Solid State Circuits 55(8):2174–2185
365. Jain A, Jiang H, Pochet C, Hall DA (2021) A 310 nW temperature sensor achieving 9.8 mK resolution using a DFLL-based readout circuit. IEEE Trans Circuits Syst II: Express Briefs 69(3):704–708
366. Shahmohammadi M, Souri K, Makinwa KA (2013) A resistor-based temperature sensor for MEMS frequency references. In: 2013 Proceedings of the ESSCIRC (ESSCIRC). IEEE, pp 225–228
367. Pan S, Luo Y, Shalmany SH, Makinwa KA (2017) A resistor-based temperature sensor with a 0.13 pJ·K2 resolution FoM. IEEE J Solid State Circuits 53(1):164–173
368. Pan S, Gürleyük Ç, Pimenta MF, Makinwa KA (2019) 10.3 A 0.12 mm 2 Wien-Bridge Temperature Sensor with 0.1° C (3σ) Inaccuracy from-40° C to 180° C. In: 2019 IEEE international solid-state circuits conference-(ISSCC). IEEE, pp 184–186
369. Pan S, Angevare JA, Makinwa KA (2021) 5.4 a hybrid thermal-diffusivity/resistor-based temperature sensor with a self-calibrated inaccuracy of±0.25° C (3 Σ) from-55° C to 125° C. In: 2021 IEEE international solid-state circuits conference (ISSCC), vol 64. IEEE, pp 78–80
370. Park P, Ruffieux D, Makinwa KA (2015) A thermistor-based temperature sensor for a real-time clock with ± 2 ppm frequency stability. IEEE J Solid State Circuits 50(7):1571–1580
371. Angevare JA, Chae Y, Makinwa KA (2021) 5.3 a highly digital 2210μm 2 resistor-based temperature sensor with a 1-point trimmed inaccuracy of±1.3° C (3 σ) from-55° C to 125° C in 65nm CMOS. In: 2021 IEEE international solid-state circuits conference (ISSCC), vol 64. IEEE, pp 76–78
372. Choi W et al (2018) A compact resistor-based CMOS temperature sensor with an inaccuracy of 0.12° C (3σ) and a resolution FoM of 0.43 pJ·K 2 in 65-nm CMOS. IEEE J Solid State Circuits 53(12):3356–3367
373. Lee Y, Kim T, Chae Y (2023) A 0.9 V 6,400-μm2 resistor-based temperature sensor with a one-point trimmed 3σ inaccuracy of 10.64°C from. 50 to 125°C. IEEE Trans Circuits Syst II: Express Briefs
374. Van Herwaarden A, Sarro P (1986) Thermal sensors based on the Seebeck effect. Sensors Actuators 10(3–4):321–346

375. Van Herwaarden A, Van Duyn D, Van Oudheusden B, Sarro P (1990) Integrated thermopile sensors. Sensors Actuators A Phys 22(1–3):621–630
376. Bataillard P, Steffgen E, Haemmerli S, Manz A, Widmer H (1993) An integrated silicon thermopile as biosensor for the thermal monitoring of glucose, urea and penicillin. Biosens Bioelectron 8(2):89–98
377. Sarro P, Van Herwaarden A, Van der Vlist W (1994) A silicon-silicon nitride membrane fabrication process for smart thermal sensors. Sensors Actuators A Phys 42(1–3):666–671
378. Jaeggi D, Funk J, Halberli A, Baltes H (1995) Overall system analysis of a CMOS thermal converter. In: Proceedings of the International Solid-State Sensors and Actuators Conference-TRANSDUCERS'95, vol 2. IEEE, pp 112–115
379. Koll A et al (1999) Micromachined CMOS calorimetric chemical sensor with on-chip low noise amplifier. In: Technical Digest. IEEE International MEMS 99 Conference. Twelfth IEEE International Conference on Micro Electro Mechanical Systems (Cat. No. 99CH36291). IEEE, pp 547–551
380. Kerness N et al (2000) N-well based CMOS calorimetric chemical sensors. In: Proceedings IEEE Thirteenth Annual International Conference on Micro Electro Mechanical Systems (Cat. No. 00CH36308). IEEE, pp 96–101
381. Voiculescu I, Zaghloul M, McGill RA (2003) Design and fabrication of a temperature sensor based on thermopile in CMOS technology. In: ASME international mechanical engineering congress and exposition, vol 37211, pp 597–601
382. Aldrete-Vidrio E, Mateo D, Altet J (2007) Differential temperature sensors fully compatible with a 0.35-um CMOS process. IEEE Trans Compon Packag Technol 30(4):618–626

Chapter 5
Advances in Electronic Biosensors

In recent years, the integration of complementary metal-oxide-semiconductor (CMOS) technology into various forms of biosensors and flexible electronics has revolutionized the landscape of healthcare, environmental monitoring, and robotics. This chapter delves into the multifaceted applications of these advanced devices, ranging from portable handheld biosensors and implantable monitoring systems to wearable electrochemical sensors and smart textiles. It also explores the innovative concept of "Body Dust", which aims to push the boundaries of in-body diagnostics through the development of ultra-miniaturized sensors. Table 5.1 compares a few recent advances in this field. This chapter provides an overview of how CMOS technology is poised to transform real-time monitoring, data analysis, and personalized medicine.

5.1 Handheld Biosensors

Handheld devices equipped with CMOS chips are designed to be portable and user-friendly, making them suitable for use in various settings outside traditional laboratory environments. Their integration into common consumer electronics, such as smartphones and tablets, enhances their accessibility for field and point-of-care (PoC) testing. CMOS handheld biosensors provide a versatile, user-friendly solution for real-time monitoring and analysis across diverse applications, including medical diagnostics, environmental monitoring, and food safety.

E. Ghafar-Zadeh et al., *Advanced CMOS Biochips*, Analog Circuits and Signal Processing, https://doi.org/10.1007/978-94-007-0099-4_5

Table 5.1 Electronic biosensors

Handheld/ Implantable/ Wearable/ Ingestible	Sensor type	Application	CMOS	Other specifications	Ref.	Year
Handheld	Thin layer chromatography	Investigations of natural extracts	NA	Analyte: Alcohol extract of Galium verum Fingerprints of individual extracts were described A standard single-lens reflex camera with CMOS chip of APS-C size was used.	[1]	2017
Handheld	NMR	Selective biologic-al target pinpointing, protein state analysis, and solvent-polymer dynamics	0.18 μm	A palm-size magnet (0.46 T, 1.25 kg) was used.	[2]	2020
Handheld	Plasmonic	Detection of H1N1 viruses, e.g., swine flu	NA	A CMOS camera was used.	[3]	2021
Handheld	Capillary electrophoresis and fluorescence detection	SARS-CoV-2 diagnostics	NA	A CMOS camera was used.	[4]	2022
Handheld	Aptamer-modified CMOS ISFET	Biomarker detection	1.2 μm	ISFET's floating gate are formed with 30 nm Ta_2O_5 LoD = 3.27 ng/mL	[5]	2024
Handheld	Potentiostat-based sensor	Electrochemical sensing	NA	Wi-Fi cloud-based portable potentiostat	[6]	2019
Implantable	Optical	In vivo neural imaging	0.35 μm	Stimulation of Schaffer-collateral pathway of the mouse hippocampus On-chip Pt electrodes with current intensities from 200 μA to 1 mA	[7]	2007
Implantable	Neural recording	Simultaneous large-scale neural recordings	0.18 μm	In-pixel gain = 45.4 ± 0.4 dB (low pass, F-3 dB = 4 kHz) Input referred noise = 7.5 ± 0.67 μVRMS (300 Hz to 7.5 kHz) Power consumption <6 μW/pixel	[8]	2019
Implantable	Thermal	NA	0.18 μm	Circuit area = 0.003 mm^2 Power = 365nW (at V_{DD} = 0.55 V) Overall inaccuracy after 2-point calibration = 0.1 °C for TT	[9]	2020

Implantable	Optical	Deep-tissue ultrasonic luminescence oxygen sensing	65 nm	Volume = 4.5 mm^3	[10]	2020
Implantable	Optical	Neural interface for computational imaging and optogenetic stimulation	5.13 µm	160 × 160 array of time-gated SPAD FoV = 5.4 × 5.4 mm^2 Frame rate = 125 fps Total power = 40 mW	[11]	2021
Ingestible	Optical	Bio-pill with in situ biomolecular sensing and quantification	65 nm	Reception energy efficiency = 28 pJ/bit at 7 Mb/s Sensitivity = −58 dBm Dc power = 196 µW	[12]	2022
Implantable	Potentiostat	Drug delivery	0.18 µm	Potential range < ±1.5 V Sensing current < ± 100 µA Data rate = 125 kbps	[13]	2021
Implantable	Stimulator SoC with an optically writable ID	Addressable cortical microimplant	0.18 µm	Received power = 1.2 V and 1 mW	[14]	2024
Implantable	Neural recording	Neuromorphic sensing of peripheral nerves	40 nm	Active area = 0.32 mm^2	[15]	2022
Implantable	MEMS pressure sensor	Readout of heart transplantation	65 nm	SNR = 53 dB BW = 4 kHz Power = 100 µW	[16]	2022
Implantable	Piezoresistive pressure sensor	Remote hemodynamic monitoring of heart failure patients	0.18 µm	3.2 × 2 × 10 mm^3	[17]	2023
Implantable	Ultrasound imager	Monitoring of body temperature	0.18 µm	A sub–0.1-mm3, sub–1-nW device	[18]	2021
Implantable	Ultrasound imager	Augmented ultrasonography	0.18 µm	Static power = 57 pW	[19]	2022
Implantable	Needle-shaped positron sensitive monolithic active pixel sensor (IMIC)	Preclinical molecular neuroimaging	NA	The probe relies on IMIC, an MAPS prototyp	[20]	2024
Implantable	Optical	Subretinal prosthetic chip	0.18 µm	256-pixel/480-pixel photovoltaic-powered chip	[21]	2020
Wearable	Potentiostatic electrochemical sensor	Real-time tracking of physical and chemical data through sweat and other body fluids	65 nm	Power = 15 µW (at V_{DD} = 1.2 V) Control range = 1.8 Vpp DR = 105 dB	[22]	2020

(continued)

Table 5.1 (continued)

Handheld/ Implantable/ Wearable/ Ingestible	Sensor type	Application	CMOS	Other specifications	Ref.	Year
Wearable	Optical	PPG, and NIRS	0.18 μm	DR = 119 dB	[23]	2020
Wearable	Optical	Chest PPG	0.18 μm	DR = 134 dB	[24]	2021
Wearable	Capacitive	Real-time blood pressure monitoring	NA	1 × 5 sensor array area of 10 × 10 mm^2 Sesitivity = 30 fF/mmHg	[25]	2020
Wearable	Nanomaterials-modified lensless imager	Simultaneous monitoring of $TcCO_2$ and pulse rates	NA	Wearable bracelet	[26]	2024
Wearable	Impedance sensor	Cardiac health monitoring, the detection, and interpretation of gestures	0.13 μm	Power = 30 μW/channel	[27]	2020
Wearable	Optical	Continuous monitoring of cerebral blood flow in freely behaving mice	NA	A combination of relative rCBF measurement, O_2 and CO_2 supplies, and behavior recording for use on conscious, freely behaving mice	[28]	2023
Wearable	Optical	Face detection, eye tracking, and gesture recognition	0.11 μm	640 × 480 pixel prototype sensor Power = 45.5 μW/pixel (at 15 fps, 320,240)	[29]	2016
Wearable	Optical	Transcutaneous oxygen sensing	0.18 μm	Power = 631 μW area = 1.04 mm^2	[30]	2020
Wearable	Optical	TD-NIRS	0.35 μm	FWHM = 300 ps DR >100 dB	[31]	2020
Wearable	Optical	Continuous blood pressure monitoring	65 nm	Power = 145.9 nW	[32]	2020
Wearable	Optical	HR, SBP, and DBP	0.35 μm	Area = 2.3 × 1.7 mm^2	[33]	2021
Wearable	Electrochemical	Glucose level monitoring	0.35 μm	Chip size = 641 × 617 $μm^2$	[34]	2021

NA Not available, *SoC* system-on-chip, *IMIC* Imageur Moléculaire Intra Cérébral, *PPG* photoplethysmography, *NIRS* Near-infrared spectroscopy, *$TcCO_2$* Transcutaneous Carbon Dioxide, *HR* Heart rate, *SBP* Systolic blood pressure, *DBP* Diastolic blood pressure, *LoD* Limit of detection, *rCBF* cerebral blood flow, *FWHM* Full-width at half-maximum, *DR* Dynamic Range

5.1.1 Electrocehmical Biosensors

Handheld electrochemical biosensors are portable devices designed for on-site detection and analysis of various biochemical substances, leveraging electrochemical reactions to quantify analyte concentrations and offering advantages such as low cost, rapid results, and ease of use. For example, the study in [6] introduces a cost-effective, portable Wi-Fi-enabled potentiostat designed for electrochemical biosensing. The system comprises a custom analog front-end (AFE) board and a development board with a system-on-chip that integrates a microcontroller and Wi-Fi network processor. This setup allows for direct transmission of data to cloud services, eliminating the need for additional software or devices for data processing. The device can store data during internet outages for later transmission. Performance validation against a conventional benchtop Autolab PGSTAT-204 workstation using ferri/ferrocyanide as a redox probe shows that the new device provides accurate, repeatable, and high-resolution measurements. The system's battery-powered design ensures enhanced portability, with an estimated battery life of 3.8 years. The device's AFE features a transimpedance amplifier (TIA) with less than 0.5% non-linearity, achieving an overall voltage measurement resolution of 0.025%. This innovative potentiostat is well-suited for both qualitative and quantitative analysis in amperometric biosensing applications.

5.1.2 FET-Based Biosensors

Handheld CMOS FET-based biosensors are cutting-edge diagnostic tools that combine biological/chemical field effect transistors (Bio/ChemFETs) with CMOS technology to enable rapid, portable, and accurate detection of various biological markers. For example, Ryazantsev et al. [5] described a portable device for PoC testing that combines ion-sensitive field-effect transistors (ISFETs) with aptamers for fast, label-free detection of various biomarkers. This PC-controlled device allows selective modification of ISFETs with different oligonucleotides and uses optimized Ta_2O_5-gated ISFET structures to reduce trapped charge and capacitive attenuation. Integrated CMOS readout circuits with a linear transfer function minimize signal distortion. An external analog signal digitizer with a constant voltage and a superimposed high-frequency sine wave enhances sensitivity. The device's performance was demonstrated with the detection of troponin I, showing a limit of detection (LoD) of 3.27 ng/mL and effective discrimination of acute myocardial infarction. This ISFET-based device offers a versatile platform for multiplexed biomarker detection in PoC applications.

5.1.3 NMR Platforms

Handheld CMOS-based nuclear magnetic resonance (NMR) biosensors are advanced portable devices that combine CMOS technology with NMR techniques to enable portable, sensitive and rapid detection of biological and chemical samples. Despite challenges such as achieving high magnetic field strength and managing power consumption, these biosensors represent a significant innovation in portable biochemical sensing technology. For instance, Mak [2] developed a portable NMR CMOS platform for biological and chemical assays, featuring a compact magnet and a 0.18 μm CMOS transceiver chip. The chip's spiral coil allows direct measurement of micro-liter droplet samples. Key components include a system printed circuit board (PCB), field-programmable gate array (FPGA), and a current driver for field stabilization. This platform excels in identifying biological targets, analyzing protein states, and studying solvent-polymer dynamics, reducing sample volume, hardware size, and weight compared to commercial products. Building on this, the author is now investigating low-cost portable magnetic resonance imaging (MRI) technology for diagnosing ligament tears, inflammation, and tumors.

5.1.4 Optical Biosensors

Handheld CMOS optical biosensors leverage CMOS technology to integrate high-efficiency cameras and advanced optical systems, such as plasmonic chips and lens-free imaging frameworks, for label-free virus detection and other analytical applications. Innovative designs, like plasmonic nanohole arrays for virus detection and micro-capillary electrophoresis (μCE) systems powered by smartphones for PoC diagnostics, overcome the limitations of traditional bulky and expensive equipment. The study in [3] outlines the development of a portable, lightweight biosensor using a plasmonic chip built on nanohole arrays, integrated with a lens-free imaging system for detecting viruses without labels in field environments. This biosensor employs a CMOS camera with high quantum efficiency to observe diffraction field patterns under light-emitting diode (LED) light tuned to the plasmonic mode. It has proven effective in detecting H1N1 viruses and includes an economical sample preparation kit for analyte binding. A user-friendly Python-based graphical interface allows for straightforward interaction with the biosensor hardware, image analysis, and virus data presentation. Weighing only 70 grams, the handheld device boasts high sensitivity with an LoD as low as 10^3 $TCID_{50}$/mL, making it ideal for rapid diagnostics in low-resource settings.

Handheld CMOS optical biosensors are particularly advantageous in low-resource settings, providing rapid, accurate, and user-friendly diagnostics for diseases such as H1N1 and SARS-CoV-2. These devices promise significant improvements in on-site molecular diagnostics and healthcare monitoring. Nguyen et al. [4] developed a compact, integrated μCE system designed for PoC molecular diagnostics, controlled and powered by a smartphone. Traditional μCE systems require bulky, high-power supplies and costly laser-induced fluorescence detectors, making them unsuitable for PoC applications. This innovative μCE system overcomes these limitations by using the smartphone to power boost converters and a laser, control the power switch, and utilize its CMOS camera for fluorescence detection of reverse transcription polymerase chain reaction (RT-PCR) amplified DNA. A custom web-based application enables the smartphone to display capillary electropherograms from fluorescence intensity data. The handheld device measures $9.6 \times 22 \times 15.5$ cm^3 and weighs approximately 1 kg, suitable for PoC DNA testing, including rapid and accurate analysis of SARS-CoV-2 genes. This μCE platform, leveraging smartphone technology and user-friendly automation, promises significant advancements in on-site molecular diagnostics.

5.1.5 Colorimetric Biosensors

CMOS handheld colorimetric biosensors use compact digital cameras, such as those found in smartphones, to assess color intensity for various assays. These tools are ideal for conducting analyses in non-laboratory settings and can achieve LoDs and sensitivity similar to those of more costly and sophisticated methods. The broad availability and decreasing prices of digital cameras, as well as their incorporation into everyday devices like smartphones and tablets, make these biosensors more accessible and practical. Although they do not directly replace traditional methods like chromatography or polymerase chain reaction (PCR), CMOS handheld colorimetric biosensors offer an affordable, portable, and convenient option for field-based testing and analysis.

For instance, Simon and colleagues [1] explored the application of thin-layer chromatography along with a compact digital camera for the analysis of natural extracts. They employed a single-lens reflex camera featuring an Advanced photo system type-C (APS-C) sized CMOS sensor to capture digital images under Ultraviolet (UV) light at 254 and 366 nm wavelengths. In a study [35], digoxigenin was detected using a lateral flow chromatography method coupled with a CMOS camera from an iPhone 5S. This test employed antibody-gold nanoparticle conjugates and reached an LoD of 14.4 nmol/l and a quantification limit of 19.1 nmol/l. Compared to a professional colorimeter, the smartphone camera demonstrated a similar level of performance while being more affordable.

5.2 Wearable Biosensors

Wearable sensors merge lab-on-a-chip (LoC) technologies, advanced microelectronics, and connected intelligence to create a data flow from analytes in body fluids to Cloud infrastructures for next-gen healthcare. Designing electrode-embedded instrumentation in advanced CMOS nodes presents challenges such as ultra-low power, small footprint, and CMOS compatibility.

Wearable patches, which merge flexible electronics with wireless systems, are transforming health monitoring and robotics. Modern embroidery tools and conductive/flexible yarns can turn ordinary textiles into smart fabrics, but a more advanced approach involves integrating electronic components and sensors directly into the fabric. This integrated method is essential for leveraging advancements in multimodal sensing and sensor fusion, which require numerous sensors and vectors. The integration with CMOS sensors enhances the patches' data processing capabilities and power efficiency, facilitating real-time health monitoring and complex data analysis. Flexible CMOS integrated circuits (ICs) can be incorporated into textile elements, enabling e-textiles to harness machine learning (ML) and artificial intelligence (AI) advancements. These e-textiles can collect diverse data and combine it with embedded electronics to generate interpretable outcomes. These patches detect strain, pressure, temperature, bending, vibration, and acoustic feedback, demonstrating their potential in applications such as shoe inserts, elbow trackers, and respiratory and heart-rate (HR) monitors. With multi-modal capabilities, these textile patches can capture extensive data on movement and environmental factors, paving the way for advanced biomedical and robotic applications through sensor fusion and ML integration [36].

Flexible sensors, such as strain, pressure, temperature, imaging, pH, inertial, and gas sensors, are essential for gathering critical sensory information from diverse environments due to their mechanical flexibility and stretchability. These sensors can be deployed on curvilinear and dynamic surfaces, making them ideal for integration with quadrupedal robots. For example, electronic skins combining thermal and tactile sensing are well-documented, offering functionalities similar to human skin [37, 38]. Imaging sensors, demonstrated by Torres Sevilla et al. [39], and organic imaging sensors presented by Wu et al. [40], improve environmental awareness and obstacle detection by transforming light stimuli into real-time data. Environmental sensors, like the chemical-sensitive FET-based gas sensors, can detect toxic gases and humidity, making them crucial for rescue missions and hazardous environment assessments [41]. Furthermore, underwater sensors, such as the Bluefin developed by Shaikh et al. [42], measure temperature, pressure, and salinity, enhancing the capabilities of marine exploration robots. Integrating these flexible sensors into quadrupedal robots can significantly expand their applications in various environments, including hazardous and underwater terrains [37, 43, 44].

5.2.1 Optical Sensors

Lin et al. [23] introduced a flexible, low-energy, high dynamic range light-to-digital converter (LDC) tailored for near-infrared spectroscopy (NIRS) and photoplethysmogram (PPG) assessments, converting photocurrent to digital code using current integration and charge counting, thus reducing noise. This LDC was tested with on-body PPG and NIRS using a photodiode and silicon photomultiplier, respectively, benefiting wearable optical sensors like smartwatches and health patches by improving long-term monitoring and spatial resolution. In a subsequent study, the same team [24] developed another energy-efficient, high dynamic range LDC for chest PPG devices, employing a second-order noise-shaping slope architecture and a high-resolution dual-slope quantizer to directly convert photocurrent to digital. Compared to traditional TIA-based systems that need high-resolution analog-to-digital converter (ADCs) and consume more power, integrator-based LDCs provide better noise efficiency and power savings. This LDC shows promise for compact, efficient medical patches for long-term monitoring of vital signs in patients with respiratory diseases such as COVID-19.

The study in [33] introduced a low-power, high-sensitivity PPG sensor designed for continuous health monitoring in wearable devices. The sensor's power efficiency is enhanced through low-duty cycling of LED lighting and automatic light control (ALC). Tested on nine subjects, it showed a mean absolute error (MAE) and standard deviation (SD) of 1.95 ± 2.13 beats per minute (BPM) for HR, 6.00 ± 4.18 mmHg for systolic blood pressure, and 6.13 ± 3.93 mmHg for diastolic blood pressure.

A study in [31] introduced a large-area, digitally controlled single-photon detector for high-sensitivity time-domain near-infrared spectroscopy (TD-NIRS). This detector integrates a time-gated digital silicon photomultiplier (dSiPM) with a programmable active area, an internal gate generator, and a time-to-digital converter (TDC) with a built-in histogram builder. This technology removes the need for external timing electronics and optomechanical signal attenuators, paving the way for compact, portable, and wearable TD-NIRS systems. These systems can perform at levels comparable to larger units and are suitable for non-invasive applications like breast cancer diagnostics, monitoring muscle and brain hemodynamics, and evaluating fruit maturity.

Daily monitoring of psychological parameters, including chemical and physical signals, is increasingly crucial for managing chronic diseases. Among vital signs, carbon dioxide exchange and pulse rate (PR) are key indicators for assessing the cardiopulmonary system. However, simultaneous monitoring of these signals non-invasively is challenging. The study in [26] introduced a wearable bracelet for simultaneous monitoring of transcutaneous carbon dioxide ($TcCO_2$) and PR using a nanomaterials-modified lensless CMOS imager (see Fig. 5.1). The bracelet demonstrates high sensitivity, selectivity, and resistance to humidity in $TcCO_2$ detection, and effectively tracks $TcCO_2$ and PR fluctuations due to daily activities, showing potential for cardiopulmonary system assessment.

Liu et al. [28] introduced a wearable, fiber-free optical sensor for continuous monitoring of cerebral blood flow (CBF) in freely behaving mice. This innovative system integrates diffuse speckle contrast flowmetry (DSCF) technology with behavioral recording capabilities, allowing for non-invasive assessment of CBF variations during natural behaviors without the need for anesthesia or immobilization. The wearable sensor, optimized for small subject applications, provides reliable measurements of relative CBF (rCBF) and successfully detects responses to CO_2-induced hypercapnia in both anesthetized and freely behaving mice. By combining real-time CBF monitoring with behavioral observations, this system offers new insights into cognitive processing, adaptive behavior, and neurological

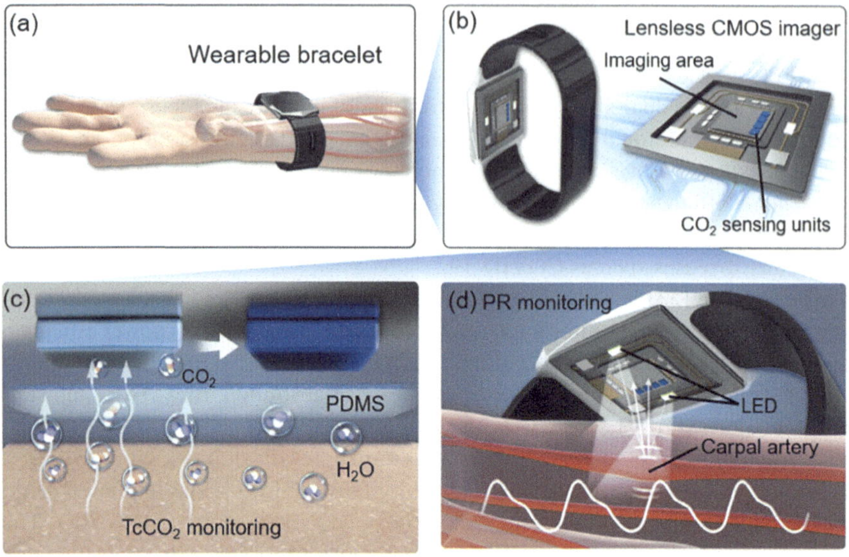

Fig. 5.1 (**a**) Schematic representation of the wearable bracelet, (**b**) Diagram illustrating the nanomaterial-modified lensless CMOS imager, (**c**) Operational principle of the wearable bracelet for $TcCO_2$, (**d**) Operational principle of the wearable bracelet for PR, with the CMOS imager capturing the fluctuation of pulsatile blood volume through the central unmodified imaging area, and the pulse waveform derived from analyzed reflected light [26]

disorders in animal studies, facilitating advancements in neuroscience research and clinical applications.

The integration of CIS in mobile and wearable devices has become commonplace for capturing high-resolution images, yet there is an increasing demand for these devices to support smart sensing functionalities such as face detection and gesture recognition. To meet this need, Choi et al. [29] introduced a novel low-power always-on CMOS image sensor tailored for such applications. This sensor continuously captures images for smart sensing tasks while also offering high-resolution image capture capability. Operating in a switchable dual mode of always-on (AO) for low-power operation and photo-shooting (PS) for high signal-to-noise ratio (SNR), the sensor employs dynamic voltage scaling to achieve high energy efficiency. Key features include the implementation of a conventional four-transistor pixel as a charge-shared pixel for low-voltage AO mode operation and the reconfiguration of the ADC to further reduce power consumption. Experimental results showcase the sensor's effectiveness, operating at 45.5 μW in AO mode and significantly extending battery life for always-on sensing applications. Furthermore, the paper includes successful application testing with a mobile eye-tracking algorithm.

Costanzo et al. [30] presented an integrated readout circuit for transcutaneous oxygen sensing in a wearable device, utilizing a fluorescence-based method to detect oxygen molecules through the skin. This innovative approach employs a platinum porphyrin thin film excited by a blue LED, with a photodiode capturing the emitted red light, which is quenched by oxygen presence. The readout IC, fabricated in a 0.18 μm 5 V CMOS process, converts the photodiode current to a voltage with variable gain and pulses the LED to conserve power. Consuming 631 μW and occupying 1.04 mm^2, the IC demonstrates the feasibility of non-invasive oxygen measurement within the 0–150 mmHg range, covering human partial pressure levels.

5.2.2 *Capacitive Textile*

In an effort, Rohit and Kaya [36] investigated capacitive textile patches featuring engineered dielectrics for strain and piezoelectric sensing with multi-modal capabilities. These patches employ a parallel plate capacitive design with highly stretchable textile electrodes and silicone or Polydimethylsiloxane (PDMS) elastomers, enhancing their functionality with high-*k* Barium Titanate (BTO) nanoparticles. This inclusion doubles the gauge factor without compromising linearity or durability, exceeding 2000 cycles. Additionally, the study explores the piezoelectric properties induced by additives like PZT and PVDF-TrFE, and corona poling boosts the voltage output.

Luo et al. [25] presented a cost-effective, paper-based, flexible tactile sensor array designed for monitoring human health, particularly cardiovascular conditions (see Fig. 5.2). Utilizing a paper substrate and spray-deposited metal electrodes, this sensor array features a capacitive sensing scheme with a deformable PDMS membrane for high sensitivity and no DC power consumption. The optimal design includes a 1 × 5 sensor array occupying 10 × 10 mm^2, each sensor with approximately 1 pF nominal capacitance and 30 fF/mmHg sensitivity. Designed for comfortable attachment to the temporal region and ankle, it accurately monitors blood pressure pulse waveforms, HR, and variability, and can detect atrial fibrillation. This affordable and user-friendly sensor offers high signal quality, addressing the cost and comfort issues of existing wearable technologies like smartwatches.

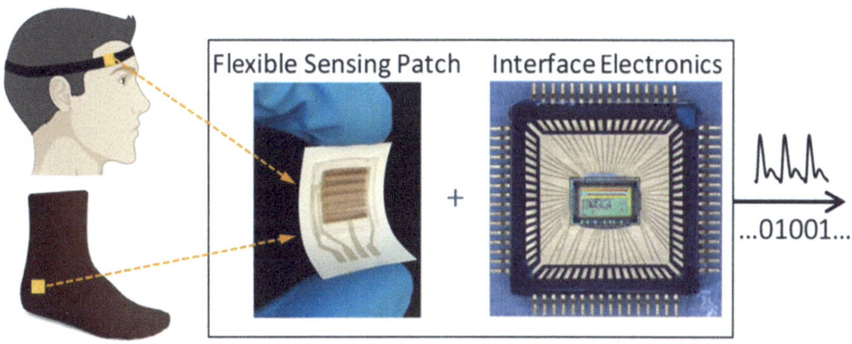

Fig. 5.2 A wearable system for monitoring human blood pressure pulse waveforms [25]

5.2.3 Potentiostatic Sensors

The work reported in [22] introduced a low-power frontend with extended amperometric dynamic and wide potentiostatic ranges for electrochemical transducers, featuring a delta-sigma modulator with digital output. The differential potentiostat achieves 1.8 V_{pp} control range on a 1.2 V supply, integrated in TSMC 65 nm CMOS technology, occupying 0.07 mm^2, achieving 80 dB signal-to-noise-and-distortion ratio (SNDR) and 105 dB multi-scale dynamic range with 15 μW power consumption. This innovative design targets wearable applications for real-time tracking of physical and chemical data, particularly through sweat and other body fluids, enhancing the potential of wearable technology.

5.2.4 Impedance and Resistance Sensor

Hedayatipour et al. [27] presented a novel non-invasive wearable impedance sensor implemented in CMOS technology, featuring impedance to frequency measurement with resistance and capacitance modes. This sensor, with low power consumption, operates in two applications: thoracic impedance for fluid accumulation detection and hand gesture recognition through tissue impedance sensing. It offers the potential for continuous monitoring of heart failure by detecting intra-thoracic impedance changes and enables real-time hand gesture recognition for interactive interfaces. The system is compact, lightweight, and cost-effective, demonstrating promising applications in healthcare and human-computer interaction. It utilizes conductive paint electrodes and is validated for accuracy with tissue models. The impedance measurement system operates efficiently, offering significant advancements in wearable sensing technology for various biomedical and interactive applications.

Seo et al. [45] discussed three designs of energy-resolution scalable time-based resistance-to-digital converters (RDCs) aimed at minimizing energy per conversion step or maximizing bit-resolution. Each RDC design uses a current-starved differential ring oscillator, differential to single-ended amplifier, and off-chip counter. The first design prioritizes low energy consumption, the second enhances oscillator phase noise to improve bit-resolution, and the third scales technology to reduce power while maintaining high resolution.

5.2.5 Temperature Sensor

Temperature sensors are crucial components in wearable devices, playing a vital role in various applications, including health monitoring, fitness tracking, and environmental sensing. These sensors help maintain optimal device performance by ensuring accurate thermal management, which is essential for user comfort and the reliability of the device. In the context of wearable internet of things (IoT) applications, Silverio et al. [46] presented a novel design for a wide temperature range, high linearity, and time-domain CMOS-based temperature sensor. The design focuses on achieving low voltage and low power consumption while providing a digital time-based output suitable for integration into SoC architectures. Utilizing a BJT-less current-mode bandgap core with sub-threshold MOS transistors, the sensor derives temperature-dependent voltages to drive a voltage-frequency converter (VFC).

5.2.6 *Pressure Sensor*

Wearable monitoring devices increasingly rely on advanced pressure sensors to detect subtle external pressures and mimic human tactile perception, facilitating applications in health monitoring and human-computer interaction. Yu et al. [47] introduced a high-performance multifunctional pressure sensor combining piezoresistive, piezoelectric, and thermochromic functions. The sensor, crafted from a piezoelectric film and a piezoresistive layer, exhibits a temperature-responsive color change from blue at 30 °C to white at 150 °C, driven by a thermochromic reaction involving crystal violet lactone (CVL), bisphenol A (BPA), and paraffin wax (PW). The piezoelectric layer, containing $Bi_{0.5}Na_{0.5}TiO_3$ (BNT) material, delivers an 80 V output voltage, 1.398 V/kPa sensitivity, and a 30 ms response time, while the piezoresistive layer, enhanced with MXene, shows 0.835 kPa sensitivity and a 73 ms response time over 0–300 kPa. This integrated sensor demonstrates exceptional sensitivity in monitoring human activities, breath airflow, and speech signals when applied to the body or masks, thus providing a new paradigm for multifunctional pressure sensors in wearable monitoring with temperature visualization.

5.2.7 *Electrochemical Sensor*

Wearable electrochemical sensors, which attach to the skin, enable continuous and non-invasive health monitoring by detecting metabolites in bodily fluids like sweat, offering a painless alternative to traditional methods such as finger pricking for glucose monitoring. These battery-free devices utilize energy harvesting technologies, enhancing user comfort, mobility, and real-time health data accessibility, thus advancing personalized healthcare. In an effort, Wuthibenjaphonchai et al. [34] discussed the development of wireless epidermal devices for personalized health monitoring, focusing on a battery-free model powered by optical energy transfer. The system includes an electrochemical sensor for glucose, highlighting its potential for noninvasive diabetes monitoring. The device utilizes photovoltaic cells to harvest light energy, which is then used to power an amperometric sensor that measures glucose levels in sweat. Results confirm the device's effectiveness in detecting varying glucose concentrations. The design aims to address the limitations of conventional glucose monitors by offering a pain-free and convenient alternative. The authors suggest that the technology can be adapted for detecting other metabolites by modifying the sensor and oxidation voltage, with future plans to develop a complete, attachable health monitoring package.

5.2.8 Multi-Biosignal Sensor

Sleep is a critical physiological process that impacts overall health and well-being, with disorders such as insomnia and sleep apnea affecting a significant portion of the global population. Traditional sleep monitoring methods, like Polysomnography (PSG), provide comprehensive sleep analysis but are cumbersome, requiring hospitalization and expert supervision. This complexity has driven the development of portable sleep monitoring devices that aim to offer more user-friendly and accessible solutions for sleep quality assessment. These devices typically focus on parameters like HR and body movement but often lack comprehensive analysis capabilities. In this context, advancements in wearable technology have opened new avenues for integrated, real-time sleep monitoring systems that are both accurate and comfortable for long-term use. The article by Kim et al. [48] details the creation of a wearable multi-biosignal interface designed for sleep monitoring, which integrates the capability for direct sleep-stage classification. Unlike traditional methods like Polysomnography (PSG) that demand extensive post-processing and expert oversight, this new interface streamlines the process by combining electroencephalography (EEG), electromyography (EMG), and electrooculography (EOG) in a headband-style device. The system employs a readout integrated circuit (ROIC) to collect and analyze biosignals, utilizing an innovative feature extraction circuit for immediate sleep-stage determination through a decision tree algorithm. Verified through comparison with OpenBCI post-processing results, the device showed a 74% correlation in detecting four sleep stages. This development addresses the limitations of existing portable sleep monitors by offering an all-in-one solution that minimizes the need for extensive data processing and supports real-time sleep analysis.

5.2.9 Electrocardiogram (ECG) Recording

Recent advancements in SoC-based ECG devices have garnered global acceptance for real-time health monitoring of patients. Researchers have introduced various innovations such as fully integrated wireless ECG SoC that incorporate ECG front ends, custom microcontrollers, and specialized random-access memory (RAM) configurations, achieving remarkably low power consumption [49]. These developments include context-aware wearable ECG monitors integrating smartphone sensors, facilitating health data display via bluetooth connectivity [50–52]. Additionally, advancements in ASIC-based ECG signal processors have demonstrated enhanced energy efficiency using CMOS technology, enabling real-time signal processing and transmission to smartphones for medical analysis [53]. Innovations like clockless SoCs with high input impedance AFEs aim to minimize motion artifacts and improve signal quality, crucial for accurate ECG monitoring in diverse settings [54]. Further innovations involve wearable ECG vests and dynamic power management techniques, ensuring continuous, reliable data collection suitable for long-term healthcare applications and remote monitoring systems [55, 56]. The integration of novel electrode designs and signal processing algorithms enhances the accuracy and usability of these devices, paving the way for comprehensive cardiac health monitoring solutions [57–61].

Wearable biomedical devices are increasingly vital for recording ECG to provide a comprehensive view of a patient's cardiac status. The work reported in [62] focused on designing a low-power, low-noise ECG amplifier for such smart wearable devices using 180 nm CMOS technology. The proposed AFE amplifier, which incorporates a drive right leg (DRL) circuit and notch filter, effectively suppresses noise and enhances signal quality. Simulation results demonstrate the amplifier's capability to achieve a mid-band gain of 50.75 dB, a power supply rejection ratio (PSRR) of 113 dB, and a common mode rejection ratio (CMRR) of 102 dB. The system exhibits an input-referred noise (IRN) of 1.47 μVrms, corresponding to a noise efficiency factor (NEF) of 2.74, while consuming only 1.08 μW from a 1.8 V supply.

Cardiovascular diseases (CVD) is the primary cause of death globally, necessitating consistent home monitoring of vital signs such as ECG, HR, SpO_2, and continuous blood pressure. The article reported in [49] introduced a real-time, low-power wearable cardiac monitoring device designed for displaying ECG signals and HR. The device utilizes the MAX30003 AFE and MAX32630 microcontroller, optimized for wearable applications with minimal power consumption (85 μW at 1.1 V). Electrodes are placed at specific positions on the body to capture ECG signals, which are processed by the microcontroller for real-time display and can be stored on a micro SD card or transmitted to a PC via USB. The system aims for compactness, efficiency, and user comfort, facilitating prolonged monitoring without interference with daily activities.

In another effort, Wang et al. [63] presented a compact, low-power wearable sensor that integrates an AFE IC to simultaneously monitor these parameters using ECG and two-wavelength PPG signals. The AFE IC features adjustable gain, current compensation, lead-off detection, and quick recovery functions, enhancing its practicality for varied users. This device utilizes an adaptive method for parameter adjustments, calculates HR from ECG signals, and employs a univariate quadratic equation for SpO_2 calibration with less than 1% error. It also estimates blood pressure using a support vector machine model, achieving mean errors of -2.10 ± 7.07 mmHg for systolic and 0.04 ± 7.34 mmHg for diastolic measurements.

5.3 Implantable Biosensors

Implantable CMOS biosensors are advanced devices embedded within the human body to monitor physiological parameters continuously. They enable real-time tracking of vital signs, biochemical markers, and other critical health indicators, providing valuable data for medical diagnostics and patient management. The integration of these biosensors with wireless communication systems allows for seamless data transmission to external devices, enhancing remote healthcare monitoring and personalized medicine. With advancements in microfabrication and integrated electronics, implantable devices have become a vital means of providing real-time medical diagnostics and treatments by monitoring and recording vital signs.

5.3.1 *Retinal Sensing*

The study in [64] describes a CMOS image sensor chip created for subretinal implantation, part of a retinal prosthesis system aimed at restoring vision in patients with retinal degenerative conditions such as retinitis pigmentosa and age-related macular degeneration. This chip utilizes pulse-frequency modulation (PFM) to handle both image capture and electrical stimulation, with a 16×16 pixel array that transforms light into biphasic current pulses. The system operates with a dual voltage supply, features a programmable waveform generator, and includes a control block for adjusting stimulus settings. Both the sensor and the stimulus array receive power and control signals wirelessly. Tests indicate that the chip can resolve basic shapes and generate stimulation currents exceeding retinal thresholds, indicating its promise for further miniaturization and enhancement.

Ohta et al. [65] have designed innovative neural stimulators for retinal implants using silicon large-scale integration (Si-LSI). These stimulators leverage LSI technology to provide advantages such as flexibility, reduced size, and high signal fidelity. Their creation features a Pt/Au layered bump electrode stimulator with epoxy encapsulation, which works well with standard LSI chips and effectively triggers retinal cells. Successful results were obtained in both saline environments and live experiments with detached frog retinas, indicating its promise for retinal implant uses. Their study also includes microchip-based stimulators on bendable polyimide substrates, available in broadcast and serial bus types, both showing encouraging performance.

The work reported in [21] introduced CMOS photovoltaic-powered subretinal prosthetic chips, specifically 256-pixel and 480-pixel versions, developed using CMOS image sensor (CIS) technology to assist individuals with retinal diseases like retinitis pigmentosa (RP) and age-related macular degeneration (AMD). The chips feature bi-directional and four-directional sharing electrodes, respectively, to enhance electrode size and stimulation charge within the same chip area. They incorporate an adaptive background cancellation circuit to adapt to varying light conditions and improve image dynamic range. Experimental results, including electrical measurements and ex vivo tests on mouse retinas, confirmed that both chip types effectively evoke ganglion cell responses under specific light intensities, validating their potential for retinal stimulation without invasive wires.

5.3.2 Neural Interface

Tissue-penetrating neural probes are essential for recording high-resolution brain activity, crucial for neuroscience and brain-computer interfaces (BCIs). However, their long-term efficacy is hampered by foreign body reaction (FBR), where biological responses to the implanted device degrade its performance over time. The shift from passive micro-electromechanical systems (MEMS) to active CMOS technology in these probes offers new possibilities to address FBR by customizing mechanical and physicochemical properties [66].

To advance the understanding of brain processes and validate preclinical studies in drug development, it is crucial to conduct molecular neuroimaging on awake, freely moving animals, as current procedures under anesthesia can introduce biases. The MAPSSIC initiative aims to address this by developing a pixelated intracerebral probe for implantation in conscious rats. This probe uses the IMIC (Imageur Moléculaire Intra Cérébral), a monolithic active pixel sensor (MAPS) prototype designed for direct positron detection. Produced in five configurations, IMIC sensors were optimized to enhance sensitivity and reduce cluster size, showing significant performance gains with CMOS process modifications. This approach aims to bridge the gap between preclinical and clinical studies by providing reliable real-time neuroimaging data without anesthesia-related biases [20].

Bench tests of a 512-electrode-pixel probe in [8] shown in Fig. 5.3 demonstrated impressive performance metrics, including low noise and power consumption. Post-processing of Simultaneous Neural Active Pixel Sensor (SiNAPS) probes involves shaping and thinning the probe, attaching it to a PCB, and applying suitable electrode materials for neuron interfacing. In vivo recordings showcased the ability to capture and distinguish neural activity from densely packed neurons, indicating the potential for compact and scalable brain recording systems. This technology, based on the APS concept, offers advantages in minimizing silicon area while enabling simultaneous recordings from hundreds to thousands of closely spaced microelectrodes. Future advancements aim to optimize probe architecture for monitoring neural activity in freely behaving animals, addressing design challenges in wiring, materials, packaging, and geometry.

To enhance understanding of brain connectivity, there is a push to cover larger cortical regions using implanted electrodes for direct neural interaction. Lee et al. [14] introduced addressable micro-implants with gate oxide-based anti-fuse IDs activated by a photodiode array, eliminating the need for traditional I/O pads. These ID-equipped wireless implants enable extensive bidirectional neural interfacing. An 8-channel wireless microstimulator and spike-sensor were created using CMOS

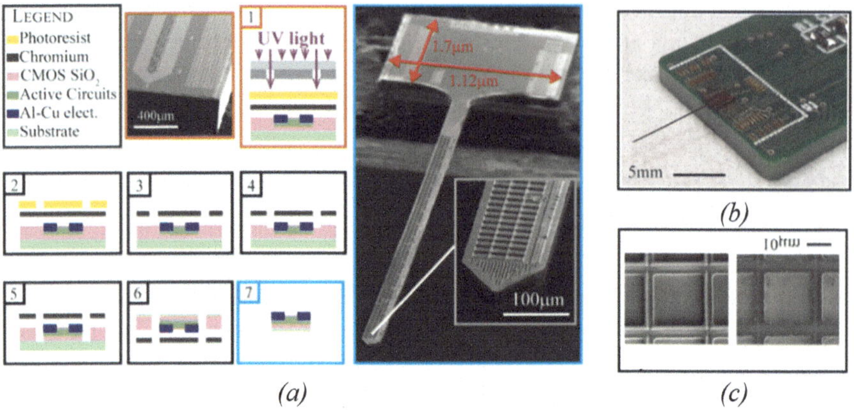

Fig. 5.3 (**a**) The microfabrication workflow (steps 1–7) includes SEM images showing the SiNAPS probe's tip and after structuring, (**b**) Structured CMOS probes are wire-bonded to a PCB, with wires protected by epoxy glue (not shown), (**c**) The sensing electrodes' native Al-Cu CMOS alloy is electroplated with platinum to lower electrode impedance, ensuring low-noise and stable neural interfacing [8]

technology, powered by radio frequency (RF) electromagnetic waves, and utilizing amplitude modulation for communication.

The study in [15] introduces a bioinspired neuromorphic sensing system (NSS) designed for peripheral nerve recording. It employs event-based sampling to leverage the sparse nature of electroneurogram signals, achieving significant data compression while maintaining signal fidelity. The system consists of three key components: a clockless level-crossing ADC for efficient data rate reduction, a spiking neural network for low-power feature extraction, and an event-driven pulse-based communication method to minimize energy use and size. Fabricated in CMOS technology, the NSS supports dual-mode operation, providing both detailed diagnostic data and energy-efficient feature extraction, making it highly suitable for miniaturized, low-power nerve implants.

Emerging optical functional imaging and optogenetics are crucial for studying neural circuits. Combining these techniques in a single implantable device allows all-optical neural interrogation, useful in freely behaving animal studies. Moazeni et al. [11] showcase such a device for optical neural recording and stimulation across large cortical areas. The device uses lens-less computational imaging and a novel packaging technique, resulting in an ultra-thin, flexible structure. Its core features a custom CMOS chip with a 160 × 160 array of single-photon avalanche photodiodes (SPADs) for low-light imaging and dual-color micro-LEDs for light sources. This innovation represents a significant step toward fully implantable, all-optical neural interfaces (see Fig. 5.4).

The research detailed in [7] presented a novel approach to in vivo imaging and electrical interfacing within the depths of the mouse brain, utilizing a sole CMOS sensor. This advanced device seamlessly integrates an imaging array, light source,

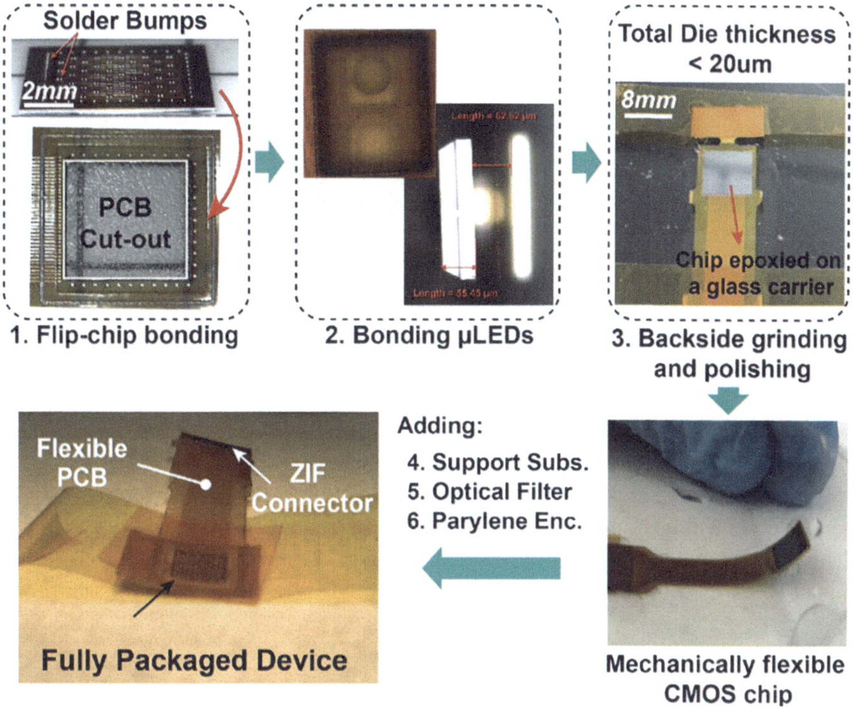

Fig. 5.4 An implantable neural interface for computational imaging and optogenetic stimulation that is mechanically flexible [11]

electrodes, and chemical delivery mechanism, facilitating concurrent fluorescence imaging and electrophysiological examinations. Employing MEMS microfabrication techniques, enhancements were made to the CMOS sensor chip, incorporating LEDs for illumination and on-chip platinum electrodes for neuron interaction. Through this device, fluorescence imaging and electrical tests were performed within the mouse brain, successfully evoking synaptic responses in the hippocampus using on-chip electrodes with currents ranging from 200 μA to 1 mA, all while ensuring minimal impact on the hippocampus.

5.3.3 Oxygen Sensing

The continuous monitoring of tissue oxygen levels is crucial for critical care patients, but existing methods rely on bulky, battery-dependent devices. The study in [10] introduced a fully implantable, wireless, battery-free sensor system for real-time deep tissue oxygen monitoring. Utilizing ultrasound (US) for power and data transmission, the device is remarkably compact at 4.5 mm^3. The sensor system

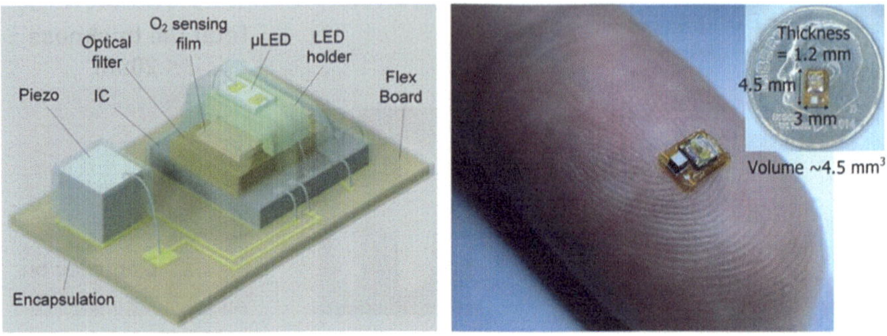

Fig. 5.5 The 4.5mm^3 fully implantable, wire-free oxygen sensing system reported in [10]

includes a luminescence sensor with a μLED, encapsulated ruthenium dyes, and a custom IC fabricated in 65 nm CMOS, all powered and communicated via a single US link. Operating safely at 50 mm depth with less than 0.76% oxygen resolution, the device consumes only 140 μW. The sensor's accuracy and efficiency make it ideal for chronic use, providing reliable oxygen level data with minimal tissue impact (see Fig. 5.5).

5.3.4 *Drug Delivery*

Implantable drug delivery systems can enable precise, personalized treatments while reducing side effects. Wang et al. [13] introduced an ultrasound-powered implantable potentiostat for controlled drug release, incorporating piezoelectric transducers for wireless power and data, a CMOS IC, and a custom drug delivery module with electro responsive nanoparticles. The chip facilitates simultaneous power and data transfer, precise potential control, and bidirectional communication. By wirelessly controlling and demonstrating fluorescein release, the system exemplifies targeted drug delivery, enhancing treatment effectiveness and minimizing adverse effects.

5.3.5 *Real-Time Temperature Sensing*

Temperature sensors are crucial for detecting issues like localized inflammation and managing electro surgeries. Implantable electronics must be low-power, often powered by wireless energy transfer, and maintain minimal heat to avoid tissue damage. Traditional temperature sensors face challenges such as high power consumption and large chip areas. A highly compact, ultra-low power, all-CMOS temperature sensor designed for implantable devices is introduced in [9], integrating an AFE, a ring oscillator, and a counter. This sensor converts temperature-modulated pulse width into a quantized signal via a pulse width modulation (PWM)-based voltage-to-time method.

Shi et al. [18] introduced a tiny implant called a mote that uses standard ultrasound imaging for wireless power and communication, enabling real-time temperature sensing, including monitoring changes from therapeutic ultrasound. This ultra-small device integrates a low-power temperature sensor chip with a microscale piezoelectric transducer, allowing minimally invasive implantation and demonstrated effectiveness in mouse neurostimulation. Another study in [19] presented a battery-free mote functioning as an electronic reporter during ultrasound imaging, transmitting data via backscattered acoustic energy captured in the image. Tested both in vitro and in vivo, this mote operates with minimal power consumption and transmits signals at depths up to 40 mm. This integration with medical sonography provides real-time, localized physiological data, offering new opportunities for advanced, miniaturized, battery-less, and biogeographically aware biosensing implants, potentially revolutionizing ultrasound diagnostics and surgical tracking.

5.3.6 Heart Implants

An implantable readout circuit has been developed by Neshatvar et al. [16] to track heart activity in post-heart transplant patients. Utilizing a MEMS pressure sensor, this circuit employs a time-domain architecture with voltage-controlled oscillators (VCOs) and phase-locked loops (PLLs), fabricated in 65 nm CMOS technology. Designed to fit within a 0.2 mm^2 area, the circuit meets stringent requirements for integration with the MEMS sensor, enabling monitoring of HR with an 8-bit resolution and a sampling frequency above 10 kHz.

Besirli et al. [17] detailed the development of a miniature implantable device for continuous remote monitoring of hemodynamics, specifically pulmonary arterial pressure (PAP) and artery cross-sectional area (CSA). The device integrates a piezoresistive pressure sensor, a custom ASIC in 180 nm CMOS, an ultrasound transducer, and a nitinol anchoring loop. The wireless system supports simultaneous power and data transfer via ultrasound, achieving a 1.8% efficiency at 8.5 cm depth and robust data transmission at 40–50 kbps. Tested in-vitro, the device accurately detects systolic and diastolic pressure peaks, presenting a promising solution for continuous hemodynamic monitoring in heart failure patients.

5.4 Smart Dust

The field of wearable and implantable sensors, particularly for human monitoring, is well-established with technologies such as FitBit for fitness tracking [67], Abbott's FreeStyle for diabetes management [68], and Medtronic's Revel LINQ for ECG monitoring [69]. Recent advancements include sensors for detecting chemicals in sweat like lactate [70], nicotine [71], and sodium [72]. The next step is Body Dust, surpassing traditional wearable and implantable models. The "Smart Dust" concept began around 1999 [73], aiming to create sub-millimeter autonomous sensing, computing, and communication systems [74]. Early prototypes focused on communication issues and energy scavenging [75]. Although initial devices were larger than expected, significant progress in miniaturization and energy efficiency has been made, promising substantial advancements in biomedical applications such as brain and metabolism monitoring over the next two decades [76].

In the early stages of research, the application of smart dust to biology was envisioned, with initial ideas including monitoring the movements of small insects [77]. More recently, there has been a shift towards in-body applications for humans, marking the third phase of smart dust research. Concepts like "Neural Dust" for brain monitoring and Body Dust for metabolic telemetry have emerged, spearheaded by researchers like Jan M. Rabaey [78], Michel Maharbiz [78], Sandro Carrara [79], and Pantelis Georgiou [79]. While progress has been made, particularly in miniaturization, challenges remain in realizing the promised applications, such as recording neural activity with sub-cranial sensory nodes and stimulating neurons with mm-scale devices [78]. Despite simulations demonstrating feasibility, actual demonstrations are limited, especially in the context of brain recording and stimulation [80].

The application of smart dust in body diagnostics holds the potential for monitoring metabolic conditions at a molecular level. Concepts like Body Dust aim to achieve extreme integration scales, allowing for diagnostic telemetry from within the human body. While simulations show promise, real device demonstrations are scarce, particularly in reaching the sizes required for integration into human blood cells [79]. However, designed architectures show feasibility in powering and sensing functionalities, suggesting that wearable, implantable, or injectable applications for monitoring and stimulating the human body could become a reality in the future, addressing a wide range of medical needs [81].

Imagining the near future reveals clear challenges surrounding Body Dust technology. These hurdles include the creation of minuscule sensors capable of long-term functionality, the design of ultrathin CMOS chips, the establishment of compact data-link systems, the development of efficient power delivery methods for tiny receivers, and the demonstration of in-body applications, such as ingestion for circulation within the bloodstream [82]. While progress has been made in sensor miniaturization and chip design, powering approaches remain a significant obstacle, with piezo-transducers currently too large for Body Dust's intended scale [83, 84]. However, advancements in electrode technology offer promise for energy-scavenging systems [85, 86]. The ultimate challenge lies in demonstrating Body Dust's in-body functionality, particularly through ingestion for circulation within the bloodstream [87]. While this remains a formidable task, early steps have been taken towards applications in the gastrointestinal tract, envisioning scenarios where patients could ingest Body Dust particles for diagnostic purposes, possibly coated with biocompatible membranes and functionalized to target specific cells [88–91]. Such advancements raise complex medical and ethical considerations, necessitating further research not only in technological development but also in the realm of medical ethics [92]. Despite the complexity, the prospect of realizing these applications with Body Dust technology looms on the horizon, promising significant advancements in medical diagnostics and treatment [76].

5.4.1 Ingestible Biosensors

Ingestible electronics capable of high-quality biomolecular analysis in a small, pill-sized format and operating at very low power with a strong wireless connection can revolutionize medical diagnostics and personalized healthcare. For example, Zhu et al. [12] presented a novel, fully-packaged biosensor system integrated with transmitter and receiver antennas on a single CMOS chip, which includes a 15-pixel fluorescence sensor array with nanoplasmonic optical filters (see Fig. 5.6). The chip operates across various ISM/MICS bands using pulse-pause-encoded amplitude-shift keying (ASK)/on-off keying (OOK) modulation, achieving high energy efficiency and sensitivity. This device enables real-time in vivo biomolecular sensing and quantification with pM sensitivity, offering wireless transmission through several inches of tissue, representing a significant advancement in ingestible electronics.

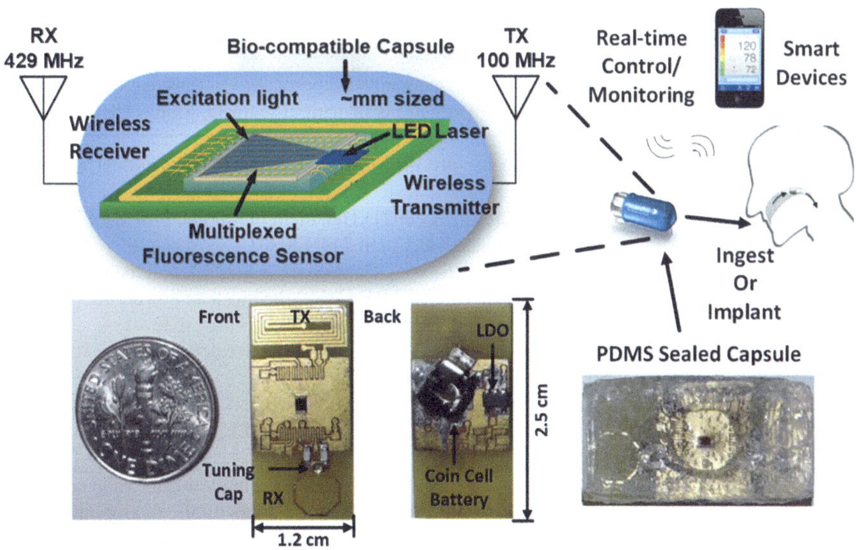

Fig. 5.6 A compact multiplexed fluorescent biomolecular sensor array with an ultra-efficient wireless interface in CMOS for swallowable electronic uses [12]

5.5 Summary

This chapter explores advancements in CMOS-based biosensors and flexible electronic technologies, emphasizing their potential in healthcare, environmental monitoring, and robotics through portable handheld devices, implantable biosensors, and wearable sensors. It also discusses integrating flexible sensors into robots and the "Body Dust" concept for in-body diagnostics, noting the importance of overcoming challenges like sensor miniaturization, energy efficiency, and ethical considerations for these technologies to reach their full potential.

While the applications covered in this chapter, such as healthcare monitoring, environmental sensing, and robotics, demonstrate the vast potential of CMOS biosensors, they represent just a fraction of the possibilities. The continued evolution of these technologies promises to unlock even more innovative applications, paving the way for a future where advanced sensing and monitoring are seamlessly integrated into everyday life. These technologies offer enhanced diagnostic accuracy, patient management, and personalized treatment through their portability, integration capabilities, and continuous monitoring features. However, to fully realize this potential, significant technological challenges such as sensor miniaturization, energy efficiency, and ethical considerations must be addressed. Continued research and development are essential to overcome these obstacles and achieve the promising advancements in medical diagnostics, environmental monitoring and other applications envisioned in this chapter.

References

1. Simion M, Cobzac S, Casoni D (2017) Image analysis approaches to improve the thin layer chromatography-chemometric-based investigations of natural extracts. Studia UBB Chemia, LXII 2:67–80
2. Mak P-I (2020) Lab-on-CMOS—An in-vitro diagnostic (IVD) tool for a healthier society. J Semicond 41(11):110301
3. Cetin AE, Kocer ZA, Topkaya SN, Yazici ZA (2021) Handheld plasmonic biosensor for virus detection in field-settings. Sensors Actuators B Chem 344:130301
4. Nguyen VD, Nguyen HQ, Bui KH, Ko YS, Park BJ, Seo TS (2022) A handheld-type total integrated capillary electrophoresis system for SARS-CoV-2 diagnostics: power, fluorescence detection, and data analysis by smartphone. Biosens Bioelectron 195:113632
5. Ryazantsev D et al (2024) A portable readout system for biomarker detection with Aptamer-modified CMOS ISFET Array. Sensors 24(10):3008
6. Bianchi V, Boni A, Fortunati S, Giannetto M, Careri M, De Munari I (2019) A Wi-Fi cloud-based portable potentiostat for electrochemical biosensors. IEEE Trans Instrum Meas 69(6):3232–3240
7. Ng DC et al (2008) An implantable and fully integrated complementary metal–oxide semiconductor device for in vivo neural imaging and electrical interfacing with the mouse hippocampus. Sensors Actuators A Phys 145:176–186
8. Angotzi GN et al (2019) SiNAPS: an implantable active pixel sensor CMOS-probe for simultaneous large-scale neural recordings. Biosens Bioelectron 126:355–364

9. De Lima JA (2020) A 0.55-V 0.1° C-Accuracy All-CMOS Temperature Sensor for Implanted Devices. In: *2020 33rd Symposium on Integrated Circuits and Systems Design (SBCCI)*. IEEE, pp 1–6
10. Sonmezoglu S, Maharbiz MM (2020) 34.4 A 4.5 mm 3 deep-tissue ultrasonic implantable luminescence oxygen sensor. In: *2020 IEEE International Solid-State Circuits Conference-(ISSCC)*. IEEE, pp 454–456
11. Moazeni S et al (2021) A mechanically flexible, implantable neural Interface for computational imaging and Optogenetic stimulation over 5.4 × 5.4 mm 2 FoV. IEEE Trans Biomed Circuits Syst 15(6):1295–1305
12. Zhu C, Hong L, Yang H, Sengupta K (2022) A packaged multiplexed fluorescent biomolecular sensor array and ultralow-power wireless interface in CMOS for ingestible electronic applications. IEEE Sensors J 22(24):24060–24074
13. Wang ML et al (2021) A wireless implantable potentiostat for programmable electrochemical drug delivery. In: *2021 IEEE biomedical circuits and systems conference (BioCAS)*. IEEE, pp 1–4
14. Lee C-E, Park J-H, Lim J, Choi C, Song Y-K (2024) A wireless stimulator system-on-chip with an optically writable ID for addressable cortical microimplants. Solid State Electron 216:108914
15. He Y et al (2022) An implantable neuromorphic sensing system featuring near-sensor computation and send-on-delta transmission for wireless neural sensing of peripheral nerves. IEEE J Solid State Circuits 57(10):3058–3070
16. Neshatvar N, Schormans M, Jiang D, Schmitt S, Detemple P, Demosthenous A (2022) An implantable phase locked loop MEMS-based readout system for heart transplantation. IEEE Trans Circuits Syst II: Express Briefs 69(10):4168–4172
17. Besirli M et al (2023) An implantable wireless system for remote hemodynamic monitoring of heart failure patients. IEEE Trans Biomed Circuits Syst 17(4):688–700
18. Shi C et al (2021) Application of a sub–0.1-mm3 implantable mote for in vivo real-time wireless temperature sensing. *Sci Adv* 7(19):eabf6312
19. Zhang Y, Muthuraman P, Andino-Pavlovsky V, Uguz I, Elloian J, Shepard KL (2022) Augmented ultrasonography with implanted CMOS electronic motes. Nat Commun 13(1):3521
20. Agnese F et al (2024) Characterization of IMIC, an implantable needle-shaped positron sensitive monolithic active pixel sensor for preclinical molecular neuroimaging. In: *Nuclear instruments and methods in physics research Section A: Accelerators, spectrometers, detectors and associated equipment*, p 169456
21. Wu C-Y et al (2020) Cmos 256-pixel/480-pixel photovoltaic-powered subretinal prosthetic chips with wide image dynamic range and bi/four-directional sharing electrodes and their ex vivo experimental validations with mice. IEEE Trans Circuits Syst I: Regular Papers 67(10):3273–3283
22. Aymerich J et al (2020) A 15-μW 105-dB 1.8-V pp Potentiostatic Delta-sigma modulator for wearable electrochemical transducers in 65-nm CMOS technology. IEEE Access 8:62127–62136
23. Lin Q et al (2020) A 119dB dynamic range charge counting light-to-digital converter for wearable PPG/NIRS monitoring applications. IEEE Trans Biomed Circuits Syst 14(4):800–810
24. Lin Q et al (2021) A 134 dB dynamic range noise shaping slope light-to-digital converter for wearable chest PPG applications. IEEE Trans Biomed Circuits Syst 15(6):1224–1235
25. Luo W, Sharma V, Young DJ (2020) A paper-based flexible tactile sensor array for low-cost wearable human health monitoring. J Microelectromech Syst 29(5):825–831
26. Cui Y et al (2024) A wearable bracelet for simultaneous monitoring of transcutaneous carbon dioxide and pulse rates. Adv Electron Mater 10:2300760
27. Hedayatipour A, Aslanzadeh S, Hesari SH, Haque MA, McFarlane N (2020) A wearable CMOS impedance to frequency sensing system for non-invasive impedance measurements. IEEE Trans Biomed Circuits Syst 14(5):1108–1121

28. Liu X et al (2022) A wearable fiber-free optical sensor for continuous monitoring of cerebral blood flow in freely behaving mice. IEEE Trans Biomed Eng
29. Choi J, Shin J, Kang D, Park D-S (2015) Always-on CMOS image sensor for mobile and wearable devices. IEEE J Solid State Circuits 51(1):130–140
30. Costanzo I, Sen D, Guler U (2020) An integrated readout circuit for a transcutaneous oxygen sensing wearable device. In: *2020 IEEE Custom Integrated Circuits Conference (CICC)*. IEEE, pp 1–4
31. Conca E et al (2020) Large-area, fast-gated digital SiPM with integrated TDC for portable and wearable time-domain NIRS. IEEE J Solid State Circuits 55(11):3097–3111
32. Singh W, Deb S, Bahubalindruni P (2020) Low-noise energy efficient readout front-end for wearable continuous blood pressure monitoring systems. IEEE Trans Consum Electron 66(4):318–326
33. Lin B, Ma Z, Atef M, Ying L, Wang G (2021) Low-power high-sensitivity photoplethysmography sensor for wearable health monitoring system. IEEE Sensors J 21(14):16141–16151
34. Wuthibenjaphonchai N, Haruta M, Sasagawa K, Tokuda T, Carrara S, Ohta J (2021) Wearable and battery-free health-monitoring devices with optical power transfer. IEEE Sensors J 21(7):9402–9412
35. Ruppert C, Phogat N, Laufer S, Kohl M, Deigner H-P (2019) A smartphone readout system for gold nanoparticle-based lateral flow assays: application to monitoring of digoxigenin. Microchim Acta 186:1–9
36. Rohit A, Kaya S (2021) A systematic study of wearable multi-modal capacitive textile patches. IEEE Sensors J 21(23):26215–26225
37. Kim MS et al (2024) Accessorizing quadrupedal robots with wearable electronics. Adv Intell Syst 6:2300633
38. Bunea A-C et al (2021) E-skin: the dawn of a new era of on-body monitoring systems. Micromachines 12(9):1091
39. Torres Sevilla GA, Qaiser N, Cordero MD, Shaikh SF, Hussain MM (2018) Fully spherical stretchable silicon photodiodes array for simultaneous 360 imaging. Appl Phys Lett 113(13)
40. Wu YL, Fukuda K, Yokota T, Someya T (2019) A highly responsive organic image sensor based on a two-terminal organic photodetector with photomultiplication. Adv Mater 31(43):1903687
41. Yuan Z et al (2020) Trace-level, multi-gas detection for food quality assessment based on decorated silicon transistor arrays. Adv Mater 32(21):1908385
42. Shaikh SF et al (2019) Noninvasive featherlight wearable compliant "marine skin": standalone multisensory system for deep-sea environmental monitoring. Small 15(10):1804385
43. Picardi G, Chellapurath M, Iacoponi S, Stefanni S, Laschi C, Calisti M (2020) Bioinspired underwater legged robot for seabed exploration with low environmental disturbance. Sci Robot 5(42):eaaz1012
44. Karimi MA et al (2019) Flexible tag design for semi-continuous wireless data acquisition from marine animals. Flex Print Electron 4(3):035006
45. Seo D-H, Chatterjee B, Scott S, Valentino D, Peroulis D, Sen S (2020) A wearable cmos biosensor with 3 designs of energy-resolution scalable time-based resistance to digital converter. arXiv preprint arXiv:2011.00649.
46. Silverio AA (2021) Design of a wide temperature range, high linearity time domain CMOS-based temperature sensor for wearable IOT applications. In: *2021 2nd International Conference on Innovative and Creative Information Technology (ICITech)*. IEEE, pp 226–230
47. Yu C et al (2023) High-performance multifunctional piezoresistive/piezoelectric pressure sensor with thermochromic function for wearable monitoring. Chem Eng J 459:141648
48. Kim S-W, Lee K, Yeom J, Lee T-H, Kim D-H, Kim JJ (2020) Wearable multi-biosignal analysis integrated interface with direct sleep-stage classification. IEEE Access 8:46131–46140
49. Khayatzadeh M, Zhang X, Tan J, Liew W-S, Lian Y (2013) A 0.7-v 17.4-/spl mu/w 3-lead wireless ecg soc. IEEE Trans Biomed Circuits Syst 7(5):583–592
50. Chen C-Y et al (2013) A low-power bio-potential acquisition system with flexible PDMS dry electrodes for portable ubiquitous healthcare applications. Sensors 13(3):3077–3091

51. Lin B-S, Chou W, Wang H-Y, Huang Y-J, Pan J-S (2013) Development of novel non-contact electrodes for mobile electrocardiogram monitoring system. IEEE J Transl Eng Health Med 1:1–8
52. Miao F, Cheng Y, He Y, He Q, Li Y (2015) A wearable context-aware ECG monitoring system integrated with built-in kinematic sensors of the smartphone. Sensors 15(5):11465–11484
53. Jain SK, Bhaumik B (2016) An energy efficient ECG signal processor detecting cardiovascular diseases on smartphone. IEEE Trans Biomed Circuits Syst 11(2):314–323
54. Zhang X, Zhang Z, Li Y, Liu C, Guo YX, Lian Y (2015) A 2.89-μW clockless wireless dry-electrode ECG SoC for wearable sensors. In: *2015 IEEE Asian Solid-State Circuits Conference (A-SSCC)*. IEEE, pp 1–4
55. Sun F, Yi C, Li W, Li Y (2017) A wearable H-shirt for exercise ECG monitoring and individual lactate threshold computing. Comput Ind 92:1–11
56. Wang T-Y, Lai M-R, Twigg CM, Peng S-Y (2013) A fully reconfigurable low-noise biopotential sensing amplifier with 1.96 noise efficiency factor. IEEE Trans Biomed Circuits Syst 8(3):411–422
57. Tseng KC, Lin B-S, Liao L-D, Wang Y-T, Wang Y-L (2013) Development of a wearable mobile electrocardiogram monitoring system by using novel dry foam electrodes. IEEE Syst J 8(3):900–906
58. Wang Y, Doleschel S, Wunderlich R, Heinen S (2015) A wearable wireless ECG monitoring system with dynamic transmission power control for long-term homecare. J Med Syst 39:1–10
59. Lin H-Y, Liang S-Y, Ho Y-L, Lin Y-H, Ma H-P (2014) Discrete-wavelet-transform-based noise removal and feature extraction for ECG signals. Irbm 35(6):351–361
60. Winokur ES, Delano MK, Sodini CG (2012) A wearable cardiac monitor for long-term data acquisition and analysis. IEEE Trans Biomed Eng 60(1):189–192
61. Singh M, Singh G, Singh J, Kumar Y (2021) Design and validation of wearable smartphone based wireless cardiac activity monitoring sensor. Wirel Pers Commun 119(1):441–457
62. Laababid Y, El Khadiri K, Tahiri A (2022) Design of a low-Power low-Noise ECG amplifier for smart wearable devices using 180nm CMOS technology. WSEAS Trans Power Syst 17:177–186
63. Wang Y, Miao F, An Q, Liu Z, Chen C, Li Y (2022) Wearable multimodal vital sign monitoring sensor with fully integrated analog front end. IEEE Sensors J 22(13):13462–13471
64. Ng DC et al (2006) Pulse frequency modulation based CMOS image sensor for subretinal stimulation. IEEE Trans Circuits Syst II: Express Briefs 53(6):487–491
65. Ohta J et al (2006) Silicon LSI-based smart stimulators for retinal prosthesis. IEEE Eng Med Biol Mag 25(5):47–59
66. Perna A, Angotzi GN, Berdondini L, Ribeiro JF (2023) Advancing the interfacing performances of chronically implantable neural probes in the era of CMOS neuroelectronics. Front Neurosci 17:1275908
67. Takacs J, Pollock CL, Guenther JR, Bahar M, Napier C, Hunt MA (2014) Validation of the Fitbit one activity monitor device during treadmill walking. J Sci Med Sport 17(5):496–500
68. Weinstein RL, Schwartz SL, Brazg RL, Bugler JR, Peyser TA, McGarraugh GV (2007) Accuracy of the 5-day FreeStyle navigator continuous glucose monitoring system: comparison with frequent laboratory reference measurements. Diabetes Care 30(5):1125–1130
69. Sanders P et al (2016) Performance of a new atrial fibrillation detection algorithm in a miniaturized insertable cardiac monitor: results from the reveal LINQ usability study. Heart Rhythm 13(7):1425–1430
70. Jia W et al (2013) Electrochemical tattoo biosensors for real-time noninvasive lactate monitoring in human perspiration. Anal Chem 85(14):6553–6560
71. Mehmeti E, Kilic T, Laur C, Carrara S (2020) Electrochemical determination of nicotine in smokers' sweat. Microchem J 158:105155
72. Wujcik EK, Blasdel NJ, Trowbridge D, Monty CN (2013) Ion sensor for the quantification of sodium in sweat samples. IEEE Sensors J 13(9):3430–3436

73. Kahn JM, Katz RH, Pister KS (1999) Next century challenges: mobile networking for "Smart Dust". In: *Proceedings of the 5th annual ACM/IEEE international conference on Mobile computing and networking*, pp 271–278
74. Warneke B, Last M, Liebowitz B, Pister KS (2001) Smart dust: communicating with a cubic-millimeter computer. Computer 34(1):44–51
75. Cook BW, Lanzisera S, Pister KS (2006) SoC issues for RF smart dust. Proc IEEE 94(6):1177–1196
76. Carrara S (2020) Body dust: well beyond wearable and implantable sensors. IEEE Sensors J 21(11):12398–12406
77. Kahn JM, Katz RH, Pister KS (2000) Emerging challenges: mobile networking for "smart dust". J Commun Net 2(3):188–196
78. Seo D, Carmena JM, Rabaey JM, Alon E, Maharbiz MM (2013) Neural dust: an ultrasonic, low power solution for chronic brain-machine interfaces. arXiv preprint arXiv:1307.2196
79. Carrara S, Georgiou P(2018) Body dust: miniaturized highly-integrated low power sensing for remotely powered drinkable CMOS bioelectronics. arXiv preprint arXiv:1805.05840
80. Seo D et al (2016) Wireless recording in the peripheral nervous system with ultrasonic neural dust. Neuron 91(3):529–539
81. Sathyan S, Pulari SR (2018) A deeper insight on developments and real-time applications of smart dust particle sensor technology. In: Computational vision and bio inspired computing. Springer, pp 193–204
82. Piech DK et al. (2018) StimDust: a mm-scale implantablewireless precision neural stimulator with ultrasonic power and communication. arXiv preprint arXiv:1807.07590
83. Charthad J, Weber MJ, Chang TC, Arbabian A (2015) A mm-sized implantable medical device (IMD) with ultrasonic power transfer and a hybrid bi-directional data link. IEEE J Solid State Circuits 50(8):1741–1753
84. Meng M, Kiani M (2016) Design and optimization of ultrasonic wireless power transmission links for millimeter-sized biomedical implants. IEEE Trans Biomed Circuits Syst 11(1):98–107
85. Rothe J, Frey O, Stettler A, Chen Y, Hierlemann A (2014) Fully integrated CMOS microsystem for electrochemical measurements on 32× 32 working electrodes at 90 frames per second. Anal Chem 86(13):6425–6432
86. Hayashi K, Arata S, Murakami S, Nishio Y, Kobayashi A, Niitsu K (2018) A 6.1-nA fully integrated CMOS supply modulated OOK transmitter in 55-nm DDC CMOS for glasses-free, self-powered, and fuel-cell-embedded continuous glucose monitoring contact lens. IEEE Trans Circuits Syst II: Express Briefs 65(10):1360–1364
87. Bermudez LE, Sangari FJ (2001) Cellular and molecular mechanisms of internalization of mycobacteria by host cells. Microbes Infect 3(1):37–42
88. Brackett DG et al (2020) Cholangiolar pattern and albumin in situ hybridisation enable a diagnosis of intrahepatic cholangiocarcinoma. J Clin Pathol 73(1):23–29
89. Wang A et al (2019) Diagnostic value of negative enrichment and immune fluorescence in situ hybridization for intraperitoneal free cancer cells of gastric cancer. Chin J Cancer Res 31(6):945–954
90. Blair E et al (2020) Test structures for developing packaging for implantable sensors. IEEE Trans Semicond Manuf 33(2):224–231
91. Manara MC, Pasello M, Scotlandi K (2018) CD99: a cell surface protein with an oncojanus role in tumors. Genes 9(3):159
92. Berglund J (2018) Technology you can swallow: moving beyond wearable sensors, researchers are creating ingestible ones. IEEE Pulse 9(1):15–18

Chapter 6
State-of -Art CMOS Biochip Technologies and Future Opportunities

This chapter provides an overview of recent advancements in CMOS sensing chips, highlighting their commercialization for various applications. The discussions emphasize the ongoing progress in CMOS sensor technology and its increasing relevance in life sciences, setting the stage for future innovations and applications. Related discussions are detailed in Sect. 6.2 of this chapter.

6.1 Recent Advances and Commercially Available CMOS Sensing Chips for Life Science Applications

The CMOS sensing chips highlight the technology's versatility and impact on life science applications, offering advanced capabilities in DNA sequencing [1], cell monitoring [2], electrochemical sensing [3] (Fig. 6.1). Their availability underscores the ongoing innovation and growing accessibility of CMOS-based solutions in both research and clinical environments. A landmark CMOS sensing chip from Ion Torrent has recently been commercialized for high-throughput DNA sequencing, as shown in Fig. 6.1a. In another example, an integrated CMOS chip for electrochemical sensing is shown in Fig. 6.1b. Although this chip is designed for electrochemical sensing and does not include integrated sensors, its on-chip electrochemical system has been commercialized for developing portable devices. Fig. 6.1c demonstrates an array of 256 integrated capacitive sensors. A more focused image of the interdigitated electrodes on the CMOS chip can also be seen in this figure.

Additionally, many other CMOS integrated sensors have been launched, featuring either integrated or off-chip sensors. This generation of CMOS chips has expanded its applications into various fields of life sciences.

E. Ghafar-Zadeh et al., *Advanced CMOS Biochips*, Analog Circuits and Signal Processing, https://doi.org/10.1007/978-94-007-0099-4_6

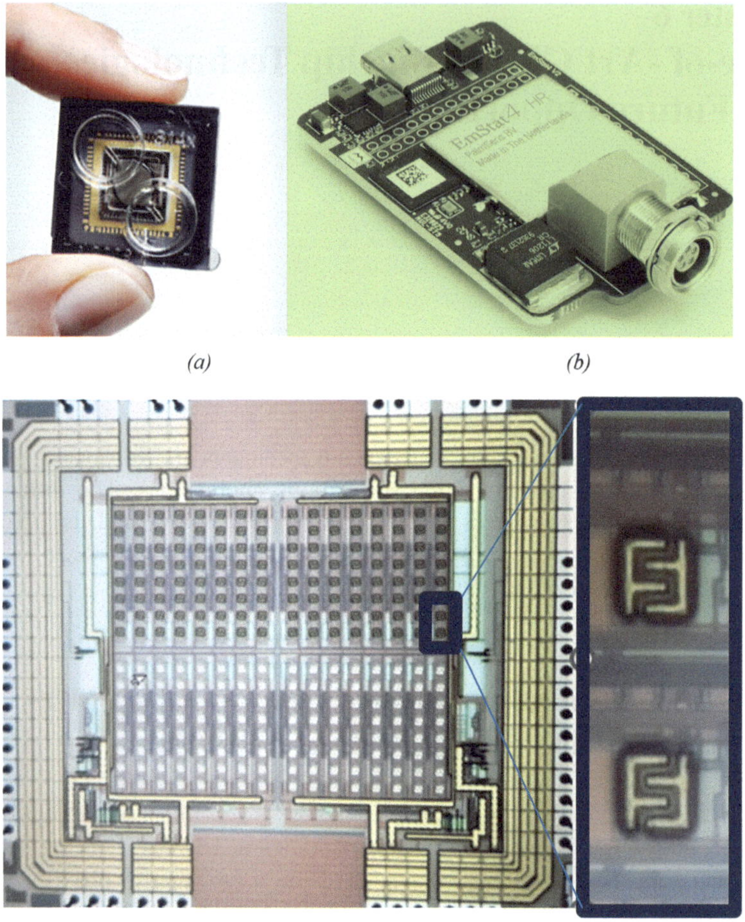

(c)

Fig. 6.1 CMOS Sensing Chips (**a**) DNA Sequencing Chip from Ion Torrent: CMOS-based chip utilizing ion-sensitive field-effect transistor (ISFET) technology for high-throughput DNA sequencing, (**b**) Electrochemical Sensing Devices Commercialized by National Instruments and PalmSense: Devices integrating CMOS technology for advanced electrochemical sensing applications, (**c**). (**b**) CMOS Capacitive Sensor Array: Array of CMOS capacitive sensors designed for high-resolution monitoring of cellular and biological samples

6.2 Future Works

CMOS sensors offer distinct advantages in various applications, providing high precision and low-cost sensing capabilities. Future improvements in this technology can be explored through several directions, as briefly described below:

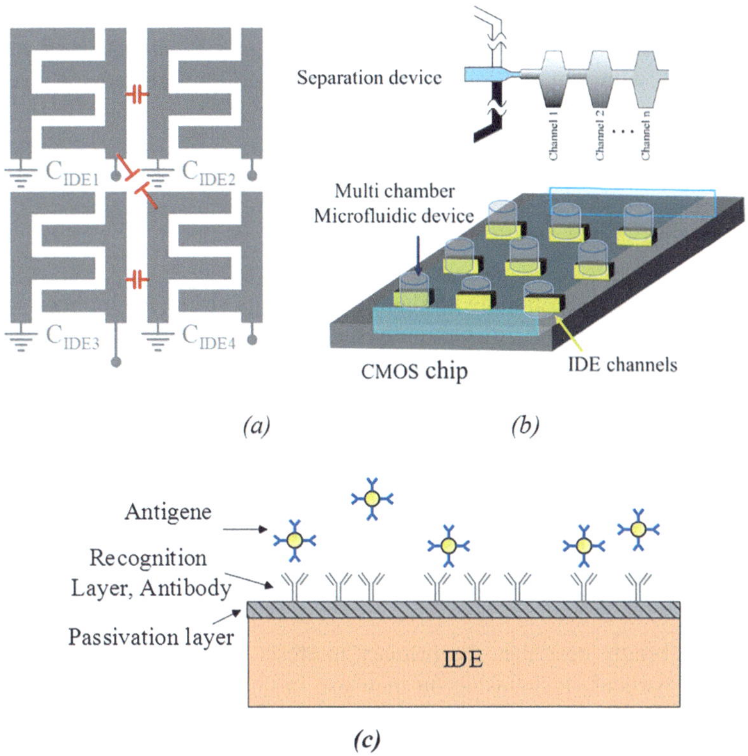

Fig. 6.2 Illustration of some future improvements of CMOS sensors: (**a**) Large sensor array, (**b**) Integrated microfluidic sensing chip, and (**c**) Selective material coating on chip

6.2.1 Highly Dense (HD) Sensing Elements

Similar to CMOS imagers, other types of sensors are advancing towards high-density (HD) sensing technologies. For instance, increasing the number of capacitive sensors on a chip allows for more extensive coverage of biological or chemical materials with minimal dead space between sensors. Figure 6.2a illustrates an array of integrated device electronics (IDEs). In designing capacitive sensors, not only should the capacitance sensing capability of each element be studied, but minimizing the cost and space between sensors is also crucial.

6.2.2 Integrated Microfluidic CMOS

Microfluidic technology is essential for CMOS sensor packaging, as it prevents direct contact between the sample and the entire chip except for the sensing area. Microfluidic devices are integrated with CMOS chips to facilitate sample preparation, such as cell separation. Despite progress, the development of sensor arrays combined with microfluidic channels capable of generating a large number of microarrays with comprehensive monitoring capabilities remains a challenge (see Fig. 6.2b).

6.2.3 Recognition Elements

Another challenge is developing recognition elements (REs) for highly selective sensing purposes (see Fig. 6.2c). Currently, methods include antibody attachment to CMOS sensors, where antibodies are used for detecting specific antigens. REs can range from antibodies to DNA with certain genetic information or other materials that can bind to target molecules. Future work includes developing new REs for a broader range of diseases or chemical monitoring applications.

6.3 Summery

This chapter briefly describes the primary interests in CMOS chips for various applications, particularly focusing on their use in diagnostic and life sciences. It also addresses the main challenges associated with utilizing CMOS technology for future disease diagnostics. In addition to these challenges, the chapter highlights additional obstacles related to the design, fabrication, characterization, and commercialization of CMOS sensors.

References

1. Rothberg JM, Hinz W, Rearick TM, Schultz J, Mileski W, Davey M et al (2011) An integrated semiconductor device enabling non-optical genome sequencing. Nature 475:348–352
2. Osouli Tabrizi H, Forouhi S, Azadmousavi T, Ghafar-Zadeh E (2024) A multidisciplinary approach toward CMOS capacitive sensor Array for droplet analysis. Micromachines 15:232
3. Jung HS, Jung W-B, Wang J, Abbott J, Horgan A, Fournier M et al (2022) CMOS electrochemical pH localizer-imager. Sci Adv 8:eabm6815

Appendix A

This appendix provides detailed software developed as a graphical user interface (GUI) and the program for the microcontroller used for the designed CMOS capacitive sensors (See Sect. 2, Design Strategy). The detailed programs and explanations offer practical guidance on developing the interface system for researchers interested in the design of CMOS-integrated sensors in particular CMOS capacitive sensors [1].

Graphical User Interface

The microcontroller and GUI communicate through four simple commands initiated via the serial port by sending 'S', 'G', 'W', and 'R' for setting the number of samples, CCO configuration, CR value, and receiving data from the SPI port, respectively.

'S'	After sending 'S', the GUI specifies the number of samples, indicating how many times the same measurement should be repeated to enhance accuracy and reduce noise.
'G'	Following 'G', the GUI sends one of the preset strings (000, 001, 011, or 111). The inherent frequency of the oscillator is at its maximum when the input is 000 and at its minimum when the input is 111. The order of the bits in these strings does not affect the outcome.
'W'	After sending 'W', a 7-bit or 8-bit string of ones and zeros is transmitted to set the value in the shift register of the capacitor bank for the left and right blocks, respectively.
'R'	The microcontroller reads the data received from the SPI port's receive buffer. The corresponding code is provided below with comments.

E. Ghafar-Zadeh et al., *Advanced CMOS Biochips*, Analog Circuits and Signal Processing, https://doi.org/10.1007/978-94-007-0099-4

Part 1: Introduction and Setup

```
// Appendix: Microcontroller Program for CMOS
Capacitive Sensors
/*
This program handles communication between a microcontroller
and a graphical user interface (GUI) via serial commands.It
enables control of a CMOS capacitive sensor system by
allowing the user to set parameters (e.g., the number of
samples, oscillator frequency, and CR values) and retrieve
data from the SPI port. The microcontroller responds to
specific commands (S, G, W, R) and outputs data to the
GUI. In this part, the serial communication is initialized,
and the digital pins required for the oscillation frequency
and capacitor bank control are set up.
*/
void setup() {
  // Setup serial communication and configure digital pins
  Serial.begin(9600);           // Initialize serial
communication at 9600 baud
  for (int i = 48; i <= 52; i += 2) {
    pinMode(i, OUTPUT);         // Set pins 48, 50, and 52 as
output (for oscillation frequency control)
  }
  pinMode(46, OUTPUT);          // Set pin 46 as output (for
capacitor bank control)}
```

Part 2: Main Loop and Sample Configuration

```
// // The main loop continuously listens for incoming serial
data from the GUI.
// Depending on the command received (S, G, W, or R), the
appropriate action is taken.
// In this part, the 'S' command sets the number of samples
for measurement.
// It reads the number of samples from the serial input and
converts it to an integer.
// The program confirms the input by sending the number of
samples back to the GUI.
```

(continued)

```
void loop() {
  char calin_i[8];              // Array to hold input values
for CR setting
  char calin_g[3];              // Array to hold input values
for oscillator frequency setting
  if (Serial.available() > 0) // Check if serial data is
available
  {
    char cmd = Serial.read(); // Read the serial command
character

    switch (cmd)
    {
      case 'S': // Set the number of samples for measurement
      {
        String N_sample_s = Serial.readStringUntil('\0'); //
Read the number of samples until null character ('\0')
        int N_sample = N_sample_s.toInt(); // Convert the
received string to an integer
        Serial.print(N_sample);             // Print the
number of samples to confirm
        Serial.print(TERMINATION_CHAR);     // Append
termination character for the GUI
        break;
```

Part 3: Oscillator and CR Value Configuration

```
// In this part, two different commands are handled:
// 1. 'G' configures the oscillator frequency by reading a
3-digit input string and setting the digital pins
accordingly.
//    The program reads each digit and either sets the pin
HIGH or LOW based on whether the digit is '1' or '0'.
// 2. 'W' configures the capacitor bank (CR values) using an
8-bit input string. The last bit determines which block of
//    the capacitor bank to control, and the inputSig
function applies the configuration. Each command is
confirmed by
//    printing the received configuration back to the GUI.
```

(continued)

```
      case 'G': // Set the oscillator frequency based on the
received string
      {
        for (int i = 0; i < 3; )
        {
          if (Serial.available() > 0)
          {
            calin_g[i] = Serial.read();       // Read each
digit of the 3-digit configuration string
            if (calin_g[i] == '1')
              digitalWrite(48 + 2*i, HIGH);  // Set
corresponding pin HIGH if '1'
            else
              digitalWrite(48 + 2*i, LOW);   // Set
corresponding pin LOW if '0'
            i++;
          }
        }
        calin_g[3] = '\0'; // Null-terminate the string for
printing
        Serial.print(calin_g);               // Print the
oscillator configuration to confirm
        Serial.print(TERMINATION_CHAR);      // Append
termination character for the GUI
        break;
      }
      case 'W': // Set the CR value by writing to the shift
register
      {
        for (int i = 0; i <= 7; )
        {
          if (Serial.available() > 0)
          {
            calin_i[i] = Serial.read(); // Read the 8-bit
configuration string
            i++;
          }
        }
        if (calin_i[7] == ' ') // Determine if the last bit
is a space (indicating left or right block)
        {
          digitalWrite(46, LOW); // Set pin 46 LOW for the
left block
```

(continued)

```
        }
        else
        {
          digitalWrite(46, HIGH); // Set pin 46 HIGH for the
right block
        }
        inputSig(calin_i);            // Apply the received
configuration via the inputSig function
        calin_i[8] = '\0';            // Null-terminate the
string for printing
        Serial.print(calin_i);        // Print the CR
configuration to confirm
        Serial.print(TERMINATION_CHAR); // Append
termination character for the GUI
        break;
      }
```

Part 4: Data Retrieval and Default Command Handling

```
// This part handles two scenarios:
// 1. The 'R' command retrieves data from the SPI port. The
program checks if data is available in the SPI receive buffer
//    and reads it into a buffer. The buffer is then formatted
as a string and sent back to the GUI for further analysis.
// 2. Any unrecognized commands are handled by printing a
default message ("Meow") to the GUI, allowing users to
identify
//    when an unsupported command is issued.
      case 'R': // Read data from the SPI port and send it
back to the GUI
      {
        int buf[N_sample]; // Buffer to store the read data
        for (int i = 0; i < N_sample; )
        {
          if (REG_SPI0_SR & 1)        // Check if data is
available in the SPI receive buffer
          {
            buf[i] = REG_SPI0_RDR;    // Read data from the
SPI port
            i++;
          }
```

(continued)

```
        }
        // Convert the buffer data to a string for serial
transmission
        char bufferr[4*N_sample+N_sample];
        int n = 0;
        for (int i = 0; i < N_sample; i++) {
            n += sprintf(&bufferr[n], "%04d,", buf[i]); //
Format the data as a string
        }
        bufferr[4*N_sample+N_sample-1] = '\0'; // Null-
terminate the string

        Serial.print(bufferr);                  // Send the
formatted data string to the GUI
        Serial.print(TERMINATION_CHAR);          // Append
termination character for the GUI
        break;
      }
      default: // Handle unknown commands
      {
        Serial.print("Meow");                    // Print a
default message for unknown commands
        Serial.print(TERMINATION_CHAR);          // Append
termination character for the GUI
        break;
      }  }}
```

Part 5: Function

```
// Function to apply the input signal configuration to the
capacitors (assumed to be implemented elsewhere)
void inputSig(char* calin_i) {
  // Implementation depends on specific hardware setup}
```

Microcontroller Design

The test bench utilizes an Arduino DUE development board. Commands are unified into a 23-bit integer array, structured as follows:

- **[0] UorD**: Determines if the up circuit (0) or down circuit (1) is measuring.
- **[1] NS{0}**: First digit of the number of samples (0-999).

- **[2] NS{1}**: Second digit of the number of samples (0-999).
- **[3] NS{2}**: Third digit of the number of samples (0-999).
- **[4] G**: IDE selection multiplexer value.
- **[5] F**: IDE selection multiplexer value.
- **[6] E**: IDE selection multiplexer value.
- **[7] D**: IDE selection multiplexer value.
- **[8] C**: IDE selection multiplexer value.
- **[9] B**: IDE selection multiplexer value.
- **[10] A**: IDE selection multiplexer value.
- **[11] ca10**: 10-bit capacitor bank value (11).
- **[12] ca9**: 10-bit capacitor bank value (12).
- **[13] ca8**: 10-bit capacitor bank value (13).
- **[14] ca7**: 10-bit capacitor bank value (14).
- **[15] ca6**: 10-bit capacitor bank value (15).
- **[16] ca5**: 10-bit capacitor bank value (16).
- **[17] ca4**: 10-bit capacitor bank value (17).
- **[18] ca3**: 10-bit capacitor bank value (18).
- **[19] ca2**: 10-bit capacitor bank value (19).
- **[20] ca1**: 10-bit capacitor bank value (20).
- **[21] Cs**: Controls the two transmission gates on R1C1 and R16C1 IDEs.
- **[22] Mode**: ASCII code for measurement mode; 'S' for sweep mode or 'R' for fixed reference.

- **MCU Flowchart and Operation**

Serial Communication	Establish a serial communication port between the MCU and the PC.
Command Decoding	Decode the received command from the GUI.
Configuration	Set the number of samples, Configure the measurement mode., Adjust multiplexers based on the decoded command.
Measurement	Perform the measurement based on the configured settings.
Data Transmission	Send the measured data to the GUI via the SPI port.

Refer to Fig. A.1 for the detailed MCU flowchart and operation process.

Note: The code modules for setting the capacitor bank, number of samples, and SPI communication are the same as those used in the non-array test bench. Below is the code with explanatory comments.

- **Pin Definitions and Initialization:**
    - The code defines several digital pins for controlling different circuits and inputs.
    - PWM is configured for three different channels with specific periods and duty cycles.
    - SPI communication is initialized with specific settings for mode and bit width.

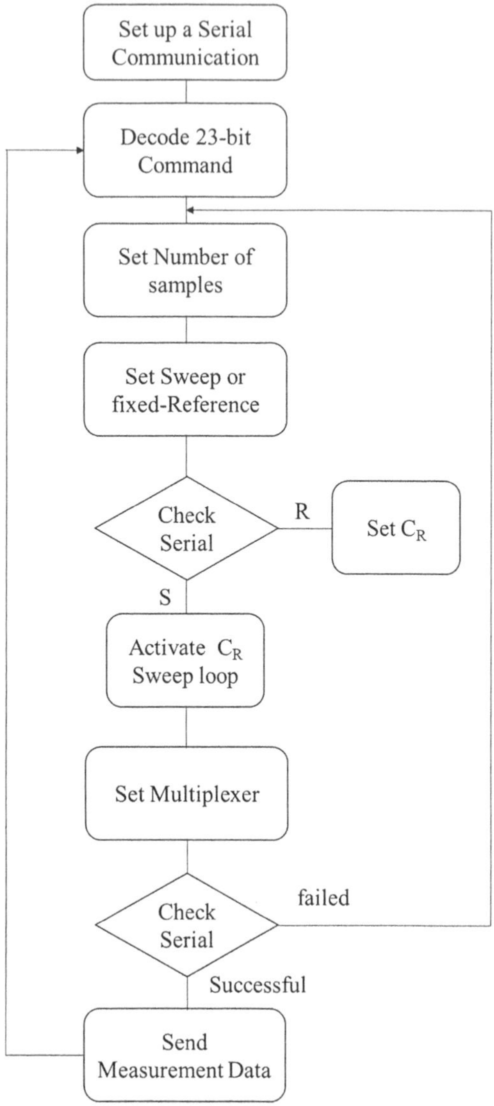

Fig. A.1 Flowchart of the MCU code for the array test bench

- **Setup Function:**
  - Serial communication is initialized.
  - Pins are set to the correct modes (input or output).
  - PWM and SPI peripherals are configured.
- **Loop Function:**
  - Reads a command from the serial input.

- Depending on the command, it configures and controls either the "Upper" or "Lower" circuit, including setting various pins high or low.
- The input sequence is applied through SPI and PWM, and the SPI communication is used to read data samples.

- **Error Handling:**
  - The code includes error checking for invalid command values and prints error codes to the serial monitor if something is wrong.
- **Data Reading:**
  - After configuring the circuit, it reads N_sample data points from the SPI device.
- Here's a summary of key components and functions:
- **Pin Definitions:**
  - Defines pins for both upper and lower circuits.
  - Sets up PWM channels for controlling clock signals.
- **Setup:**
  - Initializes serial communication.
  - Configures pins for the SPI and PWM operations.
  - Disables and re-enables the PWM channels.
- **Loop:**
  - Parses commands received via serial communication.
  - Configures either the upper or lower circuit based on the command.
  - Uses SPI to read data samples.

To use this code, one can follow these steps:

- Ensure Formatting: Make sure the code is properly formatted. If using a document editor, you might want to use a monospaced font like Courier New to preserve indentation.
- Add an Introduction: Briefly explain what this code does and its relevance. For example:

Part 1: Definitions and Global Variables

```
// Define constant characters and integers
const char TERMINATION_CHAR = '#';  // Character used to
denote the end of a command
const char OPERATION_DONE = '-';    // Character indicating
the completion of an operation
```

(continued)

```
const int MASK = 0x800;              // Mask used for bit
manipulation
int data;                            // Variable to store data
read from SPI
int satCounter = 0;                  // Counts the number of
times the output sums are mistakenly saturated
String command;                      // Stores the received
command from serial input
short result = 0;                    // Variable to store
result of operations
int N_sample = 10;                   // Number of samples to
be processed

// Pin definitions
#define SIN_U 22
#define SCLK_U 24
#define E_U 26
#define F_U 28
#define G_U 30
#define CA10_U 32
#define SEL_NOUT 40
#define SEL_PHI 42
#define SIN_D 44
#define SCLK_D 46
#define E_D 48
#define F_D 50
#define G_D 52
#define A_U 25
#define B_U 27
#define C_U 29
#define D_U 31
#define CA10_D 33
#define A_D 47
#define B_D 49
#define C_D 51
#define D_D 53
```

- **Constant Definitions:** The code defines constants to manage specific characters and values used in operations. TERMINATION_CHAR indicates the end of a command, while OPERATION_DONE signifies completion. MASK is used for bit manipulation.

- **Global Variables:** Variables are declared for storing data (data), counting saturation events (satCounter), storing commands (command), results of operations (result), and the number of samples (N_sample).
- **Pin Definitions:** Defines the pin numbers for various functions. This section assigns pin numbers to different functions and devices, including those for upper and lower circuits.

Part 2: Setup Function

```
void setup() {
  // Initialize serial communication
  Serial.begin(115200);

  // Set pin modes for Upper Circuit
  pinMode(SIN_U, OUTPUT);
  pinMode(SCLK_U, OUTPUT);
  digitalWrite(SCLK_U, LOW);
  pinMode(E_U, OUTPUT);
  pinMode(F_U, OUTPUT);
  pinMode(G_U, OUTPUT);
  pinMode(CA10_U, INPUT);
  pinMode(SEL_NOUT, OUTPUT);
  pinMode(SEL_PHI, OUTPUT);

  // Set pin modes for Lower Circuit
  pinMode(SIN_D, OUTPUT);
  pinMode(SCLK_D, OUTPUT);
  digitalWrite(SCLK_D, LOW);
  pinMode(E_D, OUTPUT);
  pinMode(F_D, OUTPUT);
  pinMode(G_D, OUTPUT);
  pinMode(A_U, OUTPUT);
  pinMode(B_U, OUTPUT);
  pinMode(C_U, OUTPUT);
  pinMode(D_U, OUTPUT);
  pinMode(CA10_D, INPUT);
  pinMode(A_D, OUTPUT);
  pinMode(B_D, OUTPUT);
  pinMode(C_D, OUTPUT);
  pinMode(D_D, OUTPUT);
```

(continued)

```
  delay(10); // Short delay for hardware stabilization

  // Configure PWM settings
  REG_PMC_PCER1 |= PMC_PCER1_PID36; // Power up PWM clock
  REG_PWM_WPCR = PWM_WPCR_WPCMD(0); // Unlock PWM user
interface
  REG_PWM_CLK = PWM_CLK_PREA(0) | PWM_CLK_DIVA(21); //
Configure PWM clock: clock A, 84/21 = 4MHz
  REG_PWM_SCM = PWM_SCM_SYNC0 | PWM_SCM_SYNC1; // Synchronize
phi1 and phi2 for same frequency

  // Configure phi1 for PWM output
  REG_PIOC_ABSR |= PIO_ABSR_P2; // Set pin PC2 for PWM
  REG_PIOC_PDR |= PIO_PDR_P2;   // Set PWM pin to an output
  REG_PWM_CMR0 = PWM_CMR_CPRE_CLKA | PWM_CMR_CPOL; // Mode
config for channel 0: clock A, left aligned, high start
  REG_PWM_CPRD0 = PWM_CPRD_CPRD(60); // PWM period
configuration
  REG_PWM_CDTY0 = PWM_CDTY_CDTY(16); // 80/3% duty cycle
  REG_PWM_ENA = PWM_ENA_CHID0; // Enable PWM channel 0

  // Configure phi1 inverted (NSS for SPI)
  REG_PIOC_ABSR |= PIO_ABSR_P3; // Set pin PC3 for PWM
  REG_PIOC_PDR |= PIO_PDR_P3;   // Set PWM pin to an output

  // Configure phi2 for PWM output
  REG_PIOC_ABSR |= PIO_ABSR_P4; // Set pin PC4 for PWM
  REG_PIOC_PDR |= PIO_PDR_P4;   // Set PWM pin to an output
  REG_PWM_CMR1 = PWM_CMR_CPRE_CLKA | PWM_CMR_DTE | PWM_CMR_
CPOL; // Mode config for channel 1: clock A, left aligned,
with dead-time generator
  REG_PWM_CPRD1 = PWM_CPRD_CPRD(60); // PWM period
configuration
  REG_PWM_DT1 = PWM_DT_DTL(4); // Dead-time configuration
(1µs delay)
  REG_PWM_CDTY1 = PWM_CDTY_CDTY(12); // 80/6% duty cycle
  REG_PWM_ENA = PWM_ENA_CHID1; // Enable PWM channel 1

  // Configure phi3 for PWM output
  REG_PIOC_ABSR |= PIO_ABSR_P6; // Set pin PC6 for PWM
  REG_PIOC_PDR |= PIO_PDR_P6;   // Set PWM pin to an output
  REG_PWM_CMR2 = PWM_CMR_CPRE_CLKA | PWM_CMR_CPOL; // Mode
```

(continued)

```
config for channel 2: clock A, left aligned, low start
  REG_PWM_CPRD2 = PWM_CPRD_CPRD(3); // PWM period
configuration
  REG_PWM_CDTY2 = PWM_CDTY_CDTY(2); // 50% duty cycle
  REG_PWM_ENA = PWM_ENA_CHID2; // Enable PWM channel 2

  // Configure SPI settings
  REG_PMC_PCER0 |= PMC_PCER0_PID24; // Power up SPI clock
  REG_SPI0_WPMR = 0 << SPI_WPMR_WPEN; // Unlock SPI user
interface
  // Configure SPI0: MISO: PA25, MOSI: PA26, SCLK: PA27,
NSS: PA28
  REG_PIOA_ABSR |= PIO_ABSR_P25; // Set pin PA25 for SPI
  REG_PIOA_PDR |= PIO_PDR_P25;    // Set MISO pin to output
  REG_PIOA_ABSR |= PIO_ABSR_P26; // Set pin PA26 for SPI
  REG_PIOA_PDR |= 0 << PIO_PDR_P26; // Set MOSI pin to input
  REG_PIOA_ABSR |= PIO_ABSR_P27; // Set pin PA27 for SPI
  REG_PIOA_PDR |= 0 << PIO_PDR_P27; // Set SCLK pin to input
  REG_PIOA_ABSR |= PIO_ABSR_P28; // Set pin PA28 for SPI
  REG_PIOA_PDR |= 0 << PIO_PDR_P28; // Set NSS pin to input
  REG_SPI0_MR = 0; // Set SPI0 to slave mode
  REG_SPI0_IER = 1 << SPI_IER_RDRF | 1 << SPI_IER_OVRES | 1
<< SPI_IER_NSSR; // Enable interrupts
  SPI0->SPI_CSR[0] = SPI_CSR_BITS_12_BIT; // Configure SPI to
capture on falling edge and transfer 12 bits
}
```

- **Serial Communication Initialization:** Begins serial communication at a baud rate of 115200 for data exchange with the host.
- **Pin Modes Setup for Upper and Lower Circuits:** Configures pins as inputs or outputs for both the upper and lower circuits. For output pins, initial states are set, and input pins are configured accordingly.
- **PWM Configuration:** Configures the PWM settings for different channels (phi1, phi2, phi3) including clock settings, duty cycles, and synchronization.
- **SPI Configuration:** Sets up SPI communication, including pin assignments for SPI functions, and enables interrupts for SPI operations.

Loop Function

```
void loop() {
  int i = 0;

  // Disable SPI for configuration
  REG_SPI0_CR = 0;

  // Check if data is available on the serial port
  if (Serial.available() > 0) {
    command = Serial.readStringUntil('\0'); // Read the
command from serial input

    // Check if command is for Upper Circuit (U) or Lower
Circuit (D)
    if (command[22] == 'R') {
      if (command[0] == 'U') {
        // Configure pins for Upper Circuit
        digitalWrite(SEL_NOUT, HIGH);
        digitalWrite(SEL_PHI, HIGH);

        // Validate command format and set sample number
```

Reference

1. Tabrizi HO, Forouhi S, Ghafar-Zadeh E (2022) A high dynamic range dual 8×16 capacitive sensor array for life science applications. IEEE Trans Biomed Circuits Syst

SPRINGER NATURE

GPSR Compliance

The European Union's (EU) General Product Safety Regulation (GPSR) is a set of rules that requires consumer products to be safe and our obligations to ensure this.

If you have any concerns about our products, you can contact us on ProductSafety@springernature.com

In case Publisher is established outside the EU, the EU authorized representative is:

Springer Nature Customer Service Center GmbH
Europaplatz 3
69115 Heidelberg, Germany

The manufacturer's authorised representative in the EU is Springer Nature Customer Service Centre GmbH, Europaplatz 3, 69115 Heidelberg, Germany. If you have any concerns regarding our products, please contact ProductSafety@springernature.com

Printed and bound by CPI Group (UK) Ltd, Croydon, CR0 4YY
31/07/2026
02182897-0004